Manchester

PATHOLOGY OF AIDS
and HIV Infection

GERALD NASH, M.D.

Professor of Pathology
University of Massachusetts Medical Center
Worcester, Massachusetts

JONATHAN W. SAID, M.D.

Associate Pathologist
Cedars Sinai Medical Center;
Clinical Professor of Pathology
University of California
Los Angeles, California

PATHOLOGY OF AIDS and HIV Infection

Volume 26 in the Series
MAJOR PROBLEMS IN PATHOLOGY

W.B. SAUNDERS COMPANY
Harcourt Brace Jovanovich, Inc.

Philadelphia, London, Toronto, Montreal, Sydney, Tokyo

W. B. SAUNDERS COMPANY
Harcourt Brace Jovanovich, Inc.

The Curtis Center
Independence Square West
Philadelphia, PA 19106

Library of Congress Cataloging-in-Publication Data

The Pathology of AIDS and HIF infection   /   [edited by] Gerald Nash.
  Jonathan W. Said; Virginia A. Livolsi, consulting editor.
      p.   cm. — (Major problems in pathology; v. 26)
    Includes bibliographical references.
    ISBN 0-7216-1540-6
    1. AIDS (Disease)   2. AIDS (Disease) — Pathophysiology.   3. AIDS
(Disease) — Diagnosis.   4. Said, Jonathan W.   I. Nash, Gerald.
II. Said, Jonathan W.   III. LiVolsi, Virginia A.   IV. Series.
    [DNLM: 1. Acquired Immunodeficiency Syndrome — pathology.   2. HIV
Infections — pathology.   W1 MA492X v. 26 / WD 308 P2965]
RC607.A26P37   1992
616.97′9207 — dc20
DNLM/DLC
For Library of Congress   91-25282
                                                                                                      CIP

Editor: Jennifer Mitchell

Pathology of AIDS and HIV Infection   ISBN   0–7216–1540–6

Last digit is the print number: 9   8   7   6   5   4   3   2   1

Contributors

ARTHUR H. COHEN, M.D.

Professor of Pathology and Medicine, University of California, Los Angeles, School of Medicine; Departments of Pathology and Medicine, Harbor—University of California, Los Angeles, Medical Center, Torrance, California

Pathology of the Kidneys

UMBERTO DE GIROLAMI, M.D.

Professor of Pathology (Neuropathology) and Neurology, University of Massachusetts Medical School; Director, Neuropathology Laboratory, University of Massachusetts Medical Center; Consultant Neuropathologist, New England Deaconess Hospital, Worcester, Massachusetts

Neuropathology; Ocular Pathology

MICHAEL C. FISHBEIN, M.D.

Adjunct Professor of Pathology, University of California, Los Angeles, School of Medicine; Associate Pathologist, Department of Pathology and Laboratory Medicine, Cedars-Sinai Medical Center, Los Angeles, California

Cardiovascular System

JEAN-JACQUES HAUW, M.D.

Professor of Pathology (Neuropathology), University of Paris; Director, R. Escourolle Neuropathology Laboratory, Hôpital de La Salpêtrière, Paris, France

Ocular Pathology

DOMINIQUE HÉNIN, M.D.

Professor of Pathology (Neuropathology), University of Paris; Director, Pathology Laboratory, Hôpital Beaujon, Paris, France

Ocular Pathology

ANTOINETTE F. HOOD, M.D.

Associate Professor, Departments of Dermatology and Pathology, Johns Hopkins University School of Medicine, Johns Hopkins Hospital, Baltimore, Maryland

Associated Cutaneous Diseases

THEODORE H. KWAN, M.D.

Assistant Professor, Harvard Medical School; Associate Pathologist, Beth Israel Hospital, Boston, Massachusetts

Associated Cutaneous Diseases

GERALD NASH, M.D.

Professor of Pathology, University of Massachusetts Medical School; Director, Division of Anatomic Pathology, University of Massachusetts Medical Center, Worcester, Massachusetts

Epidemiology of HIV Infection; Spectrum of HIV Infection; HIV Infection in Health Care Workers; Respiratory System

SHIRIN NASH, M.D.

Assistant Professor of Pathology, Harvard Medical School; Associate Pathologist, The Brigham and Women's Hospital, Boston, Massachusetts

Gastrointestinal and Hepatobiliary Disease

CYNTHIA C. NAST, M.D.

Assistant Professor of Pathology, University of California, Los Angeles, School of Medicine; Staff Pathologist, Harbor—University of California, Los Angeles, Medical Center, Torrance, California

Pathology of the Kidneys

JIAN-HUA QIAO, M.D.

Research Fellow, Department of Pathology, University of California, Los Angeles, School of Medicine, Cedars-Sinai Medical Center, Los Angeles, California

Cardiovascular System

JOHNATHAN W. SAID, M.D.

Clinical Professor of Pathology, University of California, Los Angeles, School of Medicine; Associate Pathologist, Cedars-Sinai Medical Center, Los Angeles, California

Pathogenesis of HIV Infection; Electron Microscopy in HIV Infection; Localization of Organisms in Tissue Sections; Lymphoreticular System; Miscellaneous Organ Systems

THOMAS W. SMITH, M.D.

Associate Professor of Pathology (Neuropathology) and Neurology, University of Massachusetts Medical School; Staff Neuropathologist, University of Massachusetts and St. Vincent Hospitals, Worcester, Massachusetts

Neuropathology

Foreword

The first cases of opportunistic infection associated with the condition now recognized as acquired immunodeficiency syndrome (AIDS), resulting from human immunodeficiency virus (HIV) infection, were reported by the Centers for Disease Control in 1981. Since then, 1 million people in the United States have become infected with HIV, 150,000 have developed AIDS, and nearly 100,000 have died from this disease.

This epidemic has brought many changes to the practice of pathology; most notable is the challenge of diagnosing a spectrum of unusual and frequently subtle but nevertheless life threatening lesions affecting nearly every organ and tissue in the body. The increasing frequency and expanding geographic spread of AIDS place a demand on all surgical pathologists to master a large and growing body of knowledge essential to the prompt and definitive diagnosis of AIDS-related lesions.

In *Pathology of AIDS and HIV Infection*, Drs. Jonathan Said and Gerald Nash have produced an invaluable reference source. This authoritative, up-to-date review provides detailed coverage of the epidemiology and pathophysiology of AIDS, of the application of special diagnostic procedures in this setting, and of the characteristic morphologic features and differential diagnosis of AIDS-associated lesions. This monograph will be a welcome addition to the library of pathologists and other physicians responsible for the clinical care of patients with HIV infection and AIDS.

JAMES L. BENNINGTON, M.D.
Consulting Editor

Preface

In the spring of 1981 two unusual cases of *Pneumocystis carinii* pneumonia were seen in the Department of Pathology at Cedars-Sinai Medical Center in Los Angeles, California. Both were diagnosed from lung biopsies of young adult males who had no apparent risk factors for that opportunistic organism. We were puzzled by these cases, and our curiosity increased considerably when we heard of other similar cases in the community. Further evaluation of these patients revealed that they were all homosexual men, and they appeared to have abnormalities of their T-lymphocytes. This apparently new condition was referred to locally as the gay-related immunodeficiency (GRID) syndrome. These initial cases were reported to the Centers for Disease Control (CDC), which published an account of them in June 1981.[1] Similar occurrences in San Francisco and New York, including a variety of opportunistic infections and Kaposi's sarcoma and involving groups other than homosexual and bisexual men, were reported by the CDC a month later.[2] Additional studies revealed that these individuals shared a profound cell-mediated, often fatal, immunodeficiency, and the term *acquired immunodeficiency syndrome (AIDS)* was adopted for this disorder.[3-6] As more cases were reported, it soon became apparent that AIDS had become an epidemic in this country and abroad. Over the ensuing years, the relentless spread of the epidemic, with its attendant loss of productive lives and consumption of health care resources, has had an enormous impact on our society.

AIDS is a devastating, invariably fatal disease that represents one end of the spectrum of infection with the human immunodeficiency virus (HIV).[7-9] Despite recent improvement in survival prospects resulting from antiretroviral therapy and prophylaxis against *Pneumocystis*, most victims succumb within 2 years.[10-12] The disease is characterized by recurrent bouts of opportunistic infections and often the development of malignant neoplasms. Since many of the conditions associated with AIDS and HIV infection in general require a morphologic diagnosis, the pathologist plays an important role in the care of these patients and in the postmortem assessment of what went wrong. In the early days of the epidemic, AIDS cases were clustered in only a few urban areas, and patients with the disease were treated in a limited number of medical centers. Even today, most of the cases come from five states: New York, California, Florida, Texas, and New Jersey.[13] Nevertheless, AIDS has been reported in all 50 states, and as the number of cases increases, it is likely that every hospital pathologist will become involved in diagnosing the wide range of disorders associated with HIV infection. This book is devoted to a discussion of the myriad pathologic manifestations of HIV infection and the challenging diagnostic problems this disease of acquired immunodeficiency poses for the pathologist.

For the purpose of organization, the book is divided into two sections. Section I is devoted to a general discussion of HIV infection, including epidemiology, spectrum of HIV infection, HIV and the health care worker, pathogenesis of HIV infection, ultrastructure of HIV infection, and special techniques for localization of organisms in pathologic specimens. Section II deals with the pathology of HIV infection as it relates to the major organ systems.

REFERENCES FOR PREFACE

1. Centers for Disease Control: *Pneumocystis* pneumonia—Los Angeles. MMWR 30:250-252, 1981.
2. Centers for Disease Control: Kaposi's sarcoma and *Pneumocystis* pneumonia among homosexual men—New York City and California. MMWR 30:305-308, 1981.
3. Gottlieb MS, Schroff R, Schanker HM, et al: *Pneumocystis carinii* pneumonia and mucosal candidiasis in previously healthy homosexual men: Evidence of a new acquired cellular immunodeficiency. N Engl J Med 305:1425-1431, 1981.
4. Masur H, Michelis MA, Greene JB, et al: An outbreak of community-acquired *Pneumocystis carinii* pneumonia: Initial manifestation of cellular immune dysfunction. N Engl J Med 305:1431-1438, 1981.
5. Stahl RD, Friedman-Kien A, Dubin R, et al: Immunologic abnormalities in homosexual men. Relationship to Kaposi's sarcoma. Am J Med 73:171-178, 1982.
6. Siegal FP, Lopez C, Hammer GS, et al: Severe acquired immunodeficiency in male homosexuals, manifested by chronic perianal ulcerative herpes simplex lesions. N Engl J Med 305:1439-1444, 1981.
7. Hardy AM, Curran JW: AIDS: A new kind of epidemic immunodeficiency. In Broder S (ed): AIDS. Modern concepts and therapeutic challenges. New York, Marcel Dekker, 1987, pp 75-90.
8. Selwyn PA: AIDS: What is now known. III. Clinical aspects. Hosp Prac 21:119-126, 129-131, 1986.
9. Volberding PA, Cohen PT: Clinical spectrum of HIV Infection. In Cohen PT, Sande MA, Volberding PA (eds): The AIDS knowledge base. Waltham, Mass, Medical Publishing Group, 1990, pp 1-11.
10. Fischl MA, Richman DD, Causey DM, et al: Prolonged zidovudine therapy in patients with AIDS and advanced AIDS-related complex. JAMA 262:2405-2410, 1989.
11. Lemp GF, Payne SF, Neal D, et al: Survival trends for patients with AIDS. JAMA 263:402-406, 1990.
12. Harris JE: Improved short-term survival of AIDS patients initially diagnosed with *Pneumocystis carinii* pneumonia, 1984 through 1987. JAMA 263:397-401, 1990.
13. Centers for Disease Control. HIV/AIDS Surveillance Report, August 1990, pp 1-18.

Contents

SECTION I

GENERAL CONSIDERATIONS

1

EPIDEMIOLOGY OF HIV INFECTION

Gerald Nash

DEFINITION OF AIDS

In 1982 the Centers for Disease Control (CDC) issued a case definition of acquired immunodeficiency syndrome (AIDS) for epidemiologic surveillance.[1] A case was accepted as AIDS if the patient had a disease that was moderately predictive of a defect in cell-mediated immunity and had no known cause for immunodeficiency. The indicator diseases included a list of life-threatening opportunistic infections and Kaposi's sarcoma (KS) before 60 years of age. Since then the list of opportunistic infections and neoplasms used as indicators of cellular immunodeficiency has been modified. In addition, the cause of AIDS has been identified as the human immunodeficiency virus (HIV), which can be detected by virologic and serologic techniques.[2,3] These advances made it possible to improve the definition's specificity for reporting purposes. Accordingly, a major revision of the case definition based on the status of laboratory evidence of HIV infection was introduced in 1987 (Table 1–1).[4] It broadened the spectrum of indicator diseases, allowed presumptive diagnosis of some indicator diseases in cases of known HIV infection, and eliminated exclusion of cases in which immunodeficiency may have had another cause when there was laboratory evidence for HIV infection. New indicator diseases included HIV encephalopathy and HIV wasting syndrome in adults and multiple or recurrent serious bacterial infections and lymphoid interstitial pneumonia or pulmonary lymphoid hyperplasia in children under 13 years of age. Cases that meet only the 1987 definition currently account for approximately one third of all reported cases. Compared with patients who meet the pre-1987 case definition, a higher proportion of patients who meet only the 1987 case definition are female, black, Hispanic, or intravenous drug users.[5]

The opportunistic infections and other diseases reported in AIDS are listed according to their frequency in Table 1–2. The prevalence of *Pneumocystis carinii* pneumonia, the most common opportunistic disease reported in AIDS, has remained relatively stable over the years at approximately 60%.[6,7] In contrast, the prevalence of KS has been decreasing; the cumulative percentage of AIDS patients with the disorder has fallen to less than one-third what it was in the early years of the epidemic.[6-8] One reason for this dramatic drop is that the prevalence of KS was highest in homosexual and bisexual men and the proportion of AIDS patients in that risk group has decreased significantly.[5-7] In addition, declines in HIV seroconversion rates and in prevalence of sexual behaviors associated with HIV transmission among homosexual and bisexual men suggest a reduction in their exposure to certain sexually transmitted agents such as cytomegalovirus, which may be a cofactor in the development of KS.[6,9-11] The

Table 1–1. 1987 Revision of Centers for Disease Control Case Definition for AIDS for Surveillance Purposes

---

AIDS is defined as an illness characterized by one or more of the following indicator diseases, depending on the status of laboratory evidence of HIV infection, as shown below.

I. *Without Laboratory Evidence Regarding HIV Infection*

If tests for HIV were not performed or gave inconclusive results and the patient had no other cause of immunodeficiency, any disease listed below indicates AIDS if it was diagnosed by a definitive method.

Indicator diseases diagnosed definitively

1. Candidiasis of the esophagus, trachea, bronchi, or lungs
2. Cryptococcosis, extrapulmonary
3. Cryptosporidiosis with diarrhea persisting longer than 1 month
4. Cytomegalovirus disease of an organ other than liver, spleen, or lymph nodes in a patient greater than 1 month of age
5. Herpes simplex virus infection causing a mucocutaneous ulcer that persists longer than 1 month; or bronchitis, pneumonitis, or esophagitis for any duration affecting a patient greater than 1 month of age
6. Kaposi's sarcoma affecting a patient less than 60 years of age
7. Lymphoma of the brain (primary) affecting a patient less than 60 years of age
8. Lymphoid interstitial pneumonia and/or pulmonary lymphoid hyperplasia (LIP/PLH complex) affecting a child less than 13 years of age
9. *Mycobacterium avium* complex or *M. kansasii* disease, disseminated
10. *Pneumocystis carinii* pneumonia
11. Progressive multifocal leukoencephalopathy
12. Toxoplasmosis of the brain affecting a patient greater than 1 month of age

II. *With Laboratory Evidence for HIV Infection*

Regardless of the presence of other causes of immunodeficiency, in the presence of laboratory evidence for HIV infection, any disease listed above (under I) or below (II.A or II.B) indicates a diagnosis of AIDS.

A. *Indicator diseases diagnosed definitively*

1. Bacterial infections, multiple or recurrent, affecting a child less than 13 years of age (excluding otitis media or superficial skin or mucosal abscesses)
2. Coccidioidomycosis, disseminated
3. HIV encephalopathy
4. Histoplasmosis, disseminated
5. Isosporiasis with diarrhea persisting longer than 1 month
6. Kaposi's sarcoma at any age
7. Lymphoma of the brain (primary) at any age
8. Other non-Hodgkin's lymphoma of B-cell or unknown immunologic phenotype and the following histologic types:
   (a) Small noncleaved lymphoma
   (b) Immunoblastic sarcoma
9. Any mycobacterial disease caused by mycobacteria other than *M. tuberculosis*, disseminated
10. Extrapulmonary disease caused by *M. tuberculosis*
11. *Salmonella* (nontyphoid) septicemia, recurrent
12. HIV wasting syndrome

B. *Indicator diseases diagnosed presumptively*

1. Candidiasis of the esophagus
2. Cytomegalovirus retinitis with loss of vision
3. Kaposi's sarcoma
4. LIP/PLH complex affecting a child less than 13 years of age
5. Mycobacterial disease, disseminated (species not identified by culture)
6. *Pneumocystis carinii* pneumonia
7. Toxoplasmosis of the brain affecting a patient greater than 1 month of age

III. *With Laboratory Evidence Against HIV Infection*

If laboratory tests are negative for HIV infection, a diagnosis of AIDS can still be made if (A) all other causes of immunodeficiency are excluded; AND (B) the patient has had either: 1) *Pneumocystis carinii* pneumonia diagnosed by a definitive method; OR 2) any of the other diseases indicative of AIDS listed in section I diagnosed by a definitive method AND a T-helper/inducer (CD 4) lymphocyte count less than 400/mm^3.

Modified from Centers for Disease Control: MMWR 36 (suppl):3S-15S, 1987.

frequency of cytomegalovirus infection reported in AIDS is listed as less than 10% in Table 1–2. However, the incidence of this infection reported in autopsy and clinical studies is far greater than that, indicating that active cytomegalovirus infection is underdiagnosed.[9,12]

Some general features of HIV-associated infectious diseases are noteworthy[13]:

1. The fungal, parasitic, and viral infections are rarely curable; at best they are only controlled and usually require long-term suppressive therapy.

Table 1–2. Frequency of Opportunistic Diseases Reported in AIDS

	Approximate Percentage of AIDS Patients
Pneumocystis carinii pneumonia	60
Oral/pharyngeal candidiasis (thrush)	45
Kaposi's sarcoma	10
Esophageal candidiasis	10
Extrapulmonary cryptococcosis	<10
Cytomegalovirus disease (internal organ infection)	<10
Herpes zoster	<5
Disseminated infection with *Mycobacterium avium* complex	<5
Chronic mucocutaneous herpes simplex	<5
Chronic enteric cryptosporidiosis	<5
Toxoplasmosis of the brain	<5
Tuberculosis (at any site)	<5
Immunoblastic sarcoma (other than primary of the brain)	<5
Primary lymphoma of the brain	<1
Disseminated histoplasmosis	<1
Progressive multifocal leukoencephalopathy	<1
Bronchopulmonary candidiasis	<1
Small noncleaved (Burkitt's) lymphoma	<1
Disseminated mycobacteriosis of undetermined species	<1
Chronic enteric isosporiasis	<1
Disseminated *Mycobacterium kansasii* infection	<1
Salmonella septicemia	<1
Legionella pneumonia	<1
Aspergillosis	<1
Herpes simplex virus pneumonia	<1
Coccidioidomycosis	<1
Nocardiosis	<1

Modified from Selik RM, Starcher ET, Curran JW: AIDS 1:175-182, 1987.

2. HIV-associated infections usually result from endogenous reactivation of a previously acquired organism.
3. The incidence of certain infections depends on the prevalence of asymptomatic infection with the etiologic agent in the local population. For example, more cases of coccidioidomycosis would be expected in AIDS patients from the Southwest.
4. Infections are usually severe and disseminated and are characterized by a high density of organisms.
5. Certain bacterial infections are associated with HIV disease and are probably related to defects in B-cell function.
6. Concurrent infections with different organisms are common. The pathologist should not be satisfied with finding just one infectious agent in a given specimen and should attempt to rule out the presence of additional organisms.
7. The typical morphologic response to an infectious agent may not develop in HIV disease, so the pathologist may not encounter the usual clues to the presence of a given organism. Any and all organisms should be expected in a specimen regardless of its morphologic appearance, and appropriate special stains must be used for fungi, *Pneumocystis*, mycobacteria, and bacteria.

RISK GROUPS

A small number of major risk groups were initially identified in the AIDS epidemic in the United States (Table 1–3). The distribution of reported cases in these groups has changed over the years, partly because of the 1987 revision of the case definition, but group ranking has remained constant.[5,7,14-16] AIDS was first recognized in young homosexual and bisexual men, and although the proportion of cases in this risk group (not known to have used intravenous drugs) has fallen, it still accounts for the majority of adult cases. Heterosexual intravenous drug users are the second largest risk group, and the proportion of reported cases in this group has been increasing. Homosexual or bisexual men who use intravenous drugs are the third largest group. Heterosexual sex partners of persons with

Table 1–3. AIDS Risk Groups in the United States

	Percent
Adults	
Homosexual or bisexual male	60
IV drug use	21
Homosexual or bisexual male and IV drug use	7
Heterosexual contact	5
Receipt of blood or blood components transfusion or tissue	2
Hemophilia or coagulation disorder	1
Other and undetermined	4
Children	
Mother with or at risk for HIV infection	83
Receipt of blood or blood components transfusion or tissue	10
Hemophilia or coagulation disorder	5
Undetermined	3

Centers for Disease Control: HIV/AIDS Surveillance Report, August 1990, pp. 1-18.

AIDS or at risk for AIDS, recipients of transfused blood or blood components, and persons with hemophilia or coagulation disorders are the remaining adult risk groups. Approximately 4% of adult cases cannot be assigned to a known risk group.[17] Pediatric cases (less than 13 years of age) account for a little less than 2% of the total number of AIDS cases. Of the pediatric patients, by far the largest group comes from families in which one or both parents have AIDS or are at increased risk for AIDS (Table 1–3). Blacks and Hispanics are disproportionately represented among AIDS victims, particularly among those who were intravenous drug users or sex partners or children of intravenous drug users.[5]

MODES OF TRANSMISSION

Data generated by epidemiologic studies of the AIDS epidemic suggested that AIDS is acquired through direct contact with body fluids, mainly semen and blood, infected with a transmissible agent. After the discovery of the AIDS virus, culture studies in which HIV was isolated from a variety of body fluids confirmed this hypothesis. In addition to being found in blood and semen, HIV has been isolated from saliva, tears, cerebrospinal fluid, breast milk, urine, vaginal and cervical secretions, amniotic fluid, and bronchoalveolar lavage fluid.[18] However, HIV transmission by any of these fluids other than blood and semen has not been documented. In the United States AIDS is transmitted primarily in four ways: sexual contact with HIV-infected individuals (especially receptive anal intercourse in homosexual men), sharing of contaminated needles by intravenous drug users, administration of infected blood or blood products, and perinatally from infected mothers to their fetuses or newborns.[19]

Epidemiologic studies suggest three distinct geographic patterns of transmission worldwide.[20] The first is typical of industrialized countries with large numbers of reported AIDS cases. In these countries most cases occur among homosexual and bisexual men and urban intravenous drug users, the male/female ratio is 10 to 15:1, heterosexual transmission is low but increasing, transmission through blood products is decreasing because of donor screening for HIV infection, perinatal transmission is relatively uncommon, and overall seroprevalence is less than 1%. The second pattern is observed in central, eastern, and southern Africa and in some Caribbean countries. In these areas most cases occur among heterosexuals, the male/female ratio is approximately 1:1, perinatal transmission is relatively common, intravenous drug use and homosexual transmission are uncommon, and the seroprevalence is estimated to be greater than 1%. Transmission through contaminated blood and blood products continues to be a significant problem in countries that have not implemented nationwide donor screening. The third pattern characterizes areas of the Middle East, Asia, and most of the Pacific. HIV was probably introduced into these areas in the early to mid-1980s. A relatively small number of AIDS cases have been reported in these regions, and most have occurred among persons who have traveled to endemic areas or had sexual contact with individuals from such areas.

TRENDS

As previously noted, although homosexual men remain by far the largest AIDS risk group in the United States, evidence suggests that the epidemic is slowing in that population. This phenomenon is undoubtedly related to lower seroconversion rates in homosexual men following their adoption of less risky behavior.[10,21] At the same time, reported AIDS cases among intravenous drug users and heterosexuals are increasing at alarming rates.[17,21] Although the number of cases reported in all of the high-risk groups is still increasing, the rate of increase is more than 20% greater among intravenous drug users and more than 100% greater among heterosexuals than that among homosexual men.[17] Almost all of the transfusion-associated AIDS cases are due to infected single-donor blood and blood products transfused before HIV-antibody testing became available in 1985. Transfusion-transmitted HIV infection has become rare since routine HIV antibody testing of all donations and voluntary deferral of donors at risk for HIV infection were instituted.[22] Similarly, HIV was transmitted to more than 50% of patients with hemophilia given factor VIII or factor IX concentrates in the early days of the AIDS epidemic, and these pooled concentrates are much safer today because of improved donor screening, HIV testing, and more effective methods of virus inactivation.[22]

REFERENCES

1. Centers for Disease Control: Update on acquired immune deficiency syndrome (AIDS)—United States. MMWR 31:507-514, 1982.
2. Broder S, Gallo RC: A pathogenic retrovirus (HTLV-III) linked to AIDS. N Engl J Med 311:1292-1297, 1984.
3. Coffin J, Haase A, Levy JA, et al: Human immunodeficiency viruses [letter]. Science 232:697, 1986.
4. Centers for Disease Control: Revision of the CDC surveillance case definition for acquired immunodeficiency syndrome. MMWR 36(suppl):3S-15S, 1987.
5. Centers for Disease Control: Update: Acquired immunodeficiency syndrome—United States, 1981-1988. MMWR 38:229-236, 1989.
6. Selik RM, Starcher ET, Curran JW: Opportunistic diseases reported in AIDS patients: Frequencies, associations and trends. AIDS 1:175-182, 1987.
7. Centers for Disease Control: AIDS Weekly Surveillance Report. Jan 2, 1989.
8. Centers for Disease Control: AIDS Weekly Surveillance Report. Jan 10, 1984.
9. Jacobson MA, Mills J: Cytomegalovirus infection. Clin Chest Med 9:443-448, 1988.
10. Winkelstein W, Wiley JA, Padian NS, et al: The San Francisco Men's Health Study: Continued decline in HIV seroconversion rates among homosexual/bisexual men. Am J Public Health 78:1472-1474, 1988.
11. Centers for Disease Control: Update: Acquired immunodeficiency syndrome—United States. MMWR 35:757-766, 1986.
12. Drew WL: Cytomegalovirus infection in patients with AIDS. J Infect Dis 158:449-456, 1988.
13. Glatt AE, Chirgwin K, Landesman SH: Treatment of infections associated with human immunodeficiency virus. N Engl J Med 318:1439-1448, 1988.
14. Curran JW, Jaffe HW, Hardy AM, et al: Epidemiology of HIV infection and AIDS in the United States. Science 239:610-616, 1988.
15. Selik RM, Haverkos HW, Curran JW: Acquired immune deficiency syndrome (AIDS) trends in the United States, 1978-1982. Am J Med 76:493-500, 1984.
16. Fauci AS, Macher AM, Longo DL, et al: Acquired immunodeficiency syndrome: Epidemiologic, clinical, immunologic and therapeutic considerations. Ann Intern Med 100:92-106, 1984.
17. Centers for Disease Control: HIV/AIDS Surveillance Report, August 1990, pp 1-18.
18. Hollander H: Transmission of HIV in body fluids. In Cohen PT, Sande MA, Volberding PA (eds): The AIDS Knowledge Base. Waltham, Mass, 1990, Medical Publishing Group, pp 1-3.
19. Hardy AM, Curran JW: AIDS: A new kind of epidemic immunodeficiency. In Broder S (ed): AIDS: Modern Concepts and Therapeutic Challenges. New York, Marcel Dekker, 1987, pp 75-90.
20. Centers for Disease Control: Update: Acquired immunodeficiency syndrome (AIDS)—worldwide. MMWR 37:286-295, 1988.
21. Osmond D: Prevalence of infection and projections for the future. In Cohen PT, Sande MA, Volberding PA (eds): The AIDS Knowledge Base. Waltham, Mass, Medical Publishing Group, 1990, pp 1-8.
22. Donegan E: Transmission of HIV in blood products. In Cohen PT, Sande MA, Volberding PA (eds): The AIDS Knowledge Base. Waltham, Mass, Medical Publishing Group, 1990, pp 1-5.

SPECTRUM OF HIV INFECTION

GERALD NASH

Conditions associated with HIV infection cover a wide range, and surveillance-definition AIDS represents only one end of the spectrum. In fact, AIDS accounts for only approximately 3% of people infected with the virus.[1] In addition to indicator diseases that satisfy the definition of AIDS, HIV infection may present as an acute nonspecific viral-like illness associated with initial exposure to HIV and seroconversion, an asymptomatic carrier state (accounting for the majority of infected people) diagnosed on the basis of laboratory evidence of HIV infection, persistent generalized lymphadenopathy (palpable lymphadenopathy at two or more extrainguinal sites for more than 3 months in absence of a known cause), "minor" opportunistic infections such as herpes zoster and oral candidiasis, persistent or intermittent diarrhea not caused by an opportunistic agent, a variety of hematologic manifestations including lymphopenia, granulocytopenia, thrombocytopenia, and anemia, various nonspecific constitutional symptoms, and any combination of the preceding.[1-4] Syndromes comprising combinations of these conditions and less severe than AIDS have been grouped together under the term "AIDS-related complex" (ARC) and represent HIV infection that has not yet progressed to AIDS.[2,4]

Most individuals have detectable levels of HIV antigens and antibodies within 6 months of infection.[4] During this period the patient may experience a few days of symptoms consistent with a viral illness, symptoms that are usually ignored, or may have an illness resembling infectious mononucleosis.[5,6] Some individuals do not produce antibodies for up to 3 years after infection and escape detection by the usual HIV antibody screening tests.[4,7-9] As antibody to HIV is produced, viral antigen is neutralized and disappears or greatly diminishes. The patient becomes asymptomatic and remains so for months to years, with persistence of detectable HIV antibody and with viral replication held in check.[4] Eventually viral replication accelerates and destroys the cellular immune system (see Chapter 4). The clinical condition at any time reflects the degree of immunocompromise and viral replication in target cells, particularly in the central nervous system.[4]

Attempts to predict the course of patients with HIV infection have been unsuccessful despite the vast amount of information that has been learned about the disease since the epidemic's onset. The term "AIDS" itself is no longer useful because prognoses vary among individuals who satisfy the criteria for the diagnosis and the term concentrates attention on only the latter phases of HIV infection.[4] One logical but by no means perfect staging system has been devised by the Walter Reed Army Institute (Table 2–1).[10] This system charts the course of patients from exposure to HIV (WR 0) through stages of progressive immune dysfunction to the development of AIDS (WR 6). Patients have been shown to

Table 2–1. Walter Reed Classification System for HIV Infection

Stage	HIV Antibody and/or Virus	Chronic Lymphadenopathy	T-helper Cells/mm^3	Delayed Hypersensitivity	Thrush	Opportunistic Infection
WR 0	−	−	>400	Normal	−	−
WR 1	(+)	−	>400	Normal	−	−
WR 2	(+)	(+)	>400	Normal	−	−
WR 3	(+)	+/−	(<400)	Normal	−	−
WR 4	(+)	+/−	(<400)	(Partial)	−	−
WR 5	(+)	+/−	<400	(Anergy and/or)	+	−
WR 6	(+)	+/−	<400	Anergy/partial	+/−	(+)

Modified from Redfield RR, Wright DC, Tramont EC: N Engl J Med 314:131-132, 1986.
Table entries in parentheses are essential criteria for assignment to each stage.

progress by one or two stages of this classification over 3 years. This system has been criticized because it uses lymphadenopathy as a prognostic factor, despite evidence to the contrary,[11,12] and because it fails to include thrombocytopenia as a condition that may have prognostic significance.[4,13,14]

Laboratory parameters that have been identified as correlating with a poor prognosis include elevation of the erythrocyte sedimentation rate,[11] unexplained anemia,[11] thrombocytopenia,[15,16] an absolute T4 lymphocyte count less than 150 per cubic millimeter or a falling T4 count,[17] T-helper/suppressor ratios below 0.8,[18] elevated serum and urine neopterin levels,[19] elevated serum beta$_2$-microglobulin levels,[11] and elevated serum levels of HIV p24 antigen.[4,11,20,21] Clinical factors believed to correlate with a poor prognosis include greater age at diagnosis,[11,14] exposure to an antigen that stimulates the cellular immune system, thereby presumably activating HIV replication in latently infected lymphocytes,[22] immunosuppression, and malnutrition.[4]

The number of persons infected with HIV who will ultimately have AIDS cannot be predicted. The incubation period varies from 8 months to well over 10 years.[23-25] Although progression to AIDS is rare in healthy adults during the first 2 years after seroconversion, AIDS will develop within 10 years in an estimated half of those infected with the virus.[24,25] Thus the median incubation period is approximately 10 years.

REFERENCES

1. Hardy AM, Curran JW: AIDS: A new kind of epidemic immunodeficiency. In Broder S (ed): AIDS: Modern Concepts and Therapeutic Challenges. New York, Marcel Dekker, 1987, pp 75-90.

2. Groopman JE: Spectrum of HTLV-III infection. In Broder S (ed): AIDS: Modern Concepts and Therapeutic Challenges. New York, Marcel Dekker, 1987, pp 135-142.

3. Selwyn PA: AIDS: What is now known. III. Clinical aspects. Hosp Pract 21:119-126, 1986.

4. Volberding PA: Clinical spectrum of HIV infection. In Cohen PT, Sande MA, Volberding PA (eds): The AIDS Knowledge Base. Waltham, Mass, Medical Publishing Group, 1990, pp 1-11.

5. Tindall B, Barker S, Donovan B, et al: Characterization of the acute clinical illness associated with human immunodeficiency virus infection. Arch Intern Med 148:945-949, 1988.

6. Fox R, Eldred LJ, Fuchs EJ, et al: Clinical manifestations of acute infection with human immunodeficiency virus in a cohort of gay men. AIDS 1:35-38, 1987.

7. Ranki A, Valle S, Krohn M, et al: Long latency precedes overt seroconversion in sexually transmitted human-immunodeficiency-virus infection. Lancet 2:589-593, 1987.

8. Haseltine WA: Silent HIV infections. N Engl J Med 320:1487-1489, 1989.

9. Imagawa DT, Lee MH, Wolinsky SM, et al: Human immunodeficiency virus type I infection in homosexual men who remain seronegative for prolonged periods. N Engl J Med 320:1458-1462, 1989.

10. Redfield RR, Wright DC, Tramont EC: The Walter Reed staging classification for HTLV III/LAV infection. N Engl J Med 314:131-132, 1986.

11. Moss AR, Bacchetti P, Osmond D, et al: Seropositivity for HIV and the development of AIDS or AIDS related condition: Three year follow-up of the San Francisco General Hospital cohort. Br Med J 296:745-750, 1988.

12. Osmond D, Chaisson R, Moss A, Krampf W: Lymphadenopathy in asymptomatic patients seropositive for HIV [letter]. N Engl J Med 317:246, 1987.

13. Terragna A, Dodi F, Anselmo M, et al: The Walter Reed staging classification in the follow-up of HIV infection. N Engl J Med 315:1355-1356, 1986.

14. Eyster ME, Gail MH, Ballard JO, et al: Natural history of human immunodeficiency virus infections in hemophiliacs: Effect of T-cell subsets, platelet counts, and age. Ann Intern Med 107:1-6, 1987.

15. Abrams DI, Kirpov DD, Goedert JJ, et al: Antibodies to human T-lymphotropic virus type III and development of the acquired immunodeficiency

syndrome in homosexual men presenting with immune thrombocytopenia. Ann Intern Med 104:47-50, 1986.

16. Walsh C, Krigel R, Lennette E, Karpatkin S: Thrombocytopenia in homosexual patients: Prognosis, response to therapy, and prevalence of antibody to the retrovirus associated with the acquired immunodeficiency syndrome. Ann Intern Med 103:542-545, 1985.

17. Polk BF, Fox R, Brookmeyer R, et al: Predictors of the acquired immunodeficiency syndrome developing in a cohort of seropositive homosexual men. N Engl J Med 316:61-66, 1987.

18. Taylor JM, Fahey JL, Detels R, Giorgi JV: CD4 percentage, CD4 number, and CD4:CD8 ratio in HIV infection: Which to choose and how to use. J AIDS 2:114-124, 1989.

19. Fuchs D, Reibnegger G, Wachter H, et al: Neopterin levels correlating with the Walter Reed staging classification in human immunodeficiency virus (HIV) infection. Ann Intern Med 107:784-785, 1987.

20. Allain J, Laurian Y, Paul DA, et al: Long-term evaluation of HIV antigen and antibodies to p24 and gp41 in patients with hemophilia. N Engl J Med 317:1114-1121, 1987.

21. Paul DA, Falk LA, Kessler HA, et al: Correlation of serum HIV antigen and antibody with clinical status in HIV-infected patients. J Med Virol 22:357-363, 1987.

22. Fauci AS: The human immunodeficiency virus: Infectivity and mechanisms of pathogenesis. Science 239:617-622, 1988.

23. Lui K-J, Darrow WM, Rutherford GW: A model-based estimate of the mean incubation period of AIDS in homosexual men. Science 240:1333, 1988.

24. Osmond D: Progression to AIDS in persons testing seropositive for antibody to HIV. In Cohen PT, Sande MA, Volberding PA (eds): The AIDS Knowledge Base. Waltham, Mass, Medical Publishing Group, 1990, pp 1-8.

25. Bacchetti P, Moss AR: Incubation period of AIDS in San Francisco. Nature 338:251-253, 1989.

3

HIV INFECTION IN HEALTH CARE WORKERS

Gerald Nash

RISK TO HEALTH CARE WORKERS

Even before the agent responsible for AIDS was identified, the similarity between the disease's transmission pattern and epidemiology and those of hepatitis B was apparent.[1,2] This naturally led to concern among health care workers who cared for AIDS patients or were exposed to specimens or contaminated materials from such individuals. As cases of AIDS among health care workers with no apparent risk for the disease were reported, the concern became outright anxiety. Fortunately, with the discovery of the AIDS virus, methods for detection of HIV infection were developed and the physical properties of the virus became elucidated. This led to a clearer understanding of how HIV is transmitted, a good assessment of the risk of transmission from occupational exposure, and the development of methods for preventing infection in health care settings.

Since the beginning of the AIDS epidemic numerous cases of the disease in health care workers have been reported.[3] However, investigation of such cases reported to the Centers for Disease Control (CDC) and studies of the prevalence of HIV infection in health care workers have failed to show overrepresentation of these workers among persons with AIDS or HIV infection.[1] Nevertheless, these studies have not ruled out the possibility of occupational transmission of the virus.

More direct evidence of the occurrence and risk of occupationally acquired HIV infection in health care settings has come from prospective longitudinal studies of health care workers who sustained percutaneous inoculations or exposure of mucous membranes or nonintact skin to blood or blood-containing body fluids from patients known to have HIV infection. These studies, including well over a thousand participants, have shown that the risk of acquiring HIV infection from a single percutaneous exposure (usually a needle-stick) is less than 0.5% and the risk from a mucous membrane or cutaneous exposure approaches zero.[1,4-8] This is in sharp contrast to the 6% to 30% risk of acquiring hepatitis B from a needle-stick exposure to hepatitis B surface antigen–positive blood.[9] Thus the risk of occupationally acquired HIV in the health care setting is real but small.

PREVENTION OF HIV INFECTION IN HEALTH CARE WORKERS

If percutaneous exposure to blood or other body fluids containing HIV comprises the highest risk for occupational transmission of the virus, the best way to prevent occupational infection is to minimize cutaneous (and mucous membrane) contact with infected fluids. The methods recommended for safe handling of blood and body fluids containing HIV, called "universal precautions," are essentially those that have been derived for hepatitis B and other blood-borne pathogens but depart from previous recommendations.[1] The guiding principle of universal precautions is that blood and blood-containing body fluids from all patients must be considered infectious for HIV and other blood-borne pathogens.[10,11] The rationales for this approach are that HIV carriers are often asymptomatic, knowing the HIV status of every patient is not feasible, and routine serologic tests for HIV antibody would fail to identify infected individuals who are antibody negative. Thus, if warning labels were affixed to specimens from patients with known HIV infection, unmarked specimens could engender a false sense of security and constitute a hazard. In one study of this problem in a hospital in which specimens from patients with known blood-borne infections were specially labeled "biohazard," only 36% of specimens containing antibody to HIV, hepa-

titis B surface antigen, or both were so labeled.[12] Such data are a strong argument for universal precautions.

The CDC recommended universal precautions for prevention of HIV transmission in health care settings in 1987,[10] and the Occupational Safety and Health Administration gave these guidelines de facto regulatory status by mandating compliance with them.[13] The essentials of the recommendations (Table 3–1) include routinely using barrier precautions to prevent skin and mucous membrane exposure to blood and other body fluids, handwashing, preventing needle-sticks and other injuries from sharp instruments, minimizing exposure to body fluids during resuscitation, and excusing health care workers with open skin lesions from direct contact with patients or contaminated materials.[10] In addition to universal precautions, certain recommendations have been made for individuals who work in autopsy (Table 3–2) and laboratory settings.[10,14,15]

The autopsy setting is where most hospital pathologists are at risk for occupational exposure to HIV. Geller[15] has reviewed the scientific and ethical issues, the risk to the

Table 3–1. Summary of Universal Precautions

Handwashing. Hands and other skin surfaces should be washed immediately and thoroughly if contaminated with blood or other body fluids. Hands should be washed immediately after gloves are removed.

Gloves. Gloves should be worn when soiling of the hands with blood or body fluids is likely. Double-gloving should be employed when invasive surgical (or autopsy) procedures are performed.

Masks and Protective Eyewear. Masks and protective eyewear (goggles or face shields) should be worn when splashing or splattering of blood or other body fluids is likely.

Gowns. Gowns or aprons should be worn during procedures that are likely to generate splashes of blood or other body fluids.

Prevention of Injuries from Sharp Objects. Needles, scalpels, and other sharp instruments should be handled carefully.

Contaminated needles should never be bent, clipped, or recapped.

Disposable syringes and needles, scalpel blades, and other sharp items should be placed in puncture-resistant containers for disposal.

Resuscitation. Mouthpieces, resuscitation bags, or other ventilation devices should be available to minimize need for mouth-to-mouth resuscitation.

Skin Lesions. Health-care workers who have open skin lesions should be excused from activities that might expose them to blood or other body fluids.

Sterilization and Disinfection. Germicides that are registered by the Environmental Protection Agency as "sterilants" can be used for sterilization and high-level disinfection. Germicides that are "hospital disinfectants" and are mycobactericidal may also be used for high-level disinfection. These germicides are effective in killing HIV when used in appropriate concentrations for the recommended period. All instruments should be cleaned before sterilization. Surgical instruments should be soaked in a germicidal solution and then sterilized.

Environmental Contamination. Environmental surfaces and fomites should be washed and disinfected with a hospital disinfectant that is mycobactericidal. A freshly made solution of 1:100 dilution of 5.25% sodium hypochlorite (household bleach) is an effective germicide. A 1:10 dilution should be used for heavily contaminated items.

Waste Disposal. Contaminated disposable items should be placed in waterproof bags and disposed of in accordance with local ordinances. Laboratory specimens, tissues, fluid-filled containers, and needles and other sharp objects should be decontaminated before disposal.

Laundry. Linens and hospital garments should be placed in impervious bags and laundered using standard hospital procedures. Double-bag only if outside of bag is contaminated.

Data from references 1, 10, and 22.

Table 3–2. Special Guidelines for Autopsy Personnel

I. Autopsy Facility. Since universal precautions are followed, a special isolation room is not required for the performance of autopsies on AIDS patients and there is no need to limit attendance to essential personnel.

II. Total Body Barrier Protection
- A. Water-repellent protective clothing that includes:
  1. Caps or hoods that completely cover the hair
  2. Water-protective boots
  3. Or total-body suits that include total head and foot cover
- B. Plastic face shield to cover the entire face and neck, or safety goggles with a protective seal
- C. Masks to cover mouth and nose
- D. Gloves
  1. Double surgical gloves, with frequent changes because they may become permeable with use
  2. Heavy overgloves optional
  3. Stainless-steel mesh gloves for certain procedures; these do not prevent needle-stick injuries

III. Autopsy Procedure
- A. Only one set of sharp instruments should be used.
- B. Scalpel blades should be changed when they become dull.
- C. Blades should not be passed from one prosector to another; they should be placed on a firm, stable surface and picked up from that surface.
- D. Only nonpointed scissors should be used.
- E. Bone cutting
  1. The oscillating electric saw should be used sparingly to minimize aerosolization. Techniques for containing aerosolization during removal of the calvarium and vertebral bodies may be employed but are cumbersome and not completely effective.
  2. Ribs should be cut through the cartilaginous portion to avoid producing jagged rib edges. The clavicle and sternum can be separated with a scalpel in most instances. The first rib should be severed with a rib cutter.

IV. Handling of Tissues.
- A. All tissues and organs should be fixed in at least 10 parts 4% neutral buffered formaldehyde solution for each part tissue. Bloody formaldehyde solution is not an effective fixative and should be replaced.
- B. Solid organs should be cut into slices no greater than 2 cm thick and the slices separated by absorbent paper to provide access to the fixative.

Data from references 10, 15, 23, and 24.

pathologist, and technical procedures related to the autopsy in AIDS. A few comments are appropriate, however. HIV has been isolated from a patients' blood and tissue up to 6 days after death,[16] underscoring the need for autopsy personnel to adhere to the precautions outlined previously, especially those concerning barrier protection and avoidance of percutaneous injury. Fortunately, HIV is inactivated by a variety of disinfectants, so decontamination of environmental surfaces and equipment does not pose any special problems.[17-19] Moreover, the virus requires moisture and cannot survive prolonged drying.[15,17] Occupational transmission of HIV infection has not been reported in pathologists or autopsy personnel even though autopsies were performed on AIDS patients long before the infectious nature of the disease was recognized.[15,20] Furthermore, no evidence has been found that autopsy personnel are at significant risk for transmission of any of the opportunistic infections that affect AIDS patients.[5,6,15,21] This is not surprising, since, as noted in Chapter 1, these infections are typically limited to immunocompromised individuals and arise as reactivation of latent infections.

REFERENCES

1. Henderson DK: AIDS and the health-care worker: Management of human immunodeficiency virus infection in the health-care setting. AIDS Updates 3:1-12, 1990.
2. Jaffee HW, Choi K, Thomas PA, et al: National case-control study of Kaposi's sarcoma and *Pneumocystis carinii* pneumonia in homosexual men. Ann Intern Med 99:145-151, 1983.
3. Centers for Disease Control: Update: Acquired immunodeficiency syndrome and human immunodeficiency virus infection among health-care workers. MMWR 37:229-234, 1988.
4. Marcus R, Centers for Disease Control Cooperative Needlestick Surveillance Group: Surveillance of health care workers exposed to blood from patients infected with the human immunodeficiency virus. N Engl J Med 319:1118-1123, 1988.
5. Gerberding JL, Bryant-LeBlanc CE, Nelson K, et al: Risk of transmitting the human immunodeficiency virus, cytomegalovirus, and hepatitis B virus to health care workers exposed to patients with AIDS and AIDS-related conditions. J Infect Dis 156:1-8, 1987.
6. Kuhls TL, Viker S, Parris NB, et al: Occupational risk of HIV, HBV, and HSV-2 infections in health care personnel caring for AIDS patients. Am J Public Health 77:1306-1309, 1987.
7. McEvoy M, Porter K, Mortimer P, et al: Prospective study of clinical, laboratory, and ancillary staff with accidental exposures to blood or body fluids

from patients infected with HIV. Br Med J 294: 1595-1597, 1987.

8. Elmslie K, O'Shaughnessy JV: National surveillance program on occupational exposure to HIV among health-care workers in Canada. Can Dis Week Rep 13:163-166, 1987.

9. Centers for Disease Control: Guidelines for prevention of transmission of human immunodeficiency virus and hepatitis B virus to health-care and public-safety workers. MMWR 38(suppl 6):1-37, 1989.

10. Centers for Disease Control: Recommendations for prevention of HIV transmission in health-care settings. MMWR 36(suppl):2S:1S-19S, 1987.

11. Centers for Disease Control: Update: Universal precautions for prevention of transmission of human immunodeficiency virus, hepatitis B virus, and other bloodborne pathogens in health-care settings. MMWR 37:377-388, 1988.

12. Handsfield HH, Cummings MJ, Swenson PD: Prevalence of antibody to human immunodeficiency virus and hepatitis B surface antigen in blood samples submitted to a hospital laboratory: Implications for handling specimens. JAMA 258: 3395-3397, 1987.

13. Bachner P: The epidemiology of fear: Scientific, social and political responses to the occupational risk of blood-borne infection. Arch Pathol Lab Med 114:319-323, 1990.

14. Centers for Disease Control: Agent summary statement for human immunodeficiency virus and report on laboratory-acquired infection with human immunodeficiency virus. MMWR 37(suppl 4):1-17, 1988.

15. Geller SA: The autopsy in acquired immunodeficiency syndrome: How and why. Arch Pathol Lab Med 114:324-329, 1990.

16. Nyberg M, Suni J, Haltia, M: Isolation of human immunodeficiency virus (HIV) at autopsy one to six days postmortem. Am J Clin Pathol 94: 422-425, 1990.

17. Resnick L, Veren K, Salahuddin SZ, et al: Stability and inactivation of HTLV III/LAV under clinical and laboratory environments. JAMA 255:1887-1891, 1986.

18. Spire B, Barre-Sinoussi F, Montagnier L, Chermann JC: Inactivation of lymphadenopathy associated virus by chemical disinfectants. Lancet 2:899-901, 1984.

19. Martin LS, McDougal JS, Loskoski SL: Disinfection and inactivation of the human T lymphotropic virus type III/lymphadenopathy-associated virus. J Infect Dis 152:400-403, 1985.

20. Gerberding JL, Sande MA: HIV and pathologists, persons performing necropsies, and morticians. In Cohen PT, Sande MA, Volberding PA (eds): The AIDS Knowledge Base. Waltham, Mass, Medical Publishing Group, 1990, p 1.

21. Wormser GP, Joline C, Sivak S, et al: Human immunodeficiency virus infections: Considerations for health care workers. Bull NY Acad Med 64:203-215, 1988.

22. Gerberding JL, Sande MA: Exposures to HIV in patients and laboratory specimens. In Cohen PT, Sande MA, Volberding PA (eds): The AIDS Knowledge Base. Waltham, Mass, Medical Publishing Group, 1990, pp 1-2.

23. National Committee for Clinical Laboratory Standards: Protection of laboratory workers from infectious diseases transmitted by blood, body fluids and tissue: tentative guidelines. National Committee for Clinical Laboratory Standards document M29-T. Villanova, Pa, The Committee, 1989.

24. Occupational exposure to bloodborne pathogens: proposed rule and notice of hearings (29 CFR1910). Federal Register 54 (No. 102): 23042-23139, May 30, 1989.

4

PATHOGENESIS OF HIV INFECTION

JONATHAN W. SAID

THE AIDS VIRUS

The identification of a specific etiologic agent for AIDS in 1983 by Barre-Sinoussi and associates[1] in France and Gallo and associates[2] in America followed a period of intense speculation about the true nature of the AIDS epidemic. Knowledge of the selective CD4 lymphotropic effect of the AIDS virus narrowed the search to the lymphotropic family of retroviruses (Table 4–1), of which human T-cell lymphotropic virus type I (HTLV-I) is known to be associated with human T-cell lymphoma and leukemia.[3] HTLV-II is associated with rare chronic T-cell malignancies and T-cell hairy cell leukemia. Although rarely implicated in human disease, HTLV-II has been found in a significant proportion of American intravenous drug abusers.[4] The newly discovered AIDS virus was variously named HTLV-III[2], lymphadenopathy-associated virus (LAV),[1] AIDS-related virus (ARV),[5] and human immunodeficiency virus (HIV). The Executive Committee on Taxonomy of Viruses[6] suggested the name "HIV" because it describes the host and major biologic property of the virus, recognizes the differences of the virus from HTLV-I and HTLV-II, and avoids controversy regarding the priority of discovery.[7] The AIDS virus is a retrovirus, possessing the ability to reverse the ordinary flow of genetic information with the enzyme reverse transcriptase, using viral RNA as a template for making DNA.[8-10]

The origin of HIV-1 is of more than historical interest, but the progenitor agent from which the virus either combined or mutated has not yet been identified.[11] Serologic findings implicate a retrovirus similar enough to cross react with HIV, which is widespread and

Table 4–1. Retrovirus and Disease

Virus	Subfamily	Disease
HTLV-I	Oncovirus	Adult T-cell lymphoma and leukemia
		Immunosuppression
		Tropical spastic paralysis (HTLV-I-associated myelopathy)
HTLV-II	Oncovirus	Hairy cell leukemia (rare cases)
		IV drug abusers
HIV-1	Lentivirus	AIDS-related complex and AIDS
HIV-2	Lentivirus	AIDS-like illness in West Africa
		Rare cases in the United States
SIV (STLV-III)		Simian AIDS virus

HTLV, Human T-lymphotropic virus; *SIV*, simian immunodeficiency virus; *STLV*, simian T-lymphotropic virus.

causes asymptomatic infection in African green monkeys.[11,12] Evidence suggests that HIV originated in central Africa and spread to Haiti, Europe, and North America.

STRUCTURE

HIV isolates have considerable genomic diversity, a factor that in addition to viral mutation has complicated production of an effective AIDS vaccine.[13] The virion is a sphere 100 nm in diameter that contains RNA in a truncated bullet-shaped core of which p24 is the major structural component (Fig. 4–1).[9] Knobs protrude through the viral capsule and consist of protein gp120 anchored to protein gp41. The virus is fragile, and as it leaves the host the gp120 frequently falls off the viral capsule. The gp 120 can bind to CD4, which is the receptor for HIV on the T-lymphocyte. When the immune system recognizes this complex, it destroys the cells. One infected T-cell expressing surface gp 120 may bind to other CD4-positive cells, forming a syncytium with up to 50 cells.[14]

MOLECULAR GENETICS

Only three genes encode for viral structural proteins (Fig. 4–2)[10,14]: *gag* codes for the core proteins, *env* is the envelope gene, and *pol* codes for the reverse transcriptase and DNA polymerase enzymes needed for viral replication. HIV also contains a number of genes that regulate synthesis of viral proteins. The transactivator gene *tat* is responsible for the burst of replication in CD4 cells that have been stimulated by encounter with an antigen. Other regulator genes include *rev*, a differential regulator, and *nef*, which downregulates transcription of viral DNA.[15]

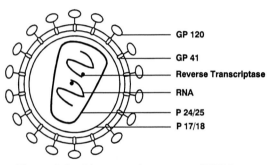

Figure 4–1. Diagrammatic structure of HIV-1.

GP 120
GP 41
Reverse Transcriptase
RNA
P 24/25
P 17/18

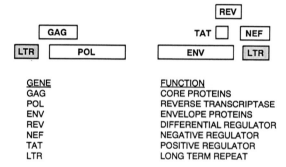

GENE	FUNCTION
GAG	CORE PROTEINS
POL	REVERSE TRANSCRIPTASE
ENV	ENVELOPE PROTEINS
REV	DIFFERENTIAL REGULATOR
NEF	NEGATIVE REGULATOR
TAT	POSITIVE REGULATOR
LTR	LONG TERM REPEAT

Figure 4–2. Molecular genetics of HIV-1. *LTR*, Long terminal repeat.

MECHANISM FOR INFECTION AND PROPAGATION

HIV has specific tropism for CD4-positive cells, which include lymphocytes, monocytes, and macrophages.[16] The CD4 antigen composes at least part of the cell surface receptor for HIV.[9] Anti-CD4 antibodies can specifically prevent HIV from binding to cells at receptor sites.[17] Cells that are pretreated with monoclonal antibody to CD4 do not replicate HIV or show a cytopathic effect. Soluble CD4 has been used to bind to virus and prevent it from infecting new cells.[18]

After specific binding to the cell membrane, HIV enters the cell, is uncoated, and injects its core into the cell.[9,19] The core includes two identical strands of RNA. DNA polymerase makes a single-strand DNA copy of viral RNA, and then a second DNA copy using the first as a template. This double-strand DNA is incorporated into the cell nucleus as a provirus and thus establishes a permanent infection. Much of the DNA of HIV remains unintegrated in the cytoplasm. The HIV replication cycle is restricted at this stage until the infected cell is activated. Activation may be achieved by other pathogens, including cytomegalovirus.[19]

Destruction of T-cells occurs by (1) replication and budding from infected cells damaging the cell membrane, (2) syncytium formation or cell fusion, in which viral envelope protein binds to the CD4 molecule on an uninfected cell, the membranes fuse, and virus cores pass into the new cell and infect it, and (3) binding of free gp120 to the CD4 receptor of uninfected cells, making them appear infected and eliciting an immune response.

The CD4-positive T-helper lymphocyte is central to the immune response, interacting with monocytes, macrophages, cytotoxic T-cells, natural killer (NK) cells, and B-cells, so that even a selective CD4 depletion can result in a multitude of immunologic defects. Monocytes and macrophages may be directly infected with HIV, causing a defect in chemotaxis. Involvement of alveolar macrophages may explain the high incidence of *Pneumocystis* infections in patients with AIDS.[19] Infected monocytes may serve as the vehicle for transport of HIV to the central nervous system. B-cell hyperplasia results from loss of the normal T-cell surveillance, and polyclonal B-cell activation may also be a direct result of HIV infection. A segment of the HIV envelope is similar to lymphokines that induce B-cell activation and immunoglobulin synthesis.[19] Enhanced release of monokines such as interleukin-2, tumor necrosis factor, and cachectin may help explain the chronic fevers and wasting of AIDS patients.

The profound depression of immune function in AIDS patients and subsequent susceptibility to opportunistic infections, oncogenic viruses, and malignant neoplasms may therefore arise from (1) quantitative deficiency of CD4 cells caused by cytopathic effect of the virus, (2) impaired function of viable T-lymphocytes that have proviral sequences incorporated into their genomes, (3) lack of inductive function for monocytes, macrophages, and other T-cells including NK cells and OKT8+ suppressor/cytotoxic cells, and (4) impaired helper function of B-cells. Many of the immune defects noted in AIDS may therefore be traced to depletion and functional defects in the CD4+ helper/inducer subset of lymphocytes following infection with HIV.

HIV persists in infected individuals, who should be considered infectious for life.[19] Not all persons with antibodies to HIV transmit the virus to their regular sexual partners, however, even over long periods, suggesting that the presence of antibody does not always indicate a high degree of infectivity.[20] Susceptibility of the host to HIV may depend on a number of factors, including genetic predisposition and the presence of HLA-DR5,[21,22] the size of the inoculum, and the route of exposure. The recipient's immune status at the time of exposure is an important factor that influences the sequelae of infection,[23] and this may be compromised by a combination of factors in individuals at risk, including effects of illicit drugs such as heroin and volatile nitrites,[24] malnutrition, and chronic infection with viruses such as cytomegalovirus, Epstein-Barr virus, and hepatitis.

Circulating HIV is present in the plasma of infected individuals,[25] and patients with more advanced disease have higher titers of circulating virus. In the early or acute phase, which lasts for weeks, the level of virus production is high. The middle or chronic phase is characterized by smoldering low levels of HIV expression that can last for years. Finally a crisis phase occurs with recrudescence of viral replication, resulting in the clinical syndrome of AIDS-related complex or AIDS, which lasts for months to years depending at least partly on the efficacy and availability of treatment. All stages involve active replication of the virus, and the infection has no totally latent phase when circulating virus is not present. The high degree of HIV viremia suggests that direct cytopathic effects of the virus are largely responsible for the pathogenesis of AIDS.[25]

REFERENCES

1. Barre-Sinoussi F, Chermann J-C, Rey F, et al: Isolation of a T-lymphotropic retrovirus from a patient at risk for acquired immune deficiency syndrome (AIDS). Science 220:868-871, 1983.
2. Gallo RC, Salahuddin SZ, Popovic M, et al: Frequent detection and isolation of cytopathic retroviruses (HTLV-III) from patients with AIDS and at risk for AIDS. Science 224:500-503, 1984.
3. Poiesz BJ, Ruscetti FW, Gazdar AF, et al: Detection and isolation of type C retrovirus particles from fresh and cultured lymphocytes of a patient with cutaneous T-cell lymphoma. Proc Natl Acad Sci USA 77:7415-7419, 1980.
4. Rosenblatt JD, Plaeger-Marshall S, Giorgi JV, et al: A clinical, hematologic, and immunologic analysis of 21 HTLV-II-infected intravenous drug users. Blood 76:409-417, 1990.
5. Levy JA, Hoffman AD, Kramer SM, et al: Isolation of lymphocytopathic retroviruses from San Francisco patients with AIDS. Science 225:840-842, 1984.
6. Coffin J, Haase A, Levy JA, et al: Human immunodeficiency virus. Science 231:697, 1986.
7. Brown F: Human immunodeficiency virus. Science 232:1486, 1986.
8. Barin F, McLane MF, Allan JS, et al: Virus envelope protein of HTLV-III represents major target antigen for antibodies in AIDS patients. Science 228:1094-1096, 1985.
9. Haseltine WA, Wong-Staal F: The molecular biology of the AIDS virus. Sci Am 259:52-63, 1988.
10. Ratner L, Haseltine W, Patarca R, et al: Complete nucleotide sequence of the AIDS virus HTLV-III. Nature 313:277-283, 1985.
11. Biggar RJ: The AIDS problem in Africa. Lancet 1:79-82, 1986.
12. Kanki PJ, Alroy J, Essex M: Isolation of T-lymphotropic retrovirus related to HTLV-III/LAV from wild-caught African green monkeys. Science 230:951-954, 1985.

13. Francis DP, Petricciani JC: The prospects for and pathways towards a vaccine for AIDS. N Engl J Med 313:1586-1590, 1985.

14. Weber JN, Weiss RA: HIV infection: The cellular picture. Sci Am 259:100-109, 1988.

15. Ahmad N, Venkatesan S: *nef* protein of HIV-1 is a transcriptional repressor of HIV-1 LTR. Science 241:1481-1485, 1988.

16. Klatzmann D, Champagne E, Chamaret S, et al: T-lymphocyte T4 molecule behaves as the receptor for human retrovirus LAV. Nature 312:767-768, 1984.

17. Dalgleish AG, Beverley PCL, Clapham PR: The CD4 (T4) antigen is an essential component of the receptor for the AIDS retrovirus. Nature 312: 763-767, 1984.

18. Smith DH, Byrn RA, Masters SA, et al: Blocking of HIV-1 infectivity by a soluble, secreted form of the CD4 antigen. Science 238:1704-1707, 1987.

19. Ho DD, Pomerantz RJ, Kaplan JC: Pathogenesis of infection with human immunodeficiency virus. N Engl J Med 317:278-286, 1987.

20. Burger H, Weiser B, Robinson WS, et al: Transmission of lymphadenopathy-associated virus/human T lymphotropic virus type III in sexual partners: Seropositivity does not predict infectivity in all cases. Am J Med 81:5-10, 1986.

21. Friedman-Kien AE, Laubenstein LJ, Rubinstein P, et al: Disseminated Kaposi's sarcoma in homosexual men. Ann Intern Med 96:693-700, 1982.

22. Metroka CE, Cunningham-Rundles S, Pollack MS, et al: Generalized lymphadenopathy in homosexual men. Ann Intern Med 99:585-591, 1983.

23. Anderson KC, Gorgone BC, Marlink RG, et al: Transfusion-acquired immunodeficiency virus infection among immunocompromised persons. Ann Intern Med 105:519-527, 1986.

24. Newell GR, Mansell PWA, Spitz MR, et al: Volatile nitrites: Use and adverse effects related to the current epidemic of the acquired immune deficiency syndrome. Am J Med 78:811-816, 1985.

25. Ho DD, Moudgil T, Alam M: Quantitation of human immunodeficiency virus type 1 in the blood of infected persons. N Engl J Med 321: 1621-1631, 1989.

5

ELECTRON MICROSCOPY IN HIV INFECTION

Jonathan W. Said

TECHNICAL CONSIDERATIONS

The usefulness of electron microscopy in identifying protozoal and viral organisms and distinguishing specific viruses is probably underestimated in the face of widely held views that information may be obtained only from fresh and optimally fixed tissue samples,[1] which are often unavailable. In many cases information may be obtained even from routine formalin-fixed tissues and paraffin-embedded blocks, particularly if replicating virions and groups of viruses are present. Hematoxylin and eosin–stained paraffin sections suspected to contain viral inclusions or protozoal organisms are particularly useful, since the structures can be identified with the light microscope and can then be embedded directly off the glass slide by orientation of sections side down over a Beem embedding capsule or embedding mold,[2] allowing the area of interest to be captured in an epoxy block. After polymerization the block is easily removed from the slide by heating on a 100° C hot plate for approximately 15 seconds.

Previously frozen tissue may also be suitable for electron microscopy, particularly if quickly frozen at low temperature to prevent ice crystal artifact. Frozen tissue blocks or cryostat sections should be plunged immediately into cold (0° C) fixative (3% glutaraldehyde or other routine electron microscopy fixative). Formalin-fixed tissue should be cut into 1 to 2 mm blocks and then fixed in glutaraldehyde

before being embedded for electron microscopy. In the case of paraffin-embedded tissues (Fig. 5–1) an area of interest should be removed from the block and trimmed into 1 to 2 mm cubes. When paraffin that contains plastic polymers (Paraplast) is used, anhydrous toluene should be the solvent. Since paraffin-embedded tissues have already been subjected to xylene (dimethylbenzene) during routine tissue processing, xylene is a natural choice as the deparaffinizing and transitional solvent for electron microscopy. Osmium tetroxide crystals can be dissolved in xylene or toluene, so that osmication and deparaffinization are carried out in one step.[2]

SPECIFIC LOCALIZATION OF HIV

Specific retrovirus-like particles can be identified in association with follicular dendritic reticulum cells (DRCs)[3-5] and in Langerhans' cells and T-zone macrophages from patients with HIV-related adenopathy.[6] Ultrastructural examination of follicles from lymph nodes in infected individuals reveals hyperplastic DRCs with elaborate labyrinthine processes, many of which show degenerative changes, including edema and vacuolar change. Between these processes are round viral particles 100 to 120 nm in diameter with a central or eccentric electron-dense core that is round, oval, or irregular in contour (Fig. 5–2). Diagnostic electron microscopy and

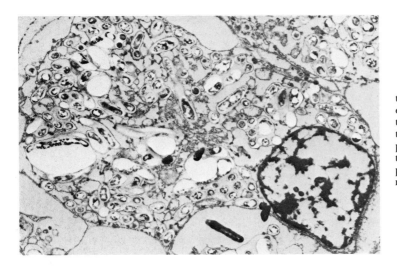

Figure 5–1. Macrophage containing rod-shaped bacilli with waxy electron-lucent walls corresponding to *Mycobacterium avium*, from rectosigmoid biopsy specimen of AIDS patient with colitis. Specimen was retrieved from paraffin block and then processed as described in text. (Uranyl acetate, lead citrate, × 7200.)

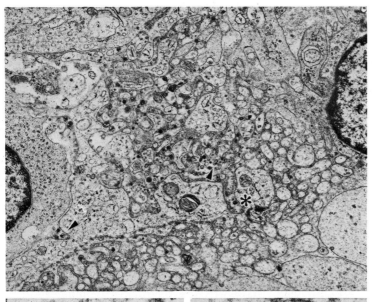

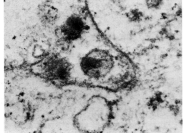
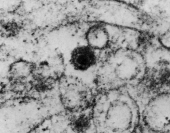

Figure 5–2. Electron micrograph from HIV-positive patient with generalized lymphadenopathy reveals labyrinthine processes from dendritic reticulum cell identified by presence of desmosome-like junctions *(asterisk)*. Numerous round viral particles are present in spaces between processes *(arrows)*. High-magnification electron micrographs *(below)* illustrate fine structure of viral particles. Note peripheral membrane and central nucleus *(right)* or rectangular eccentric nucleus with tapering apex *(left)*. (Uranyl acetate, lead citrate, × 12,000. High magnification × 75,000.)

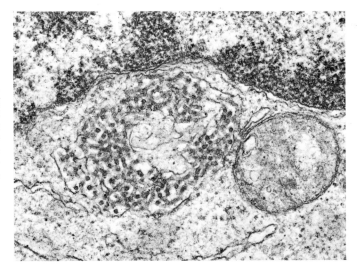

Figure 5–3. Electron micrograph showing tubuloreticular inclusion composed of 20 to 30 nm tubules. These are not specific but are frequently present in tissues from patients with AIDS and AIDS-related complex. They resemble paramyxovirus nucleocapsids and can be induced in tissue culture by exposure to alpha interferon. (Uranyl acetate, lead citrate, × 35,000.)

identification of specific viral particles may therefore play a role in evaluation of lymph nodes from patients with suspected AIDS.

NONSPECIFIC ULTRASTRUCTURAL FINDINGS

Tubuloreticular inclusions composed of 20 to 30 nm tubules are almost invariably present in tissues from HIV-infected individuals (Fig. 5–3). These structures have been associated with autoimmune disease, neoplasia, and viral infections and resemble incomplete forms of paramyxovirus nucleocapsids. Other organelles sometimes noted in lymphocytes include vesicular rosettes consisting of clusters of vesicles in and around a poorly delimited electron-opaque center[7] and test tube– and ring-shaped forms thought to arise from the fusion of cisternae of rough endoplasmic reticulum.[8] None of these structures is specific for HIV; they may be seen in biopsy specimens from HIV-negative patients, particularly in neoplastic and virus-infected cells.

POLYOMAVIRUS AND PROGRESSIVE MULTIFOCAL LEUKOENCEPHALOPATHY

Electron microscopy has played an important role in suggesting a specific viral cause for progressive multifocal leukoencephalopathy (PML).[9,10] Polyomavirus (papovavirus) can be easily identified in brain biopsies and autopsy specimens by the presence of virions 40 to 45 nm in diameter with characteristic tubular or

spherical forms. Figure 5–4 shows characteristic intranuclear virions in a brain biopsy specimen from a patient with AIDS and PML.

HERPESVIRUS

Cytomegalovirus is a herpesvirus characterized by a rod-shaped or ovoid core surrounded by a capsule. Particles develop within the nucleus and acquire a second capsule or envelope at the inner nuclear membrane.[11] Cytoplasmic dense bodies resemble lysosomes and may represent a reaction by the infected cells to virus particles (Fig. 5–5). In oral hairy leukoplakia, herpes-type virions shown by DNA hybridization studies to be Epstein-Barr viruses (Fig. 5–6) can be demonstrated ultrastructurally in keratinocytes in 63% to 100% of patients.[12]

PROTOZOAL ORGANISMS

Electron microscopy may also be helpful in characterizing protozoal organisms. The organisms causing cryptosporidiosis (Fig. 5–7) and toxoplasmosis (Fig. 5–8) have characteristic ultrastructural features,[13] trophozoites revealing nuclei, mitochondria, and other cytoplasmic organelles. Ultrastructural studies of *Pneumocystis carinii* reveal characteristic spherical or ovoid cysts with intracystic bodies (Fig. 5–9) or collapsed crescent-shaped cysts with bilayered or trilayered walls (Fig. 5–10). A complex system of anastomosing membranes surrounds the organisms and explains the eosinophilic foamy material seen by light microscopy.[14]

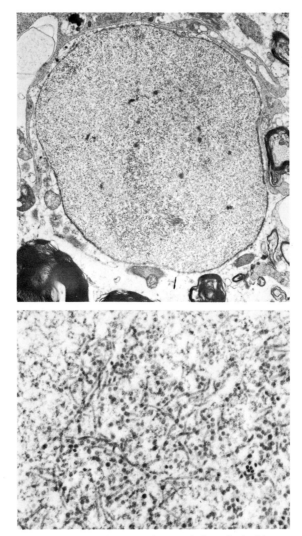

Figure 5–4. Electron micrograph from brain biopsy specimen of AIDS patient with progressive multifocal leukoencephalopathy. Intranuclear polyomavirus is identified by virions 40 to 45 nm in diameter with characteristic tubular and spherical forms. (Uranyl acetate, lead citrate; *top*, × 7000, *bottom*, × 37,000.)

Figure 5–5. *A,* Characteristic naked virions of herpesvirus group within nucleus in electron micrograph from patient with disseminated cytomegalovirus disease. This specimen was initially fixed in formalin and then fixed in gluteraldehyde before being embedded for electron microscopy. *B,* In cytoplasm, virions acquire second envelope from nuclear membrane *(arrowheads).* Dense bodies *(DB)* have lysosomal characteristics and may represent reaction by infected cell against viral particles produced in its own nucleus. (Uranyl acetate, lead citrate; *A,* × 33,000; *B,* × 41,000.)

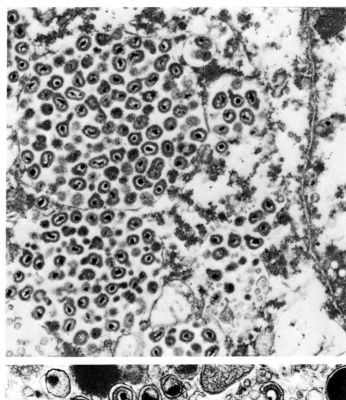

A

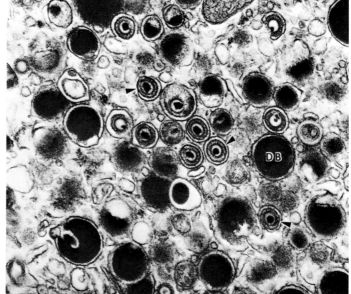

B

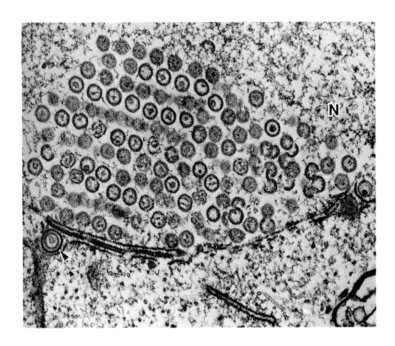

Figure 5–6. Herpes-type virions within nucleus of infected cell. These can be found in almost all patients with hairy leukoplakia and have been shown to represent Epstein-Barr virus. Nucleus *(N)* contains numerous 95 to 100 nm nucleocapsids, and cytoplasm contains enveloped viral particles *(arrowhead)*. (Uranyl acetate, lead citrate, × 55,000.)

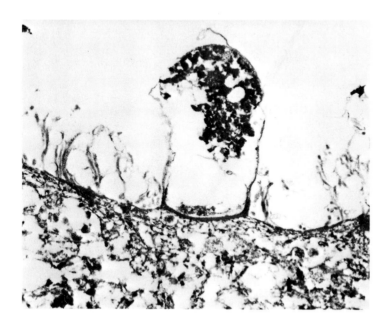

Figure 5–7. Electron micrograph showing cryptosporidiosis organisms in small bowel biopsy specimen from patient with AIDS. Tissue was reembedded in epon from glass slide as described in text. (Uranyl acetate, lead citrate, × 17,000.)

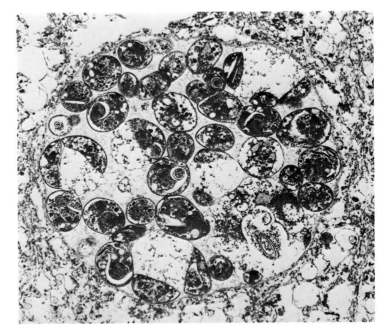

Figure 5–8. Electron micrograph showing characteristic *Toxoplasma* trophozoites with nuclei and mitochondria within a cerebral cyst (specimen retrieved from paraffin block). (Uranyl acetate, lead citrate, × 8000.)

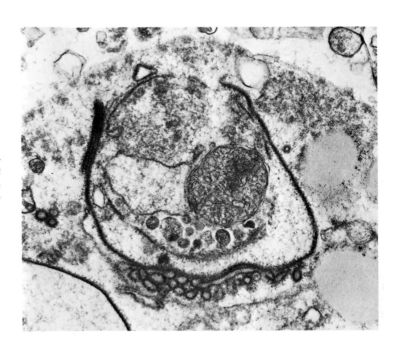

Figure 5–9. Electron micrograph of characteristic *Pneumocystis* cyst containing intracystic bodies. (Uranyl acetate, lead citrate, × 42,000.)

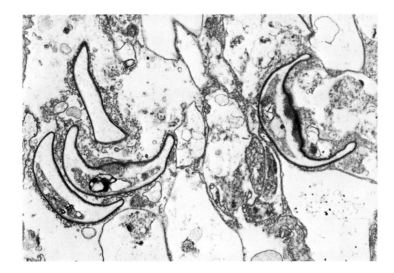

Figure 5–10. Collapsed crescent-shaped *Pneumocystis* cysts with bilayered or trilayered walls and complex system of anastomosing membranes, the ultrastructural counterpart of eosinophilic foamy material seen with light microscopy. (Uranyl acetate, lead citrate, × 8500.)

REFERENCES

1. Yunis EJ, Hashida Y, Haas JE: The role of electron microscopy in the identification of virus in human disease. Pathol Annu 12:311-330, 1977.
2. Chien K, Van de Velde RL, Heusser RC: A one step method for re-embedding paraffin embedded specimens for electron microscopy. In Bailey GW (ed): Fortieth Annual Proceedings of the Electron Microscopy Society of America. Washington, DC, The Society, 1982, p 356.
3. Armstrong JA, Horne R: Follicular dendritic cells and virus-like particles in AIDS and AIDS-related lymphadenopathy. Lancet 2:370-372, 1984.
4. Le Tourneau A, Audouin J, Diebold J, et al: LAV-like viral particles in lymph node germinal centers in patients with the persistent lymphadenopathy syndrome and the acquired immunodeficiency syndrome-related complex: An ultrastructural study of 30 cases. Hum Pathol 17:1047-1053, 1986.
5. Tenner-Racz K, Racz P, Dietrich M, et al: Altered follicular dendritic cells and virus-like particles in AIDS and AIDS-related lymphadenopathy. Lancet 1:105-106, 1985.
6. Gyorkey F, Melnick JL, Sinkovics JG, et al: Retrovirus resembling HTLV in macrophages of patients with AIDS. Lancet 1:106, 1985.
7. Ewing EP, Spira TJ, Chandler FW, et al: Unusual cytoplasmic body in lymphoid cells of homosexual men with unexplained lymphadenopathy. N Engl J Med 308:819-822, 1983.
8. Sidhu GS, Stahl RE, El-Sadr W, et al: Ultrastructural markers of AIDS. Lancet 1:990-991, 1983.
9. Anders KH, Guerra WF, Tomiyasu U, et al: The neuropathology of AIDS: UCLA experience and review. Am J Pathol 124:537-558, 1986.
10. Zu Rhein GM, Chou S-M: Particles resembling papova viruses in human cerebral demyelinating disease. Science 148:1477-1479, 1965.
11. Ruebner BH, Hirano T, Slusser RJ, et al: Human cytomegalovirus infection: Electron microscopic and histochemical changes in cultures of human fibroblasts. Am J Pathol 46:477-496, 1965.
12. Fowler CB, Reed KD, Brannon RB: Intranuclear inclusions correlate with the ultrastructural detection of herpes-type virions in oral hairy leukoplakia. Am J Surg Pathol 13:114-119, 1989.
13. Binford CH, Connor DH: Pathology of tropical and extraordinary disease. Washington, DC, Armed Forces Institute of Pathology, 1976.
14. Barton EG, Campbell WG Jr: Further observations on the ultrastructure of *Pneumocystis*. Arch Pathol 83:527-534, 1967.

6

LOCALIZATION OF ORGANISMS IN TISSUE SECTIONS

JONATHAN W. SAID

IN SITU HYBRIDIZATION TECHNIQUES FOR IDENTIFICATION OF INFECTIOUS AGENTS

With commercial DNA probes, standard in situ hybridization techniques can be used to detect infectious agents in routine fixed paraffin-embedded tissue sections. Each probe contains a specific DNA sequence that is covalently labeled with biotin and is complementary to the DNA of a particular infectious agent. Detection is based simply on the binding between biotin of the probe and avidin, which is linked to horseradish peroxidase. After the diaminobenzidine reaction, the infectious agent can be visualized with the light microscope and its exact intracellular location determined. The technique for in situ localization is described in Table 6–1.

HIV LOCALIZATION BY IMMUNOHISTOCHEMISTRY AND IN SITU HYBRIDIZATION

Commercially available monoclonal antibodies* enable detection of HIV antigens

---

* For example, commercial antibodies to HIV are obtainable from Du Pont Diagnostic Imaging Division, North Billerica, Mass.

Table 6–1. In Situ Hybridization on Formalin-Fixed Paraffin-Embedded Tissue Sections for Identification of Infectious Agents

---

Paraffin sections are placed on polylysine-coated slides and dried overnight at 55° to 60° C.

Materials:
DNA probe (for example, cytomegalovirus probe from Enzo Biochem Inc., New York, catalog no. PG-872)
3% Hydrogen peroxide in absolute methyl alcohol
Proteinase K (no. P-0390 Sigma Diagnostics, St. Louis): 0.5 mg/ml wash buffer
3,3′-Diaminobenzidine hydrochloride (2.5 mg/10 ml phosphate-buffered saline plus 1 drop of 3% hydrogen peroxide just before use)
Harris' hematoxylin

Procedure:
1. Deparaffinize the slides, place in 3% hydrogen peroxide and methyl alcohol for 10 minutes and rinse in wash buffer.
2. Drain off excess buffer, add several drops of proteinase K solution, and incubate in a humidity chamber at 37° C for 15 minutes.
3. Wash slides, apply 2% bovine serum albumin, and incubate for 20 minutes. Rinse and air-dry.
4. Place 1 drop of biotinylated DNA probe on each section and apply coverslips, excluding all air bubbles. Place slides on a 95° C hot plate for 5 minutes to denature the DNA.
5. Remove slides from hot plate and incubate in a humidity chamber for 15 minutes at 37° C.
6. Place slides in wash buffer, gently remove coverslips, and incubate for 10 minutes at 37° C.
7. Incubate with detection system (for example, avidin–horseradish peroxidase complex from Vector Laboratories, Inc., Burlingame, Calif.), followed by diaminobenzidine hydrochloride and 3% hydrogen peroxidase. Counterstain with hematoxylin.

(usually p24 or p17) in frozen, formalin-fixed, and B5-fixed tissue sections using standard immunoperoxidase techniques including the avidin-biotin complex method. Successful staining can also be achieved in tissues obtained at autopsy.[1] Use of radiolabeled cDNA probes (Du Pont Diagnostic Imaging Division) and in situ hybridization may provide greater sensitivity than the immunohistochemical method (Fig. 6–1).[2-4]

Staining in lymph nodes is seen in dendritic reticulum cells (Fig. 6–2), phagocytic and sinusoidal histiocytes, postcapillary venules, medullary and germinal center lymphocytes, and extracellular locations.[1,2] HIV is detected readily in the phase of follicular hyperplasia but with difficulty in follicular atrophy.[1] In the central nervous system, virus has been localized in capillary endothelial cells, mononuclear inflammatory cells, and giant cells (Fig. 6–3).[5] HIV has also been reported in astrocytes, vascular endothelial cells, gliomesenchymal nodules, and macrophages associated with demyelination.[1] Infected cells are most easily localized at the periphery of mass lesions and in angiocentric infiltrates.[6]

In the kidney HIV has been demonstrated in renal tubules and glomerular cells.[7] Glomerular mesangial cells have HIV receptors in the form of CD4 antigen,[8] explaining this route of infection. In the liver HIV usually can be localized in Kupffer cells, as well as in histiocytes and sinusoidal cells.[9]

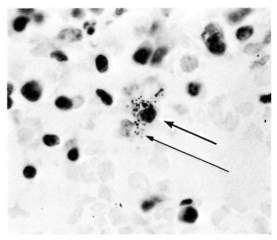

Figure 6–1. In situ hybridization for HIV using ³H-labeled cDNA probe in paraffin section of bone marrow biopsy specimen from AIDS patient. HIV nucleic acids (silver grains) are found within lymphocytes *(arrows)*. (Hematoxylin counterstain × 650. Courtesy Nora C.J. Sun, M.D., Los Angeles County Harbor–UCLA Medical Center.)

DETECTION OF CYTOMEGALOVIRUS BY IMMUNOHISTOCHEMISTRY AND IN SITU HYBRIDIZATION

Both standard immunohistochemical studies and in situ hybridization are effective in detecting cytomegalovirus (CMV) in paraffin sections from formalin-fixed surgical and

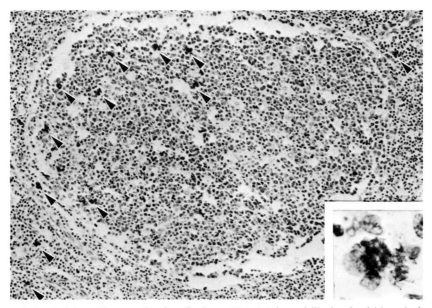

Figure 6–2. Staining with monoclonal antibody to HIV p24 shows follicular dendritic reticulum cells and a few parafollicular lymphocytes *(arrowheads)*. Inset shows dendritic reticulum cells with strong cytoplasmic staining. (Hematoxylin counterstain, × 150, inset × 800.)

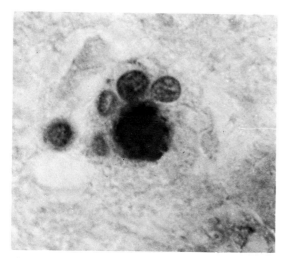

Figure 6–3. Monoclonal antibody to HIV p24 reveals strong cytoplasmic staining in multinucleated giant cell in brain specimen from AIDS patient with encephalitis. Tissue was obtained at autopsy and processed with routine formalin fixation and paraffin embedding. (Hematoxylin counterstain, × 1500.)

autopsy specimens (Fig. 6–4). Results of both techniques correlate better with culture results than does the detection of viral inclusions by routine microscopy.[10] CMV can be detected not only in cytomegalic inclusion cells, but also in histologically normal-appearing endothelial cells, pneumocytes, hepatocytes, and biliary and other epithelium.[11] Immunohistochemical studies add useful information for diagnosis of early or focal CMV colitis when few characteristic viral inclusions are present.[12] In situ hybridization may be a more sensitive tech-

nique than immunohistochemistry for demonstration of CMV,[11] although at least one study has found the two methods equally effective.[10] Hybridization stains are more difficult to prepare, however, and can be more difficult to interpret.

DIAGNOSIS OF *PNEUMOCYSTIS CARINII* WITH MONOCLONAL ANTIBODIES

Indirect immunofluorescence and immunoperoxidase stains can be used to detect *P. carinii* in tissue sections and induced sputum, in which it may be the most sensitive method.[13] Figure 6–5 shows immunoperoxidase staining for *Pneumocystis* performed with monoclonal antibodies (DAKO Corp., Carpinteria, Calif.) using standard avidin biotin complex technique. Although the methenamine silver technique is adequate for routine diagnosis, the increased sensitivity of the immunohistochemical technique is useful in detecting extrapulmonary infections in cases of disseminated disease.[14]

IMMUNOPEROXIDASE FOR DETECTION OF HERPES SIMPLEX ANTIGENS

Immunoperoxidase is a useful technique for detection of herpes simplex virus in formalin-fixed tissue sections and has a

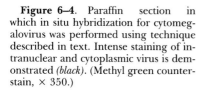

Figure 6–4. Paraffin section in which in situ hybridization for cytomegalovirus was performed using technique described in text. Intense staining of intranuclear and cytoplasmic virus is demonstrated *(black)*. (Methyl green counterstain, × 350.)

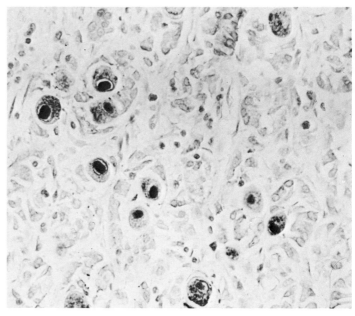

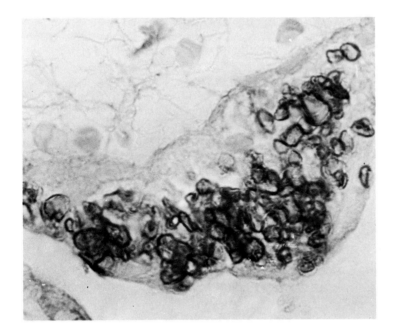

Figure 6–5. Formalin-fixed paraffin section stained for *Pneumocystis carinii* with monoclonal antibodies by ABC technique reveals intraalveolar exudate with numerous organisms stained black. Adjacent red blood cells are unstained. (Hematoxylin counterstain, × 1500.)

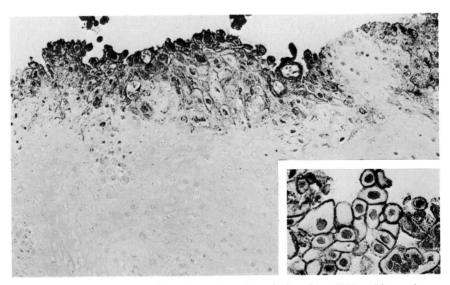

Figure 6–6. Formalin-fixed paraffin section of esophageal ulcer from HIV-positive patient reveals strong nuclear and cytoplasmic immunoreactivity for herpes simplex antigens. (Hematoxylin counterstain, × 120, inset × 250.)

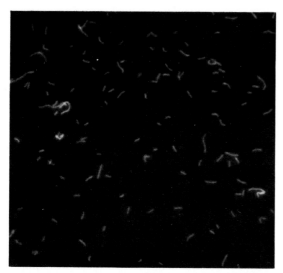

Figure 6–7. Direct fluorescent antibody stain for Legionnaires' organisms reveals numerous rod-shaped bacteria singly and in clumps. (Original magnification × 400.)

Table 6–2. Direct Fluorescent Antibody Technique for Diagnosis of Legionnaires' Disease

1. Heat-fix slides to be tested (smears or sections) at 60° C for 5 minutes.
2. Positive control slides (obtainable from the Centers for Disease Control, Atlanta, GA, 30333) are included in each run and consist of smears with Legionnaires' bacteria mixed strains. A negative control slide is run in parallel for each slide; the procedure is identical except that the specific antisera are omitted and fluorescein isothiocyanate (FITC)-conjugated normal rabbit globulin is substituted.
3. Before staining, fix slides in 10% neutral buffered formalin for 10 minutes and rinse in phosphate-buffered saline (PBS).
4. Incubate test slides with FITC-conjugated antisera to Legionnaire's bacteria (obtainable from the Centers for Disease Control) in a humidity chamber for 20 minutes.
5. After incubation, drain excess reagent onto a paper towel and rinse slides separately in PBS, mount them in glycerin, and examine with a fluorescent microscope.

greater than 80% agreement with cell culture isolation (Fig. 6–6).[15] Antibodies to herpes simplex types 1 and 2 can be obtained commercially (DAKO Corp., Carpenteria, Calif.) and can be used in combination to screen sections from suspected lesions.

DIAGNOSIS OF LEGIONNAIRES' DISEASE BY DIRECT FLUORESCENT ANTIBODY TECHNIQUE

The direct fluorescent antibody (DFA) technique can be used for rapid diagnosis of Legionnaires' disease in cytologic material (including sputum smears, endotracheal aspirates, bronchial washes, and bronchial lavage specimens), imprints or frozen sections from lung biopsy tissues, and even formalin-fixed paraffin-embedded tissues. Very few *Legionella* organisms are found in specimens from the lower respiratory tract,[16,17] and sputum appears to be more useful as a specimen than transtracheal aspirates.[17] Laboratory personnel can make tissue scrapings from formalin-fixed blocks by scraping a fresh surface with a scalpel blade and collecting the particles. Smears are then made and allowed to dry before staining. Specific polyvalent antisera that have been evaluated for detection of known strains of the bacteria can be obtained from the Centers for Disease Control, Atlanta, GA 30333. Positive control smears (also ob-

tainable from the CDC) and negative control smears with preimmune serum or conjugates prepared from the serum of unimmunized animals of the same species are run in parallel with the test slides. After immunostaining, the smears can be scanned with a 10× lens and then with a 100× oil objective. The bacteria are visible as single short rods or clumps of organisms that may be intracellular (Fig. 6–7). Visualization of five or more typical bacteria is the usual criterion for a positive result.[18] Pitfalls in interpretation include lack of preservation of the antigen in fixed specimens and problems with sampling; one strain of *Pseudomonas* has been found to stain with the Legionnaires' disease conjugate.[19] Since *Legionella* grows slowly and may be difficult to isolate, immunofluorescent staining may be the only available diagnostic test for rapid and specific diagnosis and appears superior to the Dieterle stain in this regard.[16] The staining technique is described in Table 6–2. An in situ hybridization technique for Legionnaires' bacteria has also been described.[20]

REFERENCES

1. Ward JM, O'Leary TJ, Baskin GB, et al: Immunohistochemical localization of human and simian immunodeficiency viral antigens in fixed tissue sections. Am J Pathol 127:199-205, 1987.
2. Shapshak P, Sun NCJ, Resnick L, et al: The detection of HIV by in situ hybridization. Mod Pathol 3:146-153, 1990.

3. Sun NCJ, Shapshak P, Lachant N, et al: Bone marrow studies in patients with HIV infection. Lab Invest 58:89A, 1988.

4. Sun NCJ, Shapshak P, Schmid P, et al: Comparison of HIV antigens and nucleic acids in biopsied lymph nodes from patients at risk for HIV infection. Lab Invest 58:89A, 1988.

5. Wiley CA, Schrier RD, Nelson JA: Cellular localization of human immunodeficiency virus infection within the brains of acquired immune deficiency syndrome patients. Proc Natl Acad Sci USA 83: 7089-7093, 1986.

6. Cornford ME, Said JW, Vinters HV: Immunohistochemical localization of HIV in central nervous system lymphoproliferative disorders of patients with AIDS. Mod. Pathol. In press.

7. Cohen AH, Sun NCJ, Shapshak P, et al: Demonstration of human immunodeficiency virus in renal epithelium in HIV-associated nephropathy. Mod Pathol 2:125-128, 1989.

8. Karlsson-Parra A, Dimeny E, Fellstrom B, et al: HIV receptors (CD4 antigen) in normal human glomerular cells. N Engl J Med 320:741, 1989.

9. Housset C, Boucher O, Girard PM, et al: Immunohistochemical evidence for human immunodeficiency virus-1 infection of liver Kupffer cells. Hum Pathol 21:404-408, 1990.

10. Strickler JG, Manivel JC, Copenhaver CM, et al: Comparison of in situ hybridization and immunohistochemistry for detection of cytomegalovirus and herpes simplex virus. Hum Pathol 21: 443-448, 1990.

11. Keh WC, Gerber MA: In situ hybridization for cytomegalovirus DNA in AIDS patients. Am J Pathol 131:490-496, 1988.

12. Robey SS, Gage WR, Kuhajda FP: Comparison of immunoperoxidase and DNA in situ hybridization techniques in the diagnosis of cytomegalovirus colitis. Am J Clin Pathol 89:666-672, 1988.

13. Kovacs JA, Ng VL, Masur H, et al: Diagnosis of *Pneumocystis carinii* pneumonia: Improved detection in sputum with use of monoclonal antibodies. N Engl J Med 318:589-593, 1988.

14. Radio SJ, Hansen S, Goldsmith J, et al: Immunohistochemistry of *Pneumocystis carinii* infection. Mod Pathol 3:462-469, 1990.

15. Schmidt NJ, Dennis J, Devlin V, et al: Comparison of direct immunofluorescence and direct immunoperoxidase procedures for detection of herpes simplex virus antigen in lesion specimens. J Clin Microbiol 18:445-448, 1983.

16. Cherry WB, Pittman B, Harris PP, et al: Detection of Legionnaires disease bacteria by direct immunofluorescent staining. J Clin Microbiol 8:329-338, 1978.

17. Edelstein PH, Meyer RD, Finegold SM: Laboratory diagnosis of Legionaires' disease. Am Rev Respir Dis 121:317-327, 1980.

18. Gump DW, Frank RO, Winn WC, et al: Legionnaires' disease in patients with associated serious disease. Ann Intern Med 90:538-542, 1979.

19. Jones GL, Hebert GA, Cherry WB: Fluorescent antibody techniques and bacterial applications. HEW Pub No (CDC) 78-8364, US Department of Health, Education and Welfare, Public Health Service, Centers for Disease Control, Atlanta, 1978.

20. Fain JS, Bryan RN, Cheng L, Lewin KJ, Porter DD, Grody WW: Rapid diagnosis of Legionella infection by a non-isotopic in-situ hybridization method. Am J Clin Pathol (in press).

SECTION II

ORGAN SYSTEMS IN HIV INFECTION

7

LYMPHORETICULAR SYSTEM

Jonathan W. Said

LYMPHORETICULAR SYSTEM AND HIV INFECTION

Although infection with HIV-1 inevitably results in failure of the entire immune system, the most striking alterations are noted in the T-lymphocyte subpopulations. Quantitative and functional abnormalities of T-cell subsets result in reversal of the normal T-helper/suppressor cell ratio, decreased mitogenic response in vitro, and defective reactivity in mixed lymphocyte reactions. T-lymphocytes in patients with AIDS are defective in production of lymphokines such as macrophage-inhibiting factor (MIF) and gamma-interferon.[1] In addition to diminished in vitro proliferative response, many patients exhibit cutaneous anergy.

Clinical manifestations of this defective cellular immunity include lymphopenia, marked suppression of the proliferative response to phytohemagglutinin and pokeweed mitogens, suppressed activity of natural killer cells, and decreased levels of interleukin-2. These immunologic impairments increase susceptibility to opportunistic infections and malignancies. Cutaneous anergy is exhibited toward a variety of antigens, including *Candida,* mumps, and *Trichophyton* antigens.

A decrease in the T-helper to T-suppressor/cytotoxic cell ratio in the peripheral blood is characteristic of AIDS, in which it is associated with an absolute decrease in CD4+ helper lymphocytes independent of numeric changes in other cell populations. A decreased helper/suppressor cell ratio may also arise from an increase in T-suppressor/cytotoxic lymphocytes alone, a finding that occurs in many instances, including viral infections such as cytomegalovirus (CMV), Epstein-Barr virus (EBV), and hepatitis, apparently healthy homosexual men, and otherwise healthy persons receiving factor VIII for hemophilia.[2] The combination of a decreased helper/suppressor cell ratio and an absolute decrease in T-helper cells is therefore important in distinguishing changes in AIDS from other causes of decreased T-helper/suppressor cell ratio. Absolute decrease in T-helper cells may occur in the acute phases of CMV and other infections, but in those conditions the T-helper cell changes are usually transitory.[3,4] Augmentation of T-suppressor/cytotoxic lymphocytes is uncommon in AIDS patients, most of whom have normal T-suppressor/cytotoxic cell counts, but is seen more often in AIDS patients with Kaposi's sarcoma than in those with opportunistic infections.[2]

Abnormalities in B-cell function, although less dramatic, are almost invariably present and include an early polyclonal activation of the entire B-lymphoid system with hypergammaglobulinemia, followed by decreased B-cell numbers in peripheral blood or lymph nodes and by oligoclonal and monoclonal B-cell proliferations including B-cell lymphomas. B-cell activation may be due to a direct interaction between the AIDS virus and B-lymphocytes, since isolates of the virus are potent inducers of B-cell proliferation and differentiation, which is independent of T-cells.[5] An increase in polyclonal gammaglobulins (and further fall in T-helper cell count and CD4/CD8 cell ratio) may be associated with a worsening prognosis and conversion of generalized adenopathy to AIDS.

Another serologic finding predictive of AIDS in HIV-1-seropositive persons is a high titer of CMV antibody, indicating that reactivation and systemic infection with CMV are common as cell-mediated immunity declines.[6] Paradoxically, conversion to AIDS appears to be associated with a reduced level of antibodies to HIV, presumably because the number of target cells (T-helper lymphocytes and monocytes) declines as infection progresses. Also, a high level of antibodies to HIV may confer temporary protection against progression of immunodeficiency to AIDS.[6]

Mononuclear phagocytes may be primary targets for HIV infection and agents for virus dissemination.[7] Alterations in the mononuclear phagocyte system include increase in serum lysozyme levels, decrease in cutaneous Langerhans' cells, and defective ability of peripheral blood monocytes to present antigen. Increase in natural killer (NK) cells is seen in paracortical regions of lymph nodes,[8] although the number of circulating NK cells may be normal.

PERSISTENT GENERALIZED LYMPHADENOPATHY

Persistent generalized lymphadenopathy (PGL) is part of a prodromal AIDS-related syndrome that includes such diverse clinical symptoms as fever, headaches, malaise, photophobia, night sweats, weight loss, and diarrhea. PGL is defined as lymphadenopathy (usually 1 cm or greater in size) of at least 3 months' duration and involving two or more extrainguinal noncontiguous sites in the absence of any current illness or drugs known to cause lymphadenopathy (history of intravenous drug abuse, phenytoin therapy, recent immunization, rash, or evidence of neoplastic disease). The true incidence of PGL in the homosexual population is unknown.

Adenopathy in PGL is characteristically tender and may fluctuate in size with stress and fatigue. Any or multiple lymph node groups may be involved, including unusual sites such as epitrochlear or supraclavicular

nodes. Other commonly associated findings include splenomegaly, hepatomegaly, leukopenia, hypergammaglobulinemia, and anergic response to common antigens on skin testing. In many patients these symptoms represent a prodrome of AIDS, whereas others may follow a more indolent course with waxing and waning adenopathy that does not fully resolve.

The reported incidence of the development of AIDS in patients with PGL varies but averages approximately 10% per year.[9-12] Conversion of PGL to AIDS may be accompanied by a sudden enlargement in lymph nodes,[11] lymphoid-depleted appearance in lymph node biopsy specimens, decrease in circulating CD4+ cells, increase in polyclonal hypergammaglobulinemia, and decrease in hemoglobin. Because of the incidence of malignant lymphoma and lymphadenopathic Kaposi's sarcoma (KS) in this high-risk group, and the simultaneous presence of adenopathy, malignant lymphoma, and potentially treatable infections such as tuberculosis, persistent unexplained adenopathy warrants biopsy and histologic evaluation.

Histologic Findings. Two main histologic patterns are observed in lymph nodes from patients with PGL. Follicular hyperplasia (also termed pattern A) is dominant in the early stages of the disease and leads to follicular involution in the late stages (pattern C).[13] Since the process is one of dynamic evolution from florid hyperplasia to eventual profound lymphoid depletion, a combination of findings intermediate between the two main patterns may be seen at biopsy (pattern B). Histologic patterns have prognostic significance, since progression to follicular involution is associated with development of cellular immune deficiency and AIDS. In a study of 79 patients with PGL, survival time was 54.4 months for pattern A and only 8.4 months for pattern C.[13] Almost 90% of patients with initial biopsy findings of pattern C died during the 7-year study period.

Florid follicular hyperplasia is characterized by large geographic and coalescent germinal centers (Fig. 7–1) and by disruption and absence of follicular mantles resulting in loss of the mantle zone, or so-called naked follicles (Fig. 7–2). These abnormal follicles vary greatly in size and shape and have a high cell turnover associated with numerous mitoses, abundant nuclear debris, and "tingible body" macrophages. Follicles also extend into the medulla and sometimes beyond the capsule of

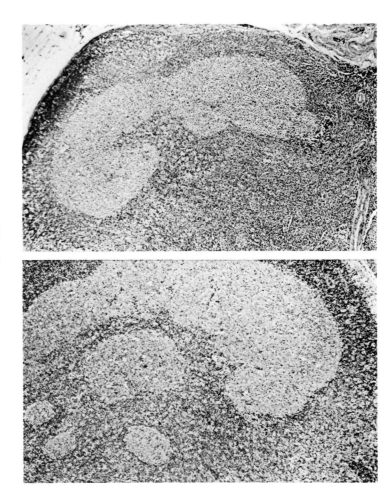

Figure 7–1. Lymph nodes from two patients with persistent generalized lymphadenopathy show explosive follicular hyperplasia with large geographic and coalescent follicles. (Hematoxylin and eosin, ×90.)

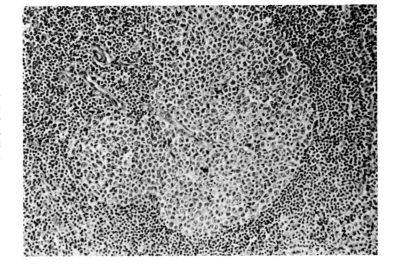

Figure 7–2. Loss of follicular mantle resulting in absent mantle zone and denuded germinal center with numerous phagocytic histiocytes ("tingible body" macrophages) and mitoses. (Hematoxylin and eosin, ×160.)

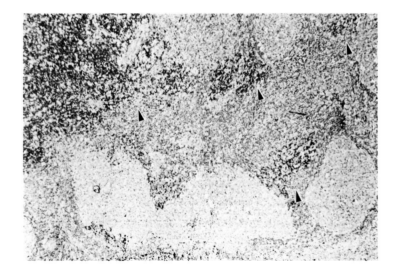

Figure 7–3. Foci of acute hemorrhage *(arrows)* adjacent to hyperplastic lymphoid follicle common in the early stages of persistent generalized lymphadenopathy. (Hematoxylin and eosin, ×90.)

the node. A prominent capillary network is present within germinal centers, and there may be areas of acute hemorrhage (Fig. 7–3). Neutrophilic aggregates are sometimes found, and multinucleate giant cells similar to Warthin-Finkeldey giant cells are observed in lymph nodes as at other sites (Fig. 7–4). Giant cells form by cell fusion, incorporating uninfected cells into HIV-infected syncytia.[14]

Monocytoid B-lymphoid cells similar to those in toxoplasmosis may be present in perisinusoidal and parafollicular lymphoid tissue.[15] Monocytoid cells usually have abundant cytoplasm, well-defined cell borders, oval or reniform nuclei with inconspicuous nucleoli, and

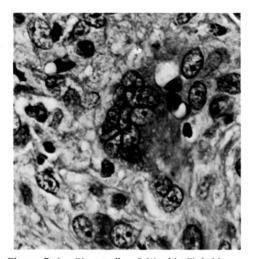

Figure 7–4. Giant cells of Warthin-Finkeldey type are occasionally numerous in lymph nodes from patient with persistent generalized lymphadenopathy and AIDS. These cells arise from fusion between infected and noninfected CD4 cells, forming a syncytium. (Hematoxylin and eosin, ×400.)

finely dispersed chromatin (Fig. 7–5). Other features of toxoplasmosis (such as prominent clusters of epithelioid cells overlying follicles) are absent. Monocytoid cells are often accompanied by small numbers of neutrophils.[15]

A peculiar dissolution of germinal centers termed follicular lysis[16-18] may accompany invagination of mantle lymphocytes into germinal centers and disruption of the dendritic cell framework of the follicle (Fig. 7–6). Follicular dendritic cells express the CD4 antigen, an essential component of the cell surface receptor necessary for HIV infection.[19] Viral particles can be found in contact with cytoplasmic processes of dendritic histiocytes,[20,21] and follicular dendritic cells from PGL and AIDS patients show intracytoplasmic reactivity with antibodies to HIV. HIV-1 mRNA has been found within dendritic cells, indicating that these cells can produce virus.[22] HIV has also been observed in multinucleated giant cells, interdigitating reticulum cells, and endothelial cells by in situ hybridization.[23]

Interfollicular areas show prominent vasculature with a mixed proliferation of small lymphoid cells, immunoblasts, occasional histiocytes, and eosinophils (Fig. 7–7). Zonal necrosis and noncaseating granulomas may be encountered. Individual nodes may show changes of dermatopathic lymphadenitis with melanin-laden macrophages and interdigitating histiocytes in the T-cell zones. Prominent histiocytic proliferation with erythrophagocytosis similar to the viral hemophagocytic syndrome[24] may also be seen.

Histologic features of HIV-related lymphadenopathy are not specific when considered alone.[25,26] However, the constellation of

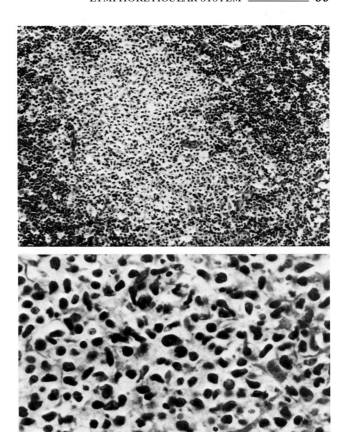

Figure 7–5. Parafollicular aggregate of monocytoid B-lymphocytes with clear cytoplasm, sharp cell borders, and oval or reniform nuclei with inconspicuous nucleoli. (Hematoxylin and eosin, *top,* ×160, *bottom,* ×240.)

histologic findings described previously is characteristic and suggestive of HIV infection in a patient with unexplained adenopathy in two or more extrainguinal sites.[15] The diagnosis should be confirmed with appropriate serologic tests, and specific tissue diagnosis can be made by localization of HIV with immunohistochemical studies, in situ hybridization, or demonstration of viral particles by electron microscopy.

Eventually the disease progresses to lymphoid depletion in which primary and secondary follicles are absent and a vascular proliferation of lymphocytes, plasma cells, and immunoblasts occurs (Figs. 7–8 to 7–10). The lymphoid proliferation in these nodes consists of mature lymphoid and plasma cells, as well as scattered large lymphoid cells (immunoblasts) and prominent capillaries and venules, some with arborization and distended lumens with flattened endothelial cells (Fig. 7–10). The remaining follicles may be fibrosed and hyalinized with a concentric layered or targetoid appearance and radially penetrating vessels (Fig. 7–11). This pattern is frequently associated with a poor prognosis and the occurrence of other features of AIDS, including opportunistic infections and KS.[13,27,28]

Immunohistochemical Findings

B-Cells. Although attention has been focused on T-cell abnormalities, in patients with PGL and AIDS the B-cell system is also greatly altered. Most striking is a polyclonal B-cell activation resulting in elevated numbers of B-cells spontaneously secreting immunoglobulin and in serum hypergammaglobulinemia.[29] Because B-cells are already maximally stimulated, the B-cell proliferative response to B-cell mitogens is decreased. Mantle B-cells express their usual phenotype, with staining for mu and delta heavy chains and polyclonal light chains. The increased interstitial immunoglobulin noted in germinal centers from patients with PGL and AIDS (Fig. 7–12) is in accordance with the polyclonal B-cell activation and immune complex deposition. Num-

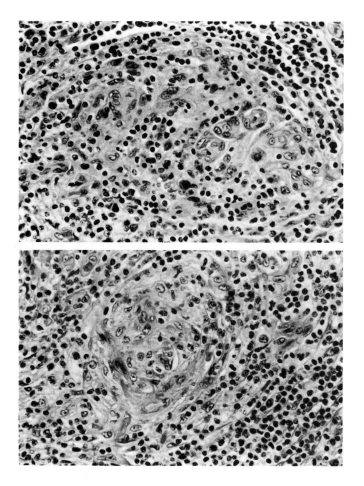

Figure 7–6. Lymphoid follicles that have undergone follicular lysis. Follicles are depleted of lymphocytes and composed predominantly of histiocytes and hyalinized stroma. Vascularity is prominent within both follicles and surrounding cortex. (Hematoxylin and eosin, ×160.)

bers of plasma cells are usually increased. Monocytoid B-cells may form prominent aggregates in parafollicular and perisinusoidal locations (Fig. 7–5).

Histiocytes. Increased serum levels of lysozyme and defective antigen presentation by peripheral blood mononuclear cells are evidence of diffuse alteration in the mononuclear phagocyte system in many patients with PGL and AIDS. Numbers of paracortical histiocytes (macrophages and reticulum cells) increase, and the follicular dendritic reticulum

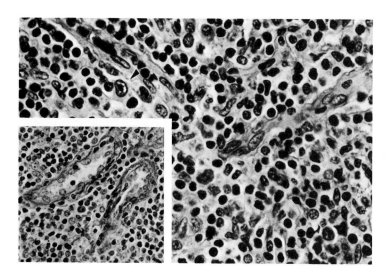

Figure 7–7. Hypervascular medullary region with mixed proliferation of small lymphoid cells, immunoblasts *(arrow),* and histiocytes. Blood vessels have prominent endothelial cells *(inset)* and may resemble immunoblastic lymphadenopathy or AILD. (Hematoxylin and eosin, × 160, inset ×230.)

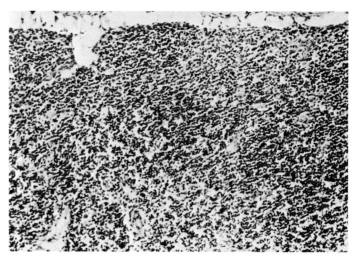

Figure 7–8. Lymph node at stage of lymphoid depletion with absence of germinal follicles and loss of distinction between cortex and medulla causing partial loss of architecture. Subcapsular sinusoid is distended. (Hematoxylin and eosin, ×90.)

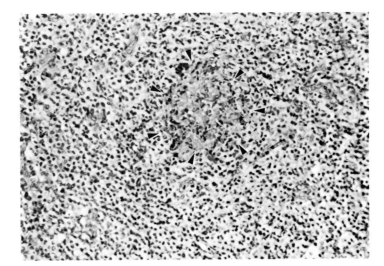

Figure 7–9. Lymph node cortex with "burnt-out" and barely discernible germinal center. (Hematoxylin and eosin, ×120.)

Figure 7–10. Diffuse lymphoid proliferation in late stage of persistent generalized lymphadenopathy with prominent vessels, decreased cellularity, and absence of follicles. (Hematoxylin and eosin, ×90.)

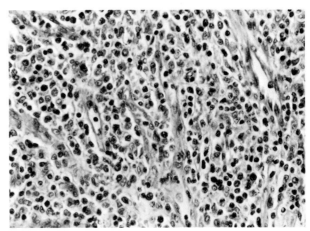

42

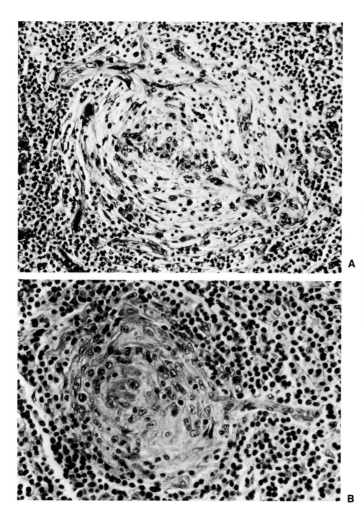

Figure 7–11. Hyaline vascular follicles with radially penetrating blood vessels. *A,* Concentric rings of sclerosis result in onion-skin appearance. *B,* Peripheral penetrating vessel results in a characteristic "lollypop" follicle. This form of hyperplasia is associated with increased incidence of lymphadenopathic Kaposi's sarcoma in same node or found in subsequent biopsy. (Hematoxylin and eosin, ×120.)

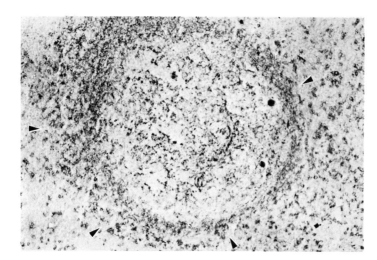

Figure 7–12. Immunoperoxidase staining for immunoglobulin M in secondary follicle from node with persistent generalized lymphadenopathy. Mantle zone lymphocytes show characteristic membrane staining *(arrows),* and there is increased interstitial immunoglobulin within the germinal center which may represent immune complex deposition on dendritic reticulum cells. (Methyl green counterstain, ×90.)

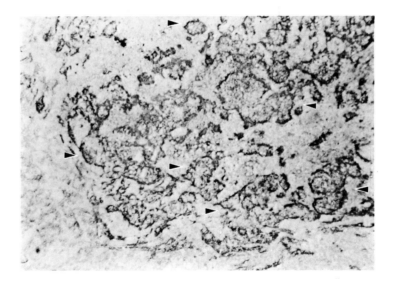

Figure 7–13. Lymph node with persistent generalized lymphadenopathy and follicular lysis stained with monoclonal antibody to dendritic reticulum cells. Darkly stained dendritic cells are fragmented into discrete aggregates *(arrows)*. (Methyl green counterstain, ×160.)

cell (DRC) framework is disrupted (Fig. 7–13). Destruction of DRCs is a characteristic early finding in PGL and may be an important factor in its pathogenesis.[30] Langerhans' cells are usually decreased in skin biopsy specimens from AIDS patients. Like DRCs, Langerhans' cells possess CD4 receptors and may be infected with HIV, serving as a reservoir for the virus.[20,31,32]

T-cells. Distribution of T-cell phenotypic subsets in hyperplastic lymph nodes from patients with PGL and AIDS is profoundly different from that of reactive nodes in most other disorders. In addition to a quantitative and qualitative defect in the CD4 inducer or helper subset within the paracortex, mantle zones, and germinal centers, the number of cells with the suppressor T-cell phenotype (CD8+) is greatly increased. Changes in helper/suppressor T-cell ratios in the paracortex usually parallel those in the peripheral blood[33] and provide evidence for progressive immunologic deterioration.[34] Studies with an antibody that dissects the CD8+ population into suppressor and cytotoxic subpopulations show that the increase is predominantly in the T-cell suppressor subset.[35] Most strikingly, suppressor/cytotoxic T-lymphocytes are also present overlying follicular centers and mantle zones (Fig. 7–14), in contrast to their virtual absence in reactive follicles from most other lymphadenopathies. Other T-cell abnormalities in HIV infection include an increase in activated T-cells in paracortical regions as identified by HLA-DR+ cells and a decrease in interleukin-2-positive cells identified with monoclonal antibody anti-TAC (CD25).

Increased percentages of suppressor/cytotoxic T-cells and decreased numbers of

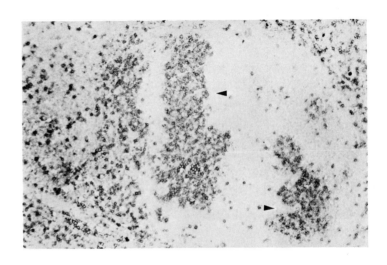

Figure 7–14. Lymph node stained for OKT8 from HIV-1-positive patient with persistent generalized lymphadenopathy contains numerous suppressor/cytotoxic T-lymphocytes, including large aggregates overlying the germinal center *(arrows)*. (Methyl green counterstain, ×90.)

helper T-cells are characteristic findings in lymph nodes from patients with HIV-related lymphadenopathy. Changes in distribution of lymphocyte subpopulations in patients with PGL are similar to those with AIDS although less severe. The immunohistochemical findings described previously, although characteristic, are not specific for HIV infection; similar findings may be encountered in nodes from HIV-negative intravenous drug abusers and patients with viral diseases such as hepatitis.

HIV-RELATED MALIGNANT LYMPHOMAS

Not surprisingly, the pool of abnormally stimulated B-lymphocytes and the impaired T-cell surveillance that characterize the AIDS-related complex and prodromal states provide fertile ground for clonal evolution of neoplastic B-lymphocytes and malignant lymphoma. The Centers for Disease Control (CDC) has expanded the definition of AIDS to include the occurrence of intermediate and high-grade non-Hodgkin's lymphomas of B and indeterminate subtype in HIV-seropositive individuals.[36] At least one third of patients with AIDS and lymphoma report prolonged periods of generalized adenopathy. Serial pathologic studies may demonstrate progressive evolution of lymphomas from generalized lymphadenopathy and abnormal lymphoid hyperplasia. This situation is not unique to AIDS but occurs in patients with other immunodysregulatory states, including renal transplant and other allograft recipients and patients with drug regimens, viral infec-

tions, and congenital abnormalities predisposing to immune defects. Individuals with AIDS in whom malignant lymphoma develops often have more severely altered immunity than other AIDS patients. As might be expected, the combination of a severely impaired immune system and high-grade malignant lymphoma indicates a poor prognosis (median survival 6 to 8 months) and a refractory response to combination chemotherapy.[10,37,38]

In a study of lymphomas in 90 homosexual men,[39] the median age at presentation was 37 years and the age distribution was identical to that of AIDS patients. Histologic subtypes and cell phenotypes have been consistent with B-cell origin in virtually all patients with AIDS-related non-Hodgkin's lymphomas, and lymphomas are predominantly high-grade or aggressive histologic types, particularly immunoblastic lymphomas of B-cells and undifferentiated or Burkitt-like (small noncleaved cell) lymphomas.[40] Intermediate-grade diffuse non-Hodgkin's lymphomas (predominantly large noncleaved cells) are less common. Rarely other types of non-Hodgkin's lymphomas, including T-cell lymphomas,[41,42] and an indolent T-cell chronic lymphocytic leukemia with suppressor cell phenotype have been described in patients with AIDS.[37] Other lymphoma types, including low-grade small cleaved cell, prolymphocytic, and lymphoplasmacytic lymphoma, as well as acute myelogenous leukemia, have been reported,[38] but their relationship to AIDS is unclear. Homosexual men with low-grade lymphomas (poorly differentiated lymphocytic lymphomas and lymphoplasmacytic lymphomas) usu-

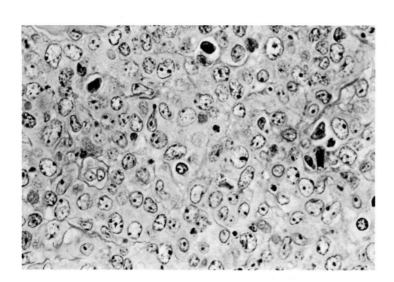

Figure 7–15. B-cell immunoblastic lymphoma from AIDS patient reveals uniform population of large transformed lymphoid cells with one to three evenly spaced nucleoli and abundant amphophilic cytoplasm. (Hematoxylin and eosin, ×400.)

ally do not have HIV antibodies,[38] suggesting that pathogenesis of this group of lymphomas is unrelated to AIDS. Similarly, low-grade follicular lymphomas, which constitute approximately half the lymphomas in otherwise healthy adults,[43] are rare in immunodeficient patients.

Immunoblastic lymphomas are characterized by diffuse nodal effacement by a proliferation of large transformed B-lymphoid cells with plasmacytoid features. Cytologic examination shows neoplastic transformed lymphocytes with uniform round or oval nuclei, one to three evenly spaced nucleoli, marginated nuclear chromatin, and prominent eosinophilic or amphophilic cytoplasm on Giemsa stain (Fig. 7–15). Methyl green–pyronine staining strongly highlights the nucleoli and cytoplasm rich in RNA. In some cases the lymphomas are more pleomorphic with multinuclear or lobated cells that resemble Reed-Sternberg cells (Fig. 7–16).

The high incidence of B-cell immunoblastic lymphomas in AIDS is common to other immune disorders, including organ transplantation, autoimmune disease, and immunoblastic lymphadenopathy. The high incidence of Burkitt or Burkitt-like lymphomas, however, is not characteristic of the other immunosuppressed groups. These tumors frequently involve the bowel wall and other extranodal sites (Fig. 7–17) and are characterized by uniform proliferation of intermediate-sized lymphocytes with round or slightly irregular nuclei, prominent, usually single nucleoli, and a small rim of pyroninophilic cytoplasm (Fig. 7–18). The high cell turnover is associated with numerous mitoses and breakdown of cells with cellular debris and "tingible body" macrophages, resulting in the characteristic "starry sky" appearance.

Most patients with HIV infections have serum antibodies against EBV, although the EBV genome usually cannot be demonstrated

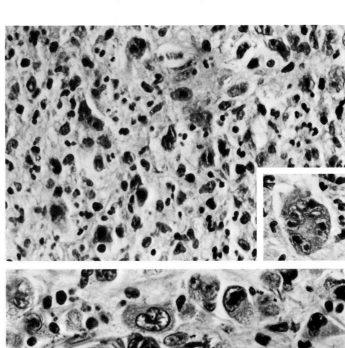

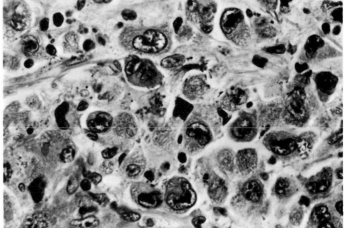

Figure 7–16. *A,* Pleomorphic B-cell immunoblastic lymphoma from AIDS patient showing variation in size and shape of transformed lymphoid cells and Reed-Sternberg-like forms *(inset). B,* Malignant lymphoma manifest as chest wall mass is composed of sheets of large polyploid Reed-Sternberg-like cells. (Hematoxylin and eosin; *A,* ×160; inset ×400; *B,* ×400.)

A

B

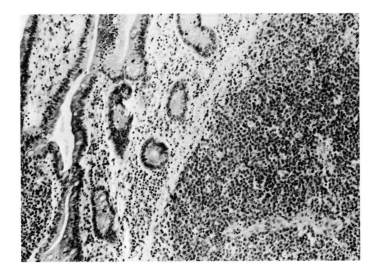

Figure 7–17. Small bowel resection from AIDS patient with Burkitt-like lymphoma reveals monomorphous infiltrate of lymphoma cells into bowel wall. (Hematoxylin and eosin, ×90.)

in lymph nodes with generalized adenopathy.[44] Since EBV-infected B-cells are long lived and may undergo many more cell divisions than noninfected B-cells, the probability of chromosomal mutations and malignant transformation in a setting of immunologic impairment is high.[45,46] In support of this theory, hyperplastic nodes from PGL sometimes contain small clonal B-cell proliferations, and AIDS-related lymphomas are often composed of multiple B-cell clones, whereas lymphomas in the general population are derived from a single neoplastic clone.[47,48]

Cytogenetic studies have revealed chromosomal abnormalities in HIV-related Burkitt's lymphoma that are similar to those in the endemic form.[49] Also an in vitro cell line has been established from a Burkitt-like lymphoma in an AIDS patient; the cells displayed a t(8;14) translocation similar to that in endemic African Burkitt's lymphoma.[50] Chromosomal translocations in Burkitt's lymphoma result in translocation of the c-*myc* oncogene to immunoglobulin gene loci on chromosomes 2, 14, or 22.[51] Unlike lymphomas in the general population, AIDS-associated lymphomas of both Burkitt's and non-Burkitt's types consistently show c-*myc* oncogene rearrangements.[48,52] Although EBV proteins and sequences are present in some HIV-related lymphomas,[48,53] the majority resemble sporadic Burkitt's lymphoma in having c-*myc* gene rearrangements without EBV sequences.[48,54] Translocations of the c-*myc* oncogene and recombination with the switch region of the immunoglobulin heavy chain locus are thought to contribute to the pathogenesis of most AIDS-associated lymphomas, analo-

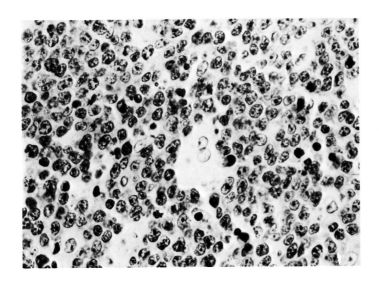

Figure 7–18. High-power photomicrograph shows characteristic cytologic features of Burkitt-like lymphoma, including uniform lymphoid cells with round or oval nuclei and "starry sky" macrophage *(center)*. (Hematoxylin and eosin, ×250.)

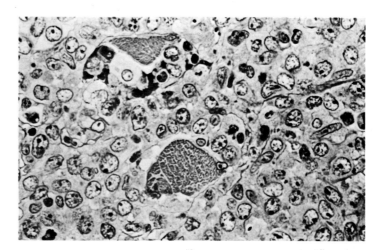

Figure 7–19. Immunoblastic lymphoma in patient with AIDS forms a soft tissue flank mass infiltrating skeletal muscle. (Hematoxylin and eosin, ×400.)

gous to the chain of events in sporadic Burkitt's lymphoma.[48]

In contrast to malignant lymphoma in the general population, in which less than 40% have stage IV disease at diagnosis,[43] extranodal lymphoma with advanced stages of disease is common in AIDS-related non-Hodgkin's lymphomas.[10,37,38,55] Lymphoma in AIDS patients most often involves the central nervous system (CNS), bone marrow, bowel, soft tissue (Fig. 7–19), and mucocutaneous areas. The frequency of presentation with intraoral or anorectal tumors (Fig. 7–20) is striking in view of similar involvement of these sites with Kaposi's sarcoma. Involvement of unusual primary sites such as kidney, heart, and adrenal glands is also seen.

The frequency of CNS involvement either with primary lymphoma or as a site of relapse mimics the pattern of lymphomatous involvement that occurs in other congenital or iatrogenic immunodeficiency syndromes. Multicentric brain mass lesions are relatively common and may resemble toxoplasmosis on radiologic studies.[56] Infiltrates in the brain are frequently perivascular (Fig. 7–21) and may result in extensive necrosis (Fig. 7–22). Onset of symptoms of CNS lymphoma in AIDS patients may be insidious, however, with nonspecific complaints such as altered mental status.[56] Cytologic examination of cerebrospinal fluid may show lymphomatous meningitis and be helpful in establishing a diagnosis.

Although non-Hodgkin's lymphomas in AIDS patients have almost invariably been of B-cell derivation, they may be devoid of B- or T-cell markers when examined by immunophenotyping techniques and may fail to express surface or cytoplasmic immunoglobulins.[48,57] This occurs most often with large cell

immunoblastic lymphomas, particularly those with pleomorphic malignant cells. In this situation immunoglobulin gene rearrangement may be extremely helpful in defining the clonal B-cell nature of the proliferation. Gene rearrangement studies are particularly useful in confirming the cytologic diagnosis of lymphoma in exfoliated cells from pleural and

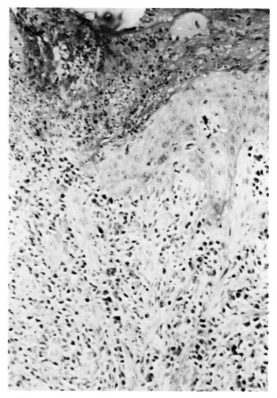

Figure 7–20. Malignant lymphoma present as anorectal mass in patient with AIDS and Kaposi's sarcoma shows ulceration of anal squamous epithelium. (Hematoxylin and eosin, ×90.)

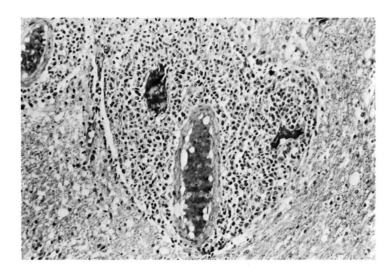

Figure 7–21. Histologic section of brain from AIDS patient with malignant lymphoma discovered at autopsy reveals characteristic multifocal and perivascular localization of malignant cells. (Hematoxylin and eosin, ×90.)

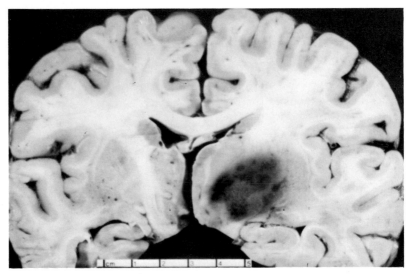

Figure 7–22. Primary immunoblastic lymphoma of brain in AIDS patient, with hemorrhagic necrosis of right basal ganglion (coronal section through brain at level of hippocampus).

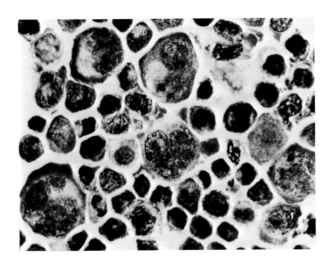

Figure 7–23. Malignant pericardial effusion from AIDS patient with large dysplastic cells having prominent nucleoli and plasmacytoid features. Cells were devoid of B- or T-cell markers when stained with extensive panel of monoclonal antibodies, but heavy chain gene rearrangement confirmed monoclonal B-cell proliferation. (Air-dried Wright-stained cytocentrifuge smear, ×800.)

pericardial effusions (Fig. 7–23). AIDS-related lymphomas may have two or more rearranged immunoglobulin gene bands, indicating more than one clonal B-cell population.[52] Also, histologically identical biopsy specimens from different anatomic sites may display different patterns of gene rearrangement, indicating derivation from clonally distinct B-cell populations. Recurrent tumors may exhibit different chromosomal breakpoints and gene rearrangements, which suggests the transformation of a second B-cell clone.[58] AIDS-related lymphomas may thus represent multiclonal B-cell expansions analogous to lymphomas in other immunosuppressed patients such as transplant recipients.[59]

HODGKIN'S DISEASE AND HIV INFECTION

The CDC does not consider the presence of Hodgkin's disease to be a criterion for the diagnosis of AIDS in HIV-positive individuals, and the existence of an association between HIV infection and Hodgkin's disease remains controversial.[60] Hodgkin's disease has, however, been reported in patients with primary immune deficiencies such as ataxia-telangiectasia.[61] The ratio of Hodgkin's to non-Hodgkin's lymphomas is higher in intravenous drug abusers with AIDS than in the homosexual population.[60] Similarly, KS is rare in intravenous drug abusers and is seldom associated with AIDS-related Hodgkin's disease.[62]

Hodgkin's disease occurring in HIV-infected patients has a number of atypical features. These include advanced clinical stage at presentation (stage III or IV disease) with frequent "B" symptoms and an aggressive clinical course similar to that of non-Hodgkin's lymphomas. Bone marrow and liver infiltration at presentation, as well as bone marrow infiltration without prior splenic disease, is sometimes found.[37] Hodgkin's disease in HIV-infected patients, unlike that in the general population, is commonly diagnosed on the basis of biopsy of bone marrow, liver, soft tissue, or other extranodal sites.

Histologic features of Hodgkin's disease in AIDS patients are the same as in Hodgkin's disease in the general population. Immuno-pathologic studies, however, reveal a decrease or depletion of helper T-lymphocytes and predominance of T-suppressor cells, which contrasts with Hodgkin's disease in the general population.[63] The lack of an appropriate T-cell immunologic response in HIV-positive patients with Hodgkin's disease may contribute to their poor prognosis and lack of response to therapy.

PEDIATRIC HIV INFECTION AND LYMPHORETICULAR DISEASE

The increased incidence of lymphoproliferative disorders in children with AIDS is not surprising considering the frequency of lymphoid neoplasms associated with congenital immune deficiency.[61] Lymphoid hyperplasia with germinal center formation occurs commonly in children with AIDS and may affect lymph nodes, lymphoid nodules in the colon, Peyer's patches in the small intestine, nodular lymphoid aggregates in the liver, and lymphoid follicles in the medulla of the thymus.[64-67]

The lungs of children with AIDS may be affected by a variety of lymphoid infiltrative disorders ranging from pulmonary lymphoid hyperplasia (PLH) and lymphoid interstitial pneumonitis (LIP) to a polyclonal and polymorphic B-cell lymphoproliferative disorder (PBLD)[68] and malignant lymphoma. PLH is characterized by peribronchiolar nodular lymphoid aggregates with or without germinal centers.[64-66] LIP is characterized by diffuse infiltration of alveolar septa and peribronchial tissue by predominantly small regular lymphocytes, with occasional plasma cells and immunoblasts. The pathogenesis and natural history of LIP in children with AIDS are still unknown, but biopsy-proven LIP is considered part of the spectrum of AIDS in children.[64,65,69,70]

PBLD, an entity intermediate between benign and malignant lymphoid proliferation, has more rarely been described in the lungs and extranodal sites.[68,71] Infiltrates in PBLD comprise a polymorphic B-cell population of lymphocytes, plasma cells, plasmacytoid lymphocytes sometimes with Russell bodies, and immunoblasts (Fig. 7–24). Despite its polymorphous nature and polyclonal staining for immunoglobulins, the infiltrate behaves in a malignant manner, causing lymphadenopathy, pulmonary nodules, and extranodal infiltrates. Whether this entity is a form of polyclonal B-cell lymphoma, similar to that described in allograft recipients, or a stage of abnormal lymphoid proliferation that may progress to lymphoma is not clear. Its patho-

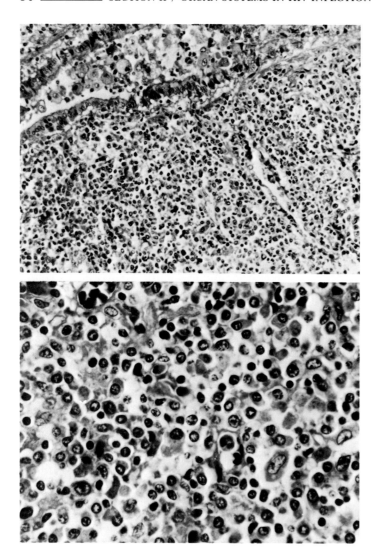

Figure 7–24. Lung section from 40-month-old girl with polyclonal polymorphic B-cell lymphoproliferative disorder and infiltration of lungs, liver, and bone marrow. Infiltrate surrounds bronchiole, extends into pulmonary parenchyma, and is composed of plasma cells, immunoblasts, and plasmacytoid lymphocytes. (Hematoxylin and eosin, *top,* ×100; *bottom,* ×250.)

genesis is presumably related to EBV infection, since EBV is known to cause polyclonal, oligoclonal, and monoclonal B-cell proliferation in immunosuppressed persons, including those with AIDS,[46] and since high titers of EBV antibodies and EBV genome are found in tissues from patients with PBLD.[71]

LYMPHADENOPATHIC KAPOSI'S SARCOMA

KS in homosexual men, like that in endemic regions of equatorial Africa, is characterized by lymphadenopathy, involvement of lungs and other viscera, and a fulminant clinical course.[72] KS predominantly affects the homosexual male population and is rare in HIV infection associated with drug abuse or blood transfu-

sions. Histopathologic findings in lymph nodes and spleen are typical of KS, with proliferation of spindle-shaped cells lining cleftlike spaces with extravasated red blood cells (Fig. 7–25). Distinctive eosinophilic globules are found in macrophages and spindle cells as in KS at other sites (Fig. 7–26). Nodal involvement may be subtle, often subcapsular and obliterating the peripheral sinus, or nodes may be replaced by tumor. KS infiltrates T-cell zones (Fig. 7–27), extending from the paracortical regions into germinal centers. Areas of the lymph node uninvolved by KS usually are lymphocyte depleted and may show foci of dermatopathic lymphadenitis.

In HIV-positive patients with KS, lymph node biopsy often shows hyaline vascular follicles (Fig. 7–11). Multicentric hyaline vascular lymphoid hyperplasia is associated with an

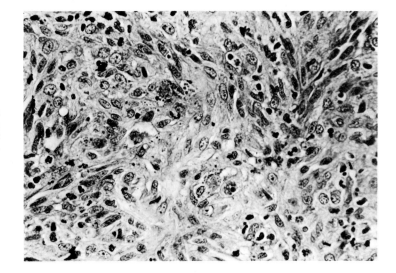

Figure 7–25. Kaposi's sarcoma in tonsillar biopsy specimen from AIDS patient shows characteristic spindle-cell proliferation. (Hematoxylin and eosin, ×260.)

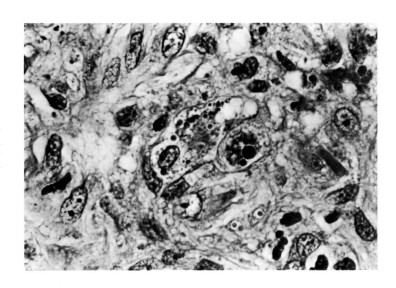

Figure 7–26. High-power photomicrograph shows eosinophilic globules characteristically present in spindle cells and macrophages in Kaposi's sarcoma. (Hematoxylin and eosin, ×400.)

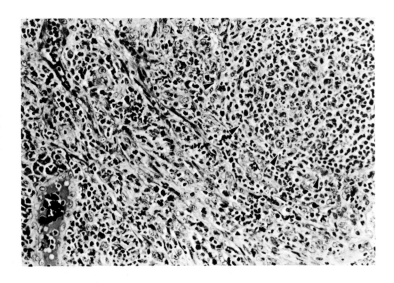

Figure 7–27. Lymph node from AIDS patient with Kaposi's sarcoma shows characteristic early involvement of T-cell zone adjacent to hyperplastic germinal center *(arrows)*. (Hematoxylin and eosin, ×120.)

increased incidence of KS in the general population[73]; in lymph node biopsies from HIV-infected persons, vascular follicles and KS may coexist in the same node or subsequent biopsy specimen.[28] In patients at risk for AIDS, lymph nodes that show hyaline vascular changes should therefore be scrutinized for KS with examination of multiple sections through the entire node.

IMMUNE THROMBOCYTOPENIC PURPURA

Patients with PGL and AIDS have an increased incidence of an immune regulatory disorder directed against platelets, which is similar to classic immune thrombocytopenic purpura (ITP) and associated with circulating immune complexes and elevated total gammaglobulin levels.[74] The finding of HIV antibodies in all homosexual men with isolated thrombocytopenia in a San Francisco series indicates that immune thrombocytopenia is part of the clinical spectrum of the AIDS-related complex.[75] The CDC does not consider thrombocytopenia a criterion for advanced disease, and it is not associated with a short-term risk of progression to AIDS.[76]

HIV-infected patients with thrombocytopenia have higher levels of platelet-bound immunoglobulin G (IgG) and complement than other patients with ITP, and thrombocytopenic purpura in HIV-infected patients may be caused by nonspecific deposition of complement and immune complexes on platelets rather than the antiplatelet IgG directed against platelet antigenic determinants that characterizes classic ITP.[77,78] In addition to autoimmune destruction of platelets, toxic effects of therapy and impaired hematopoiesis may contribute to the thrombocytopenia, and HIV may directly infect megakaryocytes.[79] Megakaryocyte numbers are normal or increased in bone marrow, and the disease is similar in its clinical course to classic ITP.[76] In addition to immune thrombocytopenia, antierythrocyte and antineutrophil antibodies may be present.[76] However, antierythrocyte antibodies are not usually associated with hemolysis. A form of thrombotic thrombocytopenic purpura has also been described in association with HIV infection.[80]

Spleens removed from HIV-positive patients with ITP have hyperplastic follicles and immunologic features (increased number of suppressor T-lymphocytes and decreased number of helper T-cells) similar to those in lymph nodes.[81] Immune complex deposition in postcapillary venules and other vessels may be found when immunofluorescence techniques are used on cryostat sections (Fig. 7–28). Although response to splenectomy is similar to that in classic ITP, sustained response to steroids is low (less than 10%) and patients have a high incidence of steroid-related side effects, including further immunosuppression.[75]

SALIVARY GLAND LYMPHOID PROLIFERATIONS IN HIV INFECTION

Salivary gland infection with HIV may occur early in the course of disease if the virus had an oral port of entry and the rate of exposure was high. HIV can be cultured from saliva of infected individuals, and salivary glands may also be infected with EBV and CMV. Lymph nodes in the parotid glands and other periductal lymphoid tissues undergo characteristic changes of HIV-related lymphadenopathy, including abnormal follicular hyperplasia and considerable enlargement. Salivary nodes may also be the site of primary non-Hodgkin's lymphomas in AIDS patients.[82]

Hyperplasia of salivary gland lymph nodes is associated with duct dilatation and cyst for-

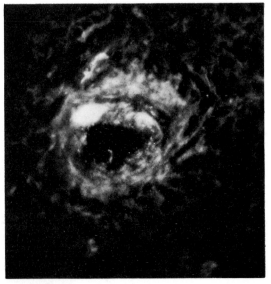

Figure 7–28. In cryostat section of spleen resected from AIDS patient with thrombocytopenic purpura, immunofluorescence microscopy shows deposition of immune complex (IgM and C3) in wall of postcapillary venule. (Original magnification × 120.)

mation. Proliferation of ductal epithelial and myoepithelial cells results in formation of myoepithelial islands identical to those in Sjögren's syndrome (Fig. 7–29).[83] Patients with HIV infections do not usually have features of sicca syndrome (xerophthalmia, keratoconjunctivitis sicca), a disease most common in middle-aged or older women with rheumatoid arthritis. HIV-related sialadenitis does not have the characteristic lymphocytic infiltration and atrophy of the salivary glands seen in Sjögren's syndrome.[82] Immunophenotypic studies reveal the same changes in CD4+ and CD8+ T-cell subsets in salivary lymphoid infiltrates in HIV-infected patients that occur in other sites, whereas in Sjögren's syndrome CD4 lymphocytes predominate.[84] Formation of myoepithelial islands and duct cysts in HIV-positive patients appears to be a reactive

process unrelated to Sjögren's syndrome in the general population. Pathogenesis may relate at least in part to duct obstruction by hyperplastic intrasalivary lymphoid tissue.[82]

BLOOD AND BONE MARROW IN HIV INFECTION

Abnormalities in the blood and bone marrow are common in patients with AIDS, even in the early stages of the disease, which suggests that the bone marrow is a target organ in HIV infection.[85] In situ hybridization studies of HIV nucleic acid have shown infection of histiocytes and lymphocytes in bone marrow specimens from patients with AIDS-related complex and AIDS.[86] The most common peripheral blood abnormalities associ-

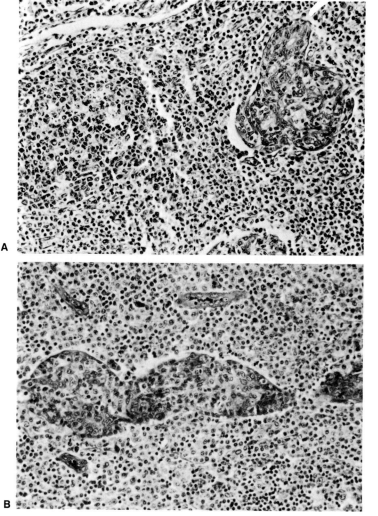

Figure 7–29. Salivary gland biopsy specimen from HIV-positive patient with bilateral salivary gland enlargement and generalized lymphadenopathy. *A,* Lymphoepithelial lesion with myoepithelial island *(right)* and denuded lymphoid follicle devoid of follicular mantle *(left)*. *B,* Large myoepithelial island surrounded by vascular lymphoid proliferation. (Hematoxylin and eosin, ×150.)

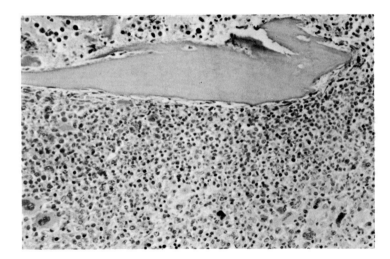

Figure 7–30. Prominent paratrabecular lymphoid infiltrate in bone marrow from patient with persistent generalized lymphadenopathy and no evidence of malignant lymphoma. (Hematoxylin and eosin, ×160.)

ated with HIV infection are granulocytopenia with a shift to immature forms in the granulocyte series, lymphopenia with circulating atypical lymphocytes, and vacuolated monocytes. Abnormal myeloid maturation with dysplastic forms and macronormoblastic erythroid maturation may occur, as well as a constellation of features similar to findings in the myelodysplastic syndromes or preleukemia.[87] Myelogenous leukemias, however, are not usually associated with HIV infection.

Normochromic normocytic anemia consistent with the anemia of chronic disease is often present with HIV infection, and reticulocyte counts are not increased, suggesting that the anemia is hypoproliferative.[85] Most patients have increased iron stores with low serum levels of iron, low or normal total iron-binding capacity, and increased ferritin levels. High ferritin and low serum iron levels have also been described in nonanemic patients with persistent generalized lymphadenopathy.[88]

In biopsy specimens cellularity of the bone marrow is frequently increased, although the marrow is hypocellular in approximately 5% of cases.[76] Eosinophils are frequently increased in number. Megaloblastoid red blood cell maturation is common, and ring sideroblasts may be present.[76] Megakaryocytes are usually normal or increased in number and may include dysplastic forms and denuded nuclei.[89]

Because increased bone marrow reticulin is common in AIDS, bone marrow aspirates may be unsatisfactory for diagnosis. Aggregates of small lymphoid cells, including irregular lymphoid forms, are frequently found in bone marrow biopsy specimens. These aggregates may be in a paratrabecular location, include

large transformed lymphoid cells or immunoblasts, and be confused with lymphomatous infiltration (Figs. 7–30 and 7–31). Primary diagnosis of malignant lymphoma based on bone marrow biopsy findings of lymphoid nodules in an HIV patient should therefore be made with caution.

Granulomatous aggregates of histiocytes often indicate marrow involvement by opportunistic organisms (usually *Mycobacterium avium-intracellulare*) (Fig. 7–32). The presence of numerous intracellular organisms within histiocytes may result in the appearance of "pseudo-Gaucher" cells.[90] As with lymph nodes, mycobacteria may be grown on cultures of bone marrow with or without granulomas. Patients with AIDS may be unable to form granulomas in response to mycobacterial infection because of impaired lymphocyte-macrophage interaction. Bone marrow and lymph node specimens from AIDS patients should be stained for acid-fast organisms regardless of the presence of granulomas.

Some patients with AIDS have numerous hemophagocytic histiocytes, similar to those in immunocompromised patients such as renal transplant recipients with viral infections.[24] Bone marrow from patients with advanced disease frequently shows damage, including a marked decrease in cellularity, myelofibrosis, areas of necrosis, and infiltration by plasma and mast cells.

Bone marrow is commonly involved early by lymphoma in AIDS patients and may be the initial site. Non-Hodgkin's lymphomas are almost invariably B-cell derived, with Burkitt-like or immunoblastic morphology. In Burkitt-type lymphoma, diffuse leukemia-like

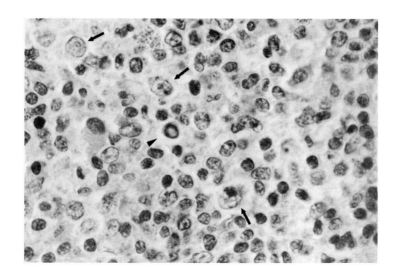

Figure 7–31. Higher power photomicrograph of lymphoid aggregate in bone marrow from patient with persistent generalized lymphadenopathy reveals small lymphoid cells and scattered immunoblasts *(arrows)*. Plasmacytoid lymphoid cell contains intranuclear inclusion *(arrowhead)*. (Hematoxylin and eosin, ×400.)

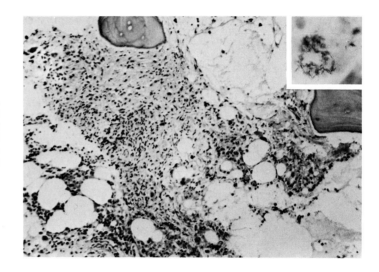

Figure 7–32. Bone marrow from AIDS patient with *Mycobacterium avium* infection shows characteristic poorly defined granulomas. Inset shows numerous acid-fast bacilli. (Hematoxylin and eosin, ×90, inset ×400.)

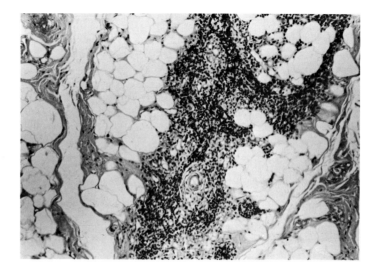

Figure 7–33. Thymus from young AIDS patient at autopsy shows profound involutional changes with absence of Hassall's corpuscles and absence of definitive cortex and medulla. (Hematoxylin and eosin, ×90.)

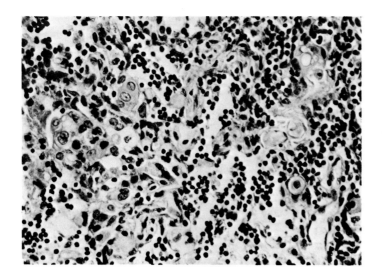

Figure 7–34. Higher power photomicrograph of involuted thymus with fibrovascular core, round or oval lymphocytes, histiocytes, and degenerated remnants of Hassall's corpuscles. (Hematoxylin and eosin, ×160.)

packing of marrow may occur in the absence of peripheral blood involvement.

THYMUS IN HIV INFECTION

Thymic involutionary changes occur in patients with advanced HIV infection, and retroviral antigens can be localized in thymic epithelium from AIDS patients.[91] Atrophy affects both cortex and medulla, with depletion or absence of Hassall's corpuscles (Fig. 7–33).[92] Definitive cortex and medulla may not be recognizable. These changes are associated with depletion of thymocytes, infiltration by plasma cells and mast cells, and fibrosis (Fig. 7–34).[93] Although the thymus involutes with age and in response to stress, this process is characterized principally by reduction of thymocytes with sparing of Hassall's corpuscles and medullary epithelium. Thymic involution in AIDS patients is therefore unlikely to result only from age or debilitating illness and resembles that sometimes noted in graft-versus-host reaction, suggesting organ-specific involutional changes. The thymic involutionary changes in AIDS are not substantially different from those in patients with congenital or acquired immunodeficiency.[91]

REFERENCES

1. Murray HW, Rubin BY, Masur H, et al: Impaired production of lymphokines and immune (gamma) interferon in the acquired immunodeficiency syndrome. N Engl J Med 310:883-889, 1984.
2. Fahey JL, Prince H, Weaver M, et al: Quantitative changes in T helper or T suppressor/cytotoxic lymphocyte subsets that distinguish acquired immune deficiency syndrome from other immune subset disorders. Am J Med 76:95-100, 1984.
3. Carney WP, Rubin RH, Hoffman RA, et al: Analysis of T lymphocyte subsets in cytomegalovirus mononucleosis. J Immunol 126:2114-2116, 1981.
4. Reinherz EL, O'Brien C, Rosenthal P, et al: The cellular basis for viral-induced immunodeficiency: Analysis by monoclonal antibodies. J Immunol 125:1269-1274, 1980.
5. Schnittman SM, Lane HC, Higgins SE, et al: Direct polyclonal activation of human B lymphocytes by the acquired immune deficiency syndrome virus. Science 233:1084-1086, 1986.
6. Polk BF, Fox R, Brookmeyer R, et al: Predictors of the acquired immunodeficiency syndrome developing in a cohort of seropositive homosexual men. N Engl J Med 316:61-66, 1987.
7. Gartner S, Markovitz P, Markovitz DM, et al: The role of mononuclear phagocytes in HTLV-III/LAV infection. Science 233:215-219, 1986.
8. Wood GS, Burns BF, Dorfman RF, et al: The immunohistology of non-T cells in the acquired immunodeficiency syndrome. Am J Pathol 120:371-379, 1985.
9. Abrams DI, Lewis BJ, Beckstead JH, et al: Persistent diffuse lymphadenopathy in homosexual men: endpoint or prodrome? Ann Intern Med 100:801:-808, 1984.
10. Levine AM, Meyer PR, Begandy MK, et al: Development of B-cell lymphoma in homosexual men. Ann Intern Med 100:7-13, 1984.
11. Mathur-Wagh U, Enlow RW, Spigland I, et al: Longitudinal study of persistent generalized lymphadenopathy in homosexual men: Relation to acquired immunodeficiency syndrome. Lancet 1:1033-1038, 1984.
12. Metroka CE, Cunningham-Rundles S, Pollack MS, et al: Generalized lymphadenopathy in homosexual men. Ann Intern Med 99:585-591, 1983.
13. Ioachim HL, Cronin W, Roy M, et al: Persistent lymphadenopathies in people at high risk for HIV infection. Am J Clin Pathol 93:208-218, 1990.
14. Lifson JD, Reyes GR, McGrath MS, et al: AIDS retrovirus induced cytopathology: Giant cell forma-

tion and involvement of CD4 antigen. Science 232:1123-1127, 1986.

15. Butler JJ, Osborne BM: Lymph node enlargement in patients with unsuspected human immunodeficiency virus infections. Hum Pathol 19:849-854, 1988.

16. Burns BF, Woods GS, Dorfman RF: The varied histopathology of lymphadenopathy in the homosexual male. Am J Surg Pathol 9:287-297, 1985.

17. Parravicini CL, Vago L, Costanzi GC, et al: Follicle lysis in lymph nodes from homosexual men. Blood 68:595-598, 1986.

18. Wood GS, Garcia C, Dorfman RF, et al: The immunohistology of follicle lysis in lymph node biopsies from homosexual men. Blood 66:1092-1097, 1985.

19. Dalgleish AG, Beverley PCL, Clapham PR, et al: The CD4 (CD4) antigen is an essential component of the receptor for the AIDS retrovirus. Nature 312:763-767, 1984.

20. Armstrong JA, Horne R: Follicular dendritic cells and virus-like particles in AIDS and AIDS-related lymphadenopathy. Lancet 2:370-372, 1984.

21. Tenner-Racz K, Racz P, Dietrich M, et al: Altered follicular dendritic cells and virus-like particles in AIDS and AIDS-related lymphadenopathy. Lancet 1:105-106, 1985.

22. Parmentier HK, van Wichen D, Sie-Go DMD, et al: HIV-1 infection and virus production in follicular dendritic cells in lymph nodes: A case report with analysis of isolated follicular dendritic cells. Am J Pathol 137:247-251, 1990.

23. Sun NCJ, Shapshak P, Schmid P, et al: Comparison of HIV antigens and nucleic acids in biopsied lymph nodes from patients at risk for HIV infection. Lab Invest 58:89A, 1988.

24. Risdall RJ, McKenna RW, Nesbit ME, et al: Virus-associated hemophagocytic syndrome. Cancer 44:993-1002, 1979.

25. O'Murchadha MT, Wolf B, Neiman RS: The histologic features of hyperplastic lymphadenopathy in AIDS-related complex are nonspecific. Am J Surg Pathol 11:94-99, 1987.

26. Stanley MW, Frizzera G: Diagnostic specificity of histologic features in lymph node biopsy specimens from patients at risk for the acquired immunodeficiency syndrome. Hum Pathol 17:1231-1239, 1986.

27. Chadburn A, Metroka C, Mouradian J: Progressive lymph node histology and its prognostic value in patients with acquired immunodeficiency syndrome and AIDS-related complex. Hum Pathol 20:579-587, 1989.

28. Harris NL: Hypervascular follicular hyperplasia and Kaposi's sarcoma in patients at risk for AIDS. N Engl J Med 310:462-463, 1984.

29. Lane HC, Masur H, Edgar LC, et al: Abnormalities of B-cell activation and immunoregulation in patients with the acquired immunodeficiency syndrome. N Engl J Med 309:453-458, 1983.

30. Janossy G, Pinching AJ, Bofill M, et al: An immunohistological approach to persistent lymphadenopathy and its relevance to AIDS. Clin Exp Immunol 59:257-266, 1985.

31. Gyorkey F, Melnick JL, Sinkovics JG, et al: Retrovirus resembling HTLV in macrophages of patients with AIDS. Lancet 1:106, 1985.

32. Kolata G: Biomedical briefings: Where is the AIDS virus harbored? Science 232:1197, 1986.

33. Said JW, Shintaku IP, Teitelbaum A, et al: Distribu-

tion of T-cell phenotypic subsets and surface immunoglobulin-bearing lymphocytes in lymph nodes from male homosexuals with persistent generalized adenopathy: An immunohistochemical and ultrastructural study. Hum Pathol 15:785-790, 1984.

34. Turner RR, Meyer PR, Taylor CR, et al: Immunohistology of persistent generalized lymphadenopathy: Evidence for progressive lymph node abnormalities in some patients. Am J Clin Pathol 88:10-19, 1987.

35. Wood GS, Burns BF, Dorfman RF, et al: In situ quantitation of lymph node helper, suppressor, and cytotoxic T cell subsets in AIDS. Blood 67:596-603, 1986.

36. Centers for Disease Control: Revision of the CDC surveillance case definition for the acquired immunodeficiency syndrome. MMWR 36(suppl):1s-15s, 1987.

37. Knowles DM, Chamaluk GA, Subar M, et al: Lymphoid neoplasia associated with the acquired immunodeficiency syndrome (AIDS): The New York University Medical Center Experience with 105 patients (1981-1986). Ann Intern Med 108:744-753, 1988.

38. Levine AM, Gill PS, Meyer PR, et al: Retrovirus and malignant lymphoma in homosexual men. JAMA 254:1921-1925, 1985.

39. Ziegler JL, Beckstead JA, Volberding PA, et al: Non-Hodgkin's lymphoma in 90 homosexual men: Relationship to generalized lymphadenopathy and the acquired immunodeficiency syndrome. N Engl J Med 311:565-570, 1984.

40. Ziegler JL, Drew WL, Miner RC, et al: Outbreak of Burkitt's-like lymphoma in homosexual men. Lancet 2:631-633, 1982.

41. Anders KH, Latta H, Chang BS, et al: Lymphomatoid granulomatosis and malignant lymphoma of the central nervous system in the acquired immunodeficiency syndrome. Hum Pathol 20:326-334, 1989.

42. Parker SC, Fenton DA, McGibbon DH: Homme rouge and the acquired immunodeficiency syndrome. N Engl J Med 321:906-907, 1989.

43. Jones SE, Fuks Z, Bull M, et al: Non-Hodgkin's lymphomas. IV. Clinicopathologic correlation in 405 cases. Cancer 31:806-823, 1973.

44. Uccini S, Monardo F, Vitolo D, et al: Human immunodeficiency virus (HIV) and Epstein-Barr virus (EBV) antigens and genome in lymph nodes of HIV-positive patients affected by persistent generalized lymphadenopathy. Am J Clin Pathol 92:729-735, 1989.

45. Birx DL, Redfield RR, Tosato G: Defective regulation of Epstein-Barr virus infection in patients with acquired immunodeficiency syndrome (AIDS) or AIDS-related disorders. N Engl J Med 314:874-879, 1986.

46. List AF, Greco A, Vogler LB: Lymphoproliferative diseases in immunocompromised hosts: The role of Epstein-Barr virus. J Clin Oncol 5:1673-1689, 1987.

47. Knowles DM, Chamaluk GA, Subar M, et al: Clinicopathologic, immunophenotypic, and molecular genetic analysis of AIDS-associated lymphoid neoplasia: Clinical and biologic implications. Pathol Annu 23:33-67, 1988.

48. Knowles DM, Inghirami G, Ubriaco A, et al: Molecular genetic analysis of three AIDS-associated neoplasms of uncertain lineage demonstrates

their B-cell derivation and the possible pathogenetic role of the Epstein-Barr virus. Blood 73:792-799, 1989.

49. Whang-Peng J, Lee EC, Sieverts H, et al: Burkitt's lymphoma in AIDS: Cytogenetic study. Blood 63:818-822, 1984.

50. Petersen JM, Tubbs RR, Savage RA: Small non-cleaved B-cell Burkitt-like lymphoma with chromosome t(8;14) translocation and Epstein-Barr virus nuclear-associated antigen in a homosexual man with acquired immune deficiency syndrome. Am J Med 78:141-148, 1985.

51. Dalla-Favera R, Bregni M, Erikson J, et al: Human c-myc onc gene is located on the region of chromosome 8 that is translocated in Burkitt lymphoma cells. Proc Natl Acad Sci USA 79: 7824-7827, 1982.

52. Pelicci P-G, Knowles II DM, Arlin ZA, et al: Multiple monoclonal B cell expansions and c-myc oncogene rearrangements in acquired immune deficiency syndrome-related lymphoproliferative disorders: Implications for lymphomagenesis. J Exp Med 164:2049-2060, 1986.

53. Borisch-Chappuis B, Nezelof C, Muller H, et al: Different Epstein-Barr virus expression in lymphomas from immunocompromised and immunocompetent patients. Am J Pathol 136:751-758, 1990.

54. Subar M, Neri A, Inghirami G, et al: Frequent c-myc oncogene activation and infrequent presence of Epstein-Barr virus genome in AIDS-associated lymphoma. Blood 72:667-671, 1988.

55. Knowles DM: Malignant lymphomas occurring in association with acquired immunodeficiency syndrome. Lab Med 17:674-678, 1986.

56. Gill PS, Levine AM, Meyer PR, et al: Primary central nervous system lymphoma in homosexual men: Clinical, immunologic and pathologic features. Am J Med 78:742-748, 1985.

57. Walts AE, Shintaku IP, Said JW: Diagnosis of malignant lymphoma in effusions from patients with AIDS by gene rearrangement. Am J Clin Pathol 94:170-175, 1990.

58. Barriga F, Whang-Pen J, Lee E, et al: Development of a second clonally discrete Burkitt's lymphoma in a human immunodeficiency virus-positive homosexual patient. Blood 72:792-795, 1988.

59. Ferry JA, Jacobson JO, Conti D, et al: Lymphoproliferative disorders and hematologic malignancies following organ transplantation. Mod Pathol 2:583-592, 1989.

60. Roithman S, Tourani J-M, Andrieu J-M: Hodgkin's disease in HIV-infected drug abusers. N Engl J Med 323:275-276, 1990.

61. Frizzera G, Rosai J, Dehner LP, et al: Lymphoreticular disorders in primary immunodeficiencies. Cancer 46:692-699, 1980.

62. Mitsuyasu RT, Colman MF, Sun NC: Simultaneous occurrence of Hodgkin's disease and Kaposi's sarcoma in a patient with the acquired immune deficiency syndrome. Am J Med 80:954-958, 1986.

63. Unger PD, Strauchen JA: Hodgkin's disease in AIDS complex patients. Cancer 58:821-825, 1986.

64. Joshi VV, Oleske JM, Minnefor AB, et al: Pathology of suspected acquired immune deficiency syndrome in children. Pediatr Pathol 2:71-87, 1984.

65. Joshi VV, Oleske JM, Minnefor AB, et al: Pathologic pulmonary findings in children with the acquired immunodeficiency syndrome. Hum Pathol 16: 241-246, 1985.

66. Joshi VV, Oleske JM: Pulmonary lesions in children with the acquired immunodeficiency syndrome: A reappraisal based on data in additional cases and follow-up study of previously reported cases. Hum Pathol 17:641-642, 1986.

67. Joshi VV, Oleske JM, Saad S, et al: Thymus biopsy in children with acquired immunodeficiency syndrome. Arch Pathol Lab Med 110:837-842, 1986.

68. Joshi VV, Kauffman S, Oleske JM, et al: Polyclonal polymorphic B-cell lymphoproliferative disorder with prominent pulmonary involvement in children with acquired immune deficiency syndrome. Cancer 59:1455-1462, 1987.

69. Goldman HS, Ziprkowski MN, Charytan M, et al: Lymphocytic interstitial pneumonitis in children with AIDS: A perfect radiographic-pathologic correlation. AJR 145:868a, 1985.

70. Scott GB, Buck BE, Leterman JG, et al: Acquired immunodeficiency syndrome in infants. N Engl J Med 310:76-81, 1984.

71. Scully RE (ed): Case records of the Massachusetts General Hospital. N Engl J Med 314:629-640, 1986.

72. Friedman-Kien AE, Laubenstein LJ, Rubinstein P, et al: Disseminated Kaposi's sarcoma in homosexual men. Ann Intern Med 96:693-700, 1982.

73. Chen KTK: Multicentric Castleman's disease and Kaposi's sarcoma. Am J Surg Pathol 8:287-293, 1984.

74. Morris L, Distenfeld A, Amorosi E, et al: Autoimmune thrombocytopenic purpura in homosexual men. Ann Intern Med 96:714-717, 1982.

75. Abrams DI, Kiprov DD, Goedert JJ: Antibodies to human T-lymphotropic virus type III and development of the acquired immunodeficiency syndrome in homosexual men presenting with immune thrombocytopenia. Ann Intern Med 104: 47-50, 1986.

76. Scadden DT, Zon LI, Groopman JE: Pathophysiology and management of HIV-associated hematologic disorders. Blood 74:1455-1463, 1989.

77. McMillan R: Chronic idiopathic thrombocytopenic purpura. N Engl J Med 304:1135-1147, 1981.

78. Walsh C, Krigel R, Lennette E, et al: Thrombocytopenia in homosexual patients: Prognosis, response to therapy, and prevalence of antibody to the retrovirus associated with the acquired immunodeficiency syndrome. Ann Intern Med 103: 542-545, 1985.

79. Zucker-Franklin D, Seremetis S, Zheng ZY: Internalization of human immunodeficiency virus type 1 and other retroviruses by megakaryocytes and platelets. Blood 75:1920-1923, 1990.

80. Nair JMG, Bellevue R, Bertoni M, et al: Thrombotic thrombocytopenic purpura in patients with the acquired immunodeficiency syndrome (AIDS)-related complex: A report of two cases. Ann Intern Med 109:209-212, 1988.

81. Rousselet M-C, Audouin J, Le Tourneau A, et al: Idiopathic thrombocytopenic purpura in patients at risk for acquired immunodeficiency syndrome: Histopathologic study, immunohistochemistry, and ultrastructural study on six spleens. Arch Pathol Lab Med 112:1242-1250, 1988.

82. Ioachim HL, Ryan JR, Blaugrund SM: Salivary gland lymph nodes: The site of lymphadenopathies and lymphomas associated with human immunodeficiency virus infection. Arch Pathol Lab Med 112:1224-1228, 1988.

83. Ulirsch RC, Jaffe ES: Sjogren's syndrome–like illness associated with the acquired immunodeficiency syndrome–related complex. Hum Pathol 18:1063-1068, 1987.

84. Kornstein MJ, Parker GA, Mills AS: Immunohistology of the benign lymphoepithelial lesion in AIDS-related lymphadenopathy: A case report. Hum Pathol 19:1359-1362, 1988.

85. Spivak JL, Bender BS, Quinn TC: Hematologic abnormalities in the acquired immune deficiency syndrome. Am J Med 77:224-228, 1984.

86. Sun NCJ, Shapshak P, Lachant N, et al: Bone marrow studies in patients with HIV infection. Lab Invest 58:89A, 1988.

87. Schneider DR, Picker LJ: Myelodysplasia in the acquired immune deficiency syndrome. Am J Clin Pathol 84:144-152, 1985.

88. Castella A, Croxson TS, Mildvan D, et al: The bone marrow in AIDS: A histologic, hematologic, and microbiologic study. Am J Clin Pathol 84:425-432, 1985.

89. Zucker-Franklin D, Termin CS, Cooper MC: Structural changes in the megakaryocytes of patients infected with the human immune deficiency virus (HIV-1). Am J Pathol 134:1295-1303, 1989.

90. Solis OG, Belmonte AH, Ramaswamy G, et al: Pseudogaucher cells in *Mycobacterium avium intracellulare* infections in the acquired immune deficiency syndrome (AIDS). Am J Clin Pathol 85:233-235, 1986.

91. Schuurman H-J, Krone WJA, Broekhuizen R, et al: The thymus in acquired immune deficiency syndrome: Comparison with other types of immunodeficiency diseases, and the presence of components of human immunodeficiency virus type 1. Am J Pathol 134:1329-1338, 1989.

92. Seemayer TA, Laroche AC, Russo P, et al: Precocious thymic involution manifest by epithelial injury in the acquired immune deficiency syndrome. Hum Pathol 15:469-474, 1984.

93. Elie R, Laroche AC, Arnoux E, et al: Thymic dysplasia in acquired immunodeficiency syndrome. N Engl J Med 308:841-843, 1983.

RESPIRATORY SYSTEM

8

GERALD NASH

Pulmonary disease develops in most AIDS patients at some point in their illness, and it may also occur in the earlier stages of HIV infection. It is a major cause of death in these individuals. Respiratory tract disorders associated with HIV infection include infections, neoplasms, inflammatory disorders, and acute lung injury (Table 8–1).

Infections are by far the most common pulmonary complications of AIDS. Profound systemic immunodeficiency and possible alterations in pulmonary defense mechanisms caused by HIV predispose AIDS patients to a variety of opportunistic infections, as well as the more usual bacterial and mycobacterial pneumonias.[1] Neoplasms that involve the lung in AIDS include Kaposi's sarcoma (KS) and lymphoma; these usually occur as part of disseminated disease. Lymphocytic interstitial pneumonitis (LIP) and nonspecific interstitial pneumonitis are idiopathic inflammatory conditions that cause pulmonary disease in AIDS patients. LIP is a common AIDS-defining condition in children and is occasionally seen in adults. An acute lung injury pattern, diffuse alveolar damage (DAD), frequently occurs in AIDS patients. As in HIV-negative individuals, DAD is typically associated with the adult respiratory distress syndrome, has a grim prognosis, and is most often observed at autopsy.

SYMPTOMS AND SIGNS

Pulmonary disease in AIDS patients produces nonspecific symptoms, the most common of which are cough and dyspnea. The cough is usually nonproductive. Pleuritic chest pain and hemoptysis also occur but much less frequently.[2,3] Acute symptoms such as fever, chills, and productive cough are common in patients with pyogenic bacterial pneumonias, whereas a more indolent presentation with weight loss, fatigue, and nonproductive cough is characteristic of opportunistic infections, especially *Pneumocystis carinii* pneumonia (PCP).[1]

RADIOGRAPHIC FINDINGS

Chest radiography is helpful in suggesting a diagnosis. A variety of radiographic patterns have been described, the most common of which are diffuse interstitial infiltrates, focal airspace consolidation, and normal lungs.[4-7] Diffuse interstitial infiltrates involving all portions of the lungs is characteristic of PCP and other opportunistic infections. Involvement of only the upper lung fields occurs when PCP develops in patients receiving aerosolized pentamidine.[8] Kaposi's sarcoma (KS)[9] or lymphoma is occasionally the sole cause of interstitial infiltrates.[7] The inflammatory conditions LIP[10] and nonspecific interstitial pneumonitis[11] are characterized by diffuse infiltrates. Focal airspace consolidation is usually caused by bacterial pneumonias[12] but may also be caused by mycobacteria, *P. carinii*, *Mycoplasma*, adenovirus, and influenza.[4,7,13,14] A normal chest roentgenogram indicates that the pulmonary symptoms are not caused by lung disease or that lung disease is present but is not severe enough to cause roentgenographic changes. Approximately 10% of patients with PCP have normal chest roent-

Table 8–1. Pulmonary Complications of HIV infection

Infections
  Viruses
    Cytomegalovirus
    Herpes simplex virus
    Varicella-zoster virus
    Epstein-Barr virus?
    Human immunodeficiency virus?
  Bacteria
    Pyogenic organisms (especially *Streptococcus
      pneumoniae, Haemophilus influenzae*)
    Mycobacterium tuberculosis
    Mycobacterium avium complex
    Other nontuberculous mycobacteria
  Fungi
    Histoplasma capsulatum
    Coccidiodes immitis
    Cryptococcus neoformans
    Candida species
    Aspergillus species
  Parasites
    Pneumocystis carinii
    Toxoplasma gondii
    Cryptosporidium
    Strongyloides stercoralis
Malignancies
  Kaposi's sarcoma
  Non-Hodgkin's lymphoma
Interstitial Pneumonias
  Diffuse alveolar damage
  Nonspecific interstitital pneumonitis
  Pulmonary lymphoid hyperplasia/lymphocytic
    interstitial pneumonitis complex
Other
  Secondary pulmonary alveolar proteinosis

Modified from Murray JF, Mills J: Am Rev Respir Dis 141:
1356-1372, 1582-1598, 1990.

genograms as do some patients with cytomegalovirus (CMV) or *Mycobacterium avium*
complex infection.[5,7]

Other radiographic findings worthy of note
include diffuse airspace consolidation, nodular lesions, cavitary lesions, pleural effusion,
intrathoracic adenopathy, and pneumothorax.[7] Diffuse airspace consolidation may be
seen when any condition that causes diffuse
interstitial infiltrates increases in severity.
Nodular lesions throughout the lungs are
most often caused by KS but may also be seen
in mycobacterial and fungal infections. Cavitation may be observed in patients with bacterial and fungal pneumonias but, in contrast to
immunocompetent individuals, rarely in mycobacterial infections. Cystic changes that represent pneumatoceles are occasionally observed in healing PCP, and true cavitation has
also been described in that infection.[15] Large
pleural effusions are most frequently caused
by KS, and smaller ones by various infections.

Intrathoracic adenopathy occurs in infectious
processes such as mycobacterial infections, as
well as in KS and lymphoma. It is rare in PCP
and is not seen in the generalized lymphadenopathy syndrome associated with HIV infection.[7] Pneumothorax has been described in
PCP[16] and is probably related to pneumato-
cele formation.

DIAGNOSTIC APPROACH

The diagnostic approach to the patient with
AIDS or HIV infection who has pulmonary disease is similar to that for the immunocompromised person without AIDS.[1,3] First, respiratory disorders that are not related to HIV
infection, such as asthma, and upper respiratory tract infection, must be ruled out. If the
patient is producing sputum, a sample should
be Gram stained for bacteria and examined for
acid-fast bacilli. Cultures of sputum, blood,
and when available pleural fluid should also be
ordered. The sequence of diagnostic studies
should then progress logically from noninvasive to more invasive modalities, and an attempt should be made to arrive at a specific
diagnosis. This is more readily accomplished
in AIDS patients than in compromised individuals without HIV infection because infectious
agents are identified more often in the former
and nonspecific findings related to therapy or
underlying disease are more commonly encountered in the latter.[17,18] Empiric treatment
is not recommended except while the results of
diagnostic studies are awaited.[1]

The diagnostic workup is oriented toward
the identification of *P. carinii* because that organism is by far the most common cause of
pulmonary disease in AIDS. Before the AIDS
pandemic the procedure used to diagnose
PCP was either an open lung biopsy or a
transbronchial biopsy performed with fiberoptic bronchoscopy. The large number of
AIDS-related cases of PCP stimulated interest
in developing less invasive and expensive diagnostic methods. Fortunately, considerable
progress has been made in this area over the
past few years.

Sputum Induction

The search for noninvasive, rapid, inexpen-
sive ways to diagnose PCP eventually led to a
reevaluation of sputum examination, a modality that was used only occasionally in the
past because most patients with PCP do not

produce sputum spontaneously.[19] Initial studies with direct smears or homogenized and centrifuged specimens of sputum induced by inhaling an aerosol of hypertonic saline generated by an ultrasonic nebulizer yielded a sensitivity of slightly more than 50%.[20,21] Refinements in the technique of specimen collection and preparation, including digestion and concentration of the sputum and heat fixation of the smear, improved the sensitivity to approximately 75%.[22] In one study the use of indirect immunofluorescent staining with monoclonal antibodies to *P. carinii* on similarly collected and prepared induced sputum samples improved the sensitivity to more than 90%.[23] Not every laboratory has had such favorable experience with sputum examination in the diagnosis of PCP.[24] Furthermore, even though the sensitivity may be high, the negative predictive value of sputum examination is approximately 60%.[20,22] Therefore a negative result does not rule out PCP and necessitates another diagnostic study.[25]

Induced sputum is not very sensitive for detecting other important viral and fungal pathogens in AIDS patients.[22,26] Routine culture of induced sputum for mycobacteria and fungi is not warranted because the yield is low and because a patient whose stained sputum is negative for *P. carinii* should not have to wait for the results of sputum cultures before undergoing bronchoscopy.[22]

Bronchoalveolar Lavage

Early in the AIDS pandemic, bronchoalveolar lavage (BAL) performed during fiberoptic bronchoscopy was found to be useful in diagnosing pulmonary infections. BAL is especially effective in diagnosing PCP, with sensitivity ranging from 79% to 98%.[27-31] The excellent results for BAL should not be surprising, considering that the alveolar area sampled by lavage is greater than that obtained even by an open lung biopsy.[32] In addition to having excellent sensitivity, BAL is less injurious to AIDS patients than transbronchial biopsy. This has led physicians in many institutions to perform only BAL during the initial bronchoscopy.[31-33] Nonbronchoscopic BAL has also been reported to be useful for the diagnosis of PCP in AIDS.[34,35]

In cases of diffuse lung disease BAL is performed by wedging the bronchoscope in the right middle or lower lobe, instilling sterile saline in 20 ml aliquots, and applying suction after each bolus. A total of 100 to 120 ml is instilled, and the return is usually 50 to 60 ml. The material obtained should be stained for *P. carinii*, acid-fast organisms, and fungi and cultured for mycobacteria and fungi. Staining and culture studies for viruses and *Legionella* species should be performed if indicated.[25]

Transbronchial Biopsy

As noted previously, in the early days of the AIDS pandemic transbronchial biopsy was the method of choice for diagnosing lung disease in individuals with or at risk for AIDS. Its role in this setting has diminished for a number of reasons[1,30]: (1) PCP is the most common pulmonary complication of HIV infection, and cytologic methods (induced sputum and BAL) have become highly sensitive for the detection of this infection. (2) Fiberoptic bronchoscopy is easier and faster to perform if transbronchial biopsy is omitted. (3) Transbronchial biopsy occasionally causes severe pulmonary hemorrhage and is responsible for an appreciable incidence of pneumothorax (9%). Moreover, an uncorrectable coagulopathy and respiratory failure necessitating mechanical ventilation are absolute and relative contraindications, respectively, for transbronchial biopsy, but BAL can be performed in these situations.[36] Thus in many centers transbronchial biopsy is not routinely performed during the initial bronchoscopy and is done only if the first procedure is nondiagnostic. Transbronchial biopsy is, however, complementary to BAL in the diagnosis of pulmonary infections in AIDS patients,[27,30] and it is superior to cytologic methods for diagnosing the inflammatory and neoplastic conditions of the lungs occurring in these patients.[11,28]

Sufficient biopsy specimens should be obtained to permit both microbiologic and histologic examinations.[25] The tissue should be cultured for mycobacteria and fungi, as well as for *Legionella* species and viruses if indicated. Staining of touch imprints of biopsy specimens have been found effective in diagnosing *P. carinii* and should be performed.[27] Histologic tissue sections should be routinely stained for *Pneumocystis,* fungi, and mycobacteria.

Open-Lung Biopsy

Open-lung biopsy plays a limited role in the evaluation of patients with HIV-related pulmonary disease. Indications for its use include patients in whom BAL was nondiagnostic and in whom a transbronchial biopsy is contraindicated or was negative.[1,25] The yield of open-lung biopsy in this selected group of difficult diagnostic problems is high, but the proportion of patients with conditions that respond to therapy is low. Therefore the appropriate role of this procedure is uncertain.[1,25]

Processing of the tissue obtained is similar for open-lung biopsy and transbronchial biopsy except that the former provides more material for the various microbiologic and histologic studies needed. In addition, if indicated, a frozen section can be prepared at the time of surgery and may yield a working diagnosis.

Other Diagnostic Procedures

A brush biopsy was originally performed as part of the bronchoscopic procedure, but because of its low yield it is no longer recommended.[36] Percutaneous needle aspiration of the lung has a high diagnostic yield in patients with diffuse lung disease but has an unacceptable complication rate (pneumothorax in 50%). However, it is useful in the evaluation of focal pulmonary lesions.[1,25]

INFECTIONS

Pneumocystis carinii

PCP is the most common pulmonary disease and opportunistic infection in AIDS patients. It is the initial manifestation of AIDS in approximately 60% of patients. If chemoprophylaxis is not administered, PCP will eventually develop in approximately 80% of HIV-infected individuals and will recur in 20% to 65%.[1,37-39] PCP is also the most common serious complication of HIV infection, with respiratory failure and death the outcome in 5% to 20% of first episodes despite appropriate therapy.[41,42]

Taxonomy and Morphology. The taxonomic position of P. carinii is uncertain. It was originally classified as a protozoan on the basis of its morphologic appearance and the identification of cyst and trophozoite phases.[43,44] However, ultrastructural and biochemical studies of *P. carinii* have revealed similarities to fungi.[45,46] The most compelling evidence favoring a relationship to fungi comes from nucleotide sequencing analyses of isolated ribosomal RNA, which demonstrated a higher degree of homology of *P. carinii* to certain fungi than to other protozoa.[47] Although *P. carinii* is definitely related to fungi, its structure and antimicrobial sensitivity are different from those of other pathogenic fungi.[1] Its exact position within the fungi remains to be determined.

P. carinii is generally believed to be an extracellular organism that develops in the pulmonary alveolus.[43] Two major forms of the organism, trophozoites and cysts, are identified in the lung.[43,48,49] Trophozoites, ameboid pleomorphic organisms 2 to 8 μm in diameter, are the more numerous. They tend to occur in clumps and are recognized by their association with the cysts.[43] Although the life cycle is not completely known, it has been established that trophozoites develop into cysts (Fig. 8–1). Diploid trophozoites selectively attach themselves to type I pneumocytes, and they become precysts by acquiring a thicker cell membrane.[50-52] The nucleus of the precyst undergoes meiotic and mitotic divisions, yielding eight haploid nuclei.[43,53,54] As the precyst matures into a cyst, the cytoplasm forms partitions around each nucleus to produce eight intracystic bodies (sporozoites), which are structurally similar to trophozoites but are 1 to 1.5 μm in diameter.[43] The precyst also increases in size and develops a wall four times thicker than the trophozoite's pellicle. The thick-walled mature cysts are cup shaped, ovoid, or crescentic and range from 5 to 7 μm in diameter. Methenamine-silver stains the cyst wall black, and single or paired, 1 to 2 μm, oval or comma-shaped, discrete foci of enhanced staining are observed (Fig. 8–2), which represent focal thickenings of the wall as demonstrated by electron microscopy.[55] Openings through which the intracystic bodies leave the cyst appear in the thickened areas. Whether the irregularly collapsed crescentic cysts represent empty forms that have released their trophozoites or are an artifact of fixation and processing is not clear.[43] The haploid trophozoites that are released undergo conjugation to form diploid trophozoites that can produce additional trophozoites by mitosis or develop into cysts, completing the cycle.

Epidemiology. The pulmonary alveolus of humans and other mammals has been considered the natural habitat of *P. carinii*.[44,56-58] Studies of outbreaks of pneumocystosis among hospital patients[59,60] and numerous animal studies suggest that the organism is transmitted by the airborne route.[31] Although *P. carinii* has been identified only in mammalian tissues and no environmental reservoir

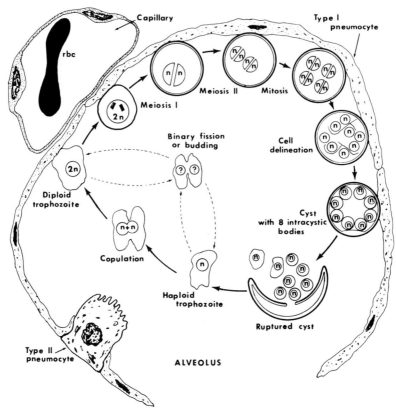

Figure 8–1. Proposed life cycle of *Pneumocystis carinii*. (From Gutierrez Y: Semin Diagn Pathol 6:203-211, 1989; modified from Matsumoto Y, Yoshida Y: Parasitol Today 2:137-142, 1986.)

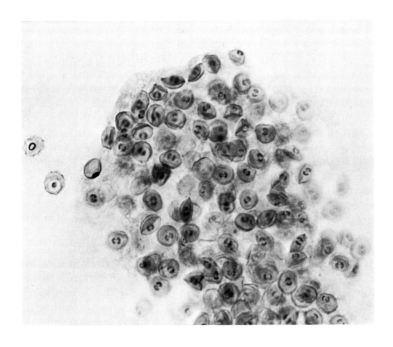

Figure 8–2. Smear of bronchoalveolar lavage sediment stained by the methenamine-silver stain showing cysts of *Pneumocystis carinii* with paired comma-shaped thickenings of their walls. Single wall thickening is evident in cyst at left of group. (×250.)

has been found, recent evidence of the organism's relationship to fungi suggests that soil is a possible reservoir.[1]

Serologic surveys have revealed that antibodies to *P. carinii* are present in up to 80% of children by 4 years of age and persist in adulthood.[61,62] This evidence suggests that latent infection with *P. carinii* is common in the population. Additional support for this idea comes from studies in which small numbers of the organism were found in the lungs of patients who did not have clinical evidence of pneumonia.[63,64] However, *P. carinii* could not be found in the lungs of a group of individuals, 18% of whom were HIV seropositive, who died unexpectedly in San Francisco,[65] and another study failed to reveal the organism in BAL specimens from HIV-positive patients without pulmonary disease.[66] Perhaps the strongest evidence that PCP results from reactivation of a latent infection comes from an animal study in which immunosuppression induced the infection in almost all animals even under conditions that limited the organism's transmission.[67]

Clinical Features. PCP occurs in the late stages of HIV infection when the patient is significantly immunodeficient. More than 90% of HIV-infected patients with PCP have CD4 counts less than 200/mm^3, and the median count is less than 100/mm^3.[42,68] In fact, PCP is not likely to develop until the CD4 count falls below 200/mm^3, and primary prophylaxis is not recommended for asymptomatic individuals unless the count is below that level.[42,69]

A number of important differences between PCP in AIDS patients and in immunocompromised individuals without AIDS have been documented. The attack rate of PCP in AIDS is approximately 30% per year compared with 1% in patients with lymphoproliferative disorders or renal transplants.[19,41] PCP is usually a subacute and insidious illness in AIDS patients, who have a longer duration of symptoms than the rapidly progressive respiratory compromise that occurs in other immunocompromised hosts.[31,41,70] However, PCP may be fulminant in some AIDS patients, with respiratory failure developing within 1 week.[71] AIDS patients with pneumocystosis also have a much higher incidence of adverse reactions to therapy, more than 50% compared with approximately 10% in patients without AIDS.[41,70] Although an adverse reaction requires a change in the initial therapeutic agent, it does not appear to affect survival. PCP in AIDS has a slower clinical and roentgenographic response to therapy, necessitat-

ing longer treatment. However, a number of studies have shown that the rate of response to therapy is about the same in both groups of patients, with 50% to more than 90% responding favorably.[41,70-72] Recurrent episodes of PCP are two to three times more common in AIDS patients than in other immunodeficient individuals if suppressive therapy is not used, and they are attended by an increased mortality rate.[41,70-72]

Poor short-term survival of AIDS patients with PCP is associated with severe abnormalities on initial chest roentgenograms, alveolar-arterial oxygen differences greater than 30 mm Hg,[73] high serum lactate dehydrogenase levels,[74] neutrophilia in BAL,[75] failure to respond to initial therapy,[27] development of respiratory failure requiring mechanical ventilation, and concurrent infection with CMV.[2]

AIDS patients may have atypical pulmonary manifestations of *P. carinii* infection, including localized involvement of upper lobes,[8,76] pulmonary nodules with and without cavitation,[15,77-79] and spontaneous pneumothorax.[15,16,77-81] Many of these cases have been associated with administration of aerosolized pentamidine for secondary prophylaxis. In one AIDS treatment center two thirds of relapses in patients given this prophylaxis involved predominantly the lung apices.[76] This is probably because the aerosolized drug is poorly distributed to the upper lung zones under certain conditions, such as use of an ultrasonic nebulizer that produces large particles and delivery of the drug with the patient in a sitting position.[8,82]

Extrapulmonary involvement with *P. carinii* is a rare but well-documented complication of pulmonary pneumocystosis in immunocompromised patients without AIDS.[83,84] However, many AIDS patients have been reported to have extrapulmonary *P. carinii* infection, including both widespread dissemination and localized involvement, especially of the reticuloendothelial organs and skin.[85-92, 94] In some of the localized infections concurrent pulmonary pneumocystosis was not evident but could not be ruled out.[87,92,94] Vascular invasion[87] and transportation outside the lung by macrophages[85] have been suggested as mechanisms of dissemination. Possibly the numerous cases of extrapulmonary pneumocystosis encountered in AIDS patients are just a reflection of the high incidence of PCP in that population and of increased ability to detect the organism. However, many of these cases were in patients treated with aerosolized pentamidine, and systemic absorption of the drug administered in this fashion is minimal.[95] Therefore this therapy would not be expected to eradicate the organism systemically and might predispose to dissemination.[96]

Pathogenesis and Pathology. Even before the AIDS pandemic, PCP was known to occur characteristically in individuals with defects in T-cell function, suggesting that an altered cellular immunity predisposes to activation of latent infection and proliferation of the organism in alveoli.[19,97,98] The humoral immune system may also play some role, since PCP has been found in a few individuals with isolated B-cell defects,[99,100] and since antibodies facilitate uptake and destruction of *P. carinii* by alveolar macrophages.[101]

Pneumocystis trophozoites selectively attach themselves to type I pneumocytes apparently without fusion of cell membranes or intracellular penetration.[50-52] The organisms somehow change the permeability of the air-blood membrane, causing the formation of subepithelial blebs, which triggers degenerative changes in type I pneumocytes, eventual denudation of the epithelial basement membrane, and exudation of fibrin and other plasma proteins into the alveolar space.[50,52]

Eosinophilic intraalveolar foam, believed to be composed of the organisms and serum proteins, is the histologic hallmark of PCP in hematoxylin and eosin preparations (Fig. 8–3).[48,50,58,102] This is superimposed on a background of changes consistent with a mild degree of the proliferative (organizing) phase of DAD characterized by interstitial edema, a mild interstitial infiltrate of lymphocytes, plasma cells, and histiocytes, and hypertrophy and hyperplasia of type II pneumocytes.[17,102,103] The last is undoubtedly a regenerative response to the injury to type I cells caused by trophozoites. Occasionally the findings are those of the acute (exudative) phase of DAD, with hyaline membranes and less interstitial inflammation.[104,105]

The foamy eosinophilic material has a granular three-dimensional honeycomb architecture of enmeshed cysts and trophozoites, and the cyst walls may impart a refractile quality to it. Dark blue punctate bodies less than 1 μm in diameter, believed to be nuclei of intracystic bodies, may also be discerned and contribute to the material's granular appearance.[105-107] The foamy material is quite different from other eosinophilic intraalveolar substances such as homogeneous "watery" pulmonary edema, fibrillar strands of fibrin in a fibrinous exudate, and dense strongly periodic acid–Schiff (PAS)-positive material with cholesterol clefts seen in pulmonary alveolar proteinosis.[105]

The pathologic changes of PCP in AIDS are generally similar to those in non-AIDS patients.[108] However, AIDS patients have greater numbers of organisms in their lungs,[109] and the number of organisms and intensity of the histologic reaction do not decrease as rapidly as they do in patients without AIDS.[110] This correlates with the slower clinical response to therapy and the propensity to recurrence noted previously. Even if clinically recovered from an episode of PCP, up to 90%

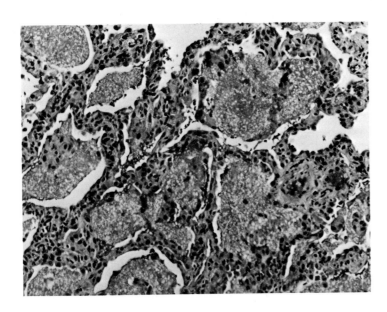

Figure 8–3. *Pneumocystis carinii* pneumonia exhibiting foamy material in alveolar spaces and proliferative phase of diffuse alveolar damage. (Hematoxylin and eosin, ×50.)

of AIDS patients have persistent organisms demonstrated on repeat bronchoscopy after 2 to 3 weeks of therapy, and in approximately 25% organisms persist after 6 to 7 weeks of therapy.[29,110,111] Nevertheless, treatment eventually eradicates the organism in many cases. In one clinical study the mean time until eradication in successfully treated patients was 36 days.[73] Additional evidence for eradication of *P. carinii* comes from autopsy studies, in which the frequency of PCP in AIDS patients was considerably less than that documented during life.[18,112]

Atypical histologic responses to *P. carinii* occur in AIDS patients just as they do in other compromised hosts but probably with greater frequency (Table 8–2). Many of these reactions would not suggest a diagnosis of PCP on routine preparations, underscoring the necessity of using special stains for *Pneumocystis* on all pulmonary specimens from HIV-infected individuals. PCP with minimal or absent alveolar foam has been well documented in individuals with[18,113] and without AIDS.[102,104] In some instances, especially after treatment for PCP, organisms may be few and difficult to find.[18,114] In cases of nonresolving PCP associated with respiratory failure and clinical signs and symptoms of the adult respiratory distress syndrome for more than a week, a marked proliferative phase of DAD may be observed, with striking interstitial thickening and extensive alveolar collapse.[18,114] In such cases persistent alveolar foam is often scanty, compacted, and deeply eosinophilic (Fig.

Table 8–2. Atypical Patterns of Pneumocystosis in AIDS

Clinical
Dissemination
Localized extrapulmonary involvement with or without pulmonary pneumocystosis
Localized involvement of upper lobes
Pulmonary nodules with or without cavitation
Spontaneous pneumothorax
Rapid progression to respiratory failure

Pathological
Minimal or absent alveolar foam
Rare organisms
Severe organizing diffuse alveolar damage (associated with acute respiratory failure)
Granulomatous inflammation
    Epithelioid granulomas
    Multinucleated giant cell reaction to alveolar foam
Calcification of alveolar foam
Necrotizing and cavitary pulmonary lesions
Lymphocytic interstitial pneumonitis–like interstitial inflammation
Extrapulmonary infection, localized and disseminated

8–4).[114] Calcification of the foamy material and a multinucleated giant cell reaction to the foam (Fig. 8–4) may also develop in this setting.[105,115] PCP may be manifest as pulmonary nodules, and about half of these patients show histologic features of granuloma formation (Fig. 8–5).[15,77,116-118] The granulomas may undergo central necrosis and suggest tuberculosis except that they contain cysts. Necrotizing PCP with cavity formation has been reported,[116] with vascular invasion by the organisms implicated as a

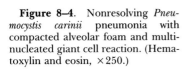

Figure 8–4. Nonresolving *Pneumocystis carinii* pneumonia with compacted alveolar foam and multinucleated giant cell reaction. (Hematoxylin and eosin, ×250.)

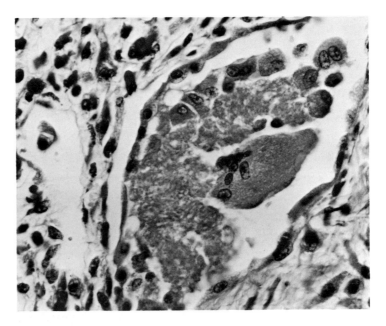

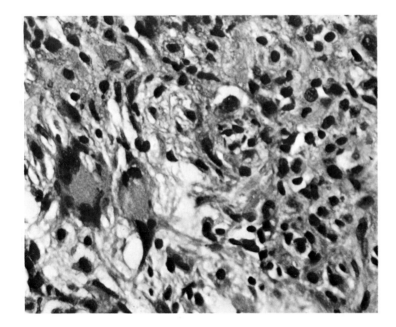

Figure 8–5. Granulomatous inflammatory response in patient with *Pneumocystis carinii* pneumonia. (Hematoxylin and eosin, ×100.)

cause of infarctlike necrosis in some of these patients.[79,119] PCP may be characterized by a marked lymphoplasmacytic interstitial infiltrate. This is especially prevalent in pediatric AIDS and resembles the endemic cases of pediatric PCP in central European countries at the end of World War II.[116] When alveolar foam is minimal or absent in such a case, a mistaken diagnosis of lymphocytic interstitial pneumonitis could be made if staining for *Pneumocystis* is not performed.

Extrapulmonary pneumocystosis is characterized by the typical eosinophilic foamy material, which may be overlooked in this situation but demonstrates the organisms when appropriately stained. The response in tissue, as in the lung, ranges from nil[86,89,92] to necrotizing[85] and may include mild chronic inflammation[87] and granulomatous inflammation.[87,92]

Diagnosis. The usual microbiologic techniques for diagnosing infectious diseases, such as isolation of the etiologic agent on cell-free

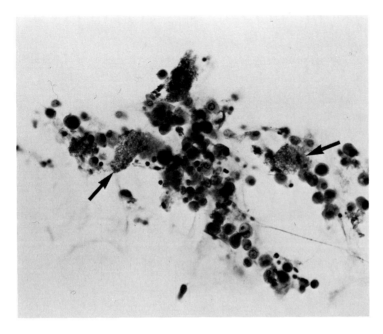

Figure 8–6. Papanicolaou-stained smear of bronchoalveolar lavage sediment showing alveolar foam *(arrows).* (×50.)

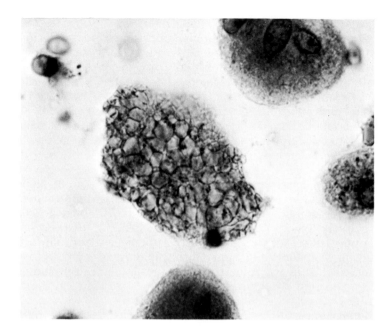

Figure 8–7. Higher power of alveolar foam in bronchoalveolar lavage sediment that virtually establishes diagnosis of *Pneumocystis carinii* pneumonia. (Papanicolaou's stain, ×250.)

medium or detection of antibodies or antigens, are not reliable for detection of *P. carinii*. Diagnosis of PCP still requires morphologic identification of the organism in pulmonary specimens. Rapid cytologic diagnosis of PCP has essentially replaced tissue diagnosis and has confronted pathologists with a new challenge: how to identify the organism without the benefit of the familiar histologic findings of alveolar foam and interstitial pneumonitis. Fortunately, alveolar foam is usually present as foamy masses in cytologic specimens, especially BAL fluid, and can be easily identified on Papanicolaou-stained smears even at the magnification used for screening cytologic material (Fig.

8–6).[32,120-124] The foamy masses generally have the size and shape of distended alveolar sacs (Fig. 8–7) and may stain as amphophilic, eosinophilic, basophilic, or mixtures of these colors. Although observation of the characteristic foamy material in routine histologic and cytologic preparations virtually establishes the diagnosis of PCP,[124] confirmation by visualization of the organism is recommended.

Special stains are necessary because the various forms of *Pneumocystis* cannot be visualized with hematoxylin and eosin or Papanicolaou's stains. A variety of histochemical stains that can be used for this purpose are listed in Table 8–3. Some of these stain the cyst form, and others demonstrate trophozoites and in-

Table 8–3. Histochemical Stains for *Pneumocystis*

	Type of Preparation		Form of Organism	
	Cytologic*	Paraffin Sections	Cyst Walls	Sporozoites and Trophozoites
Methenamine-silver	+	+	+	−
Cresyl violet	+	+	+	−
Gram-Weigert	+	+	+	+/−
Toluidine blue O	+	+	+	+/−
Periodic acid – Schiff	+	+	+/−	−
Giemsa	+	−	−	+
Polychrome methylene blue	+	−	−	+
Wright (Diff-Quik)	+	−	−	+
Gram	+	−	−	+
Acridine orange	+	−	−	+

Modified from Nash G: Hum Pathol 13:841-858, 1982.
*Includes sputum, bronchial brushings and washings, bronchoalveolar lavage, lung aspirates, and tissue imprints.

tracystic bodies. In addition, some stains are effective only in histologic preparations and others in cytologic specimens. Most pathologists prefer stains that demonstrate cysts, the largest and most easily recognized form of the organism, over those that identify trophozoites and sporozoites. Inexperienced observers should be especially cautious when using the latter stains, such as Wright's (Diff-Quik) and Giemsa, because trophozoites and sporozoites are difficult to distinguish from background material and because debris and platelets can be mistaken for the small forms of the organism.[31,48,125,126] In addition, therapy may quickly destroy sporozoites and trophozoites,[127-129] whereas empty cysts persist for many days and can confirm the diagnosis if therapy was initiated before morphologic identification of the organism.[130]

The Grocott modification of Gomori's methenamine-silver stain,[131] which stains cyst walls black, has long been the "gold standard" for identification of *P. carinii*, but the time required for this technique (about 3 hours) precludes rapid diagnosis. Modifications of the Grocott technique that shorten the staining time to 20 to 30 minutes have contributed significantly to the timely and accurate diagnosis of PCP. Particularly useful modifications include that of Mahan and Sale[132] and a microwave technique.[133] The methenamine-silver stain has a number of advantages worthy of note: (1) It stains the cyst form of the organism. (2) It detects fungi, as well as *P. carinii*. (3) It creates a sharp contrast between the organism and its background. (4) It can be applied to all types of preparations, histologic as well as cytologic.

A number of pitfalls to the diagnosis of PCP with the methenamine-silver stain should be kept in mind. Using a *Pneumocystis* control instead of a fungus control is important because the former may not stain when the latter does.[132] Pneumocystis look-alikes may be troublesome in the evaluation of cytologic specimens. A variety of elements may be confused with *P. carinii* cysts because they are approximately the same size and shape and also stain with methenamine-silver. These include fungal yeast and conidial forms[134-136] and noncellular structures such as corpora amylacea, starch granules, and aspirated foreign material.[137] In addition, in overstained specimens erythrocytes and nuclei of inflammatory cells may take the silver stain and mimic cysts (Fig. 8–8*A*).[19,138] Identification of the capsular thickenings noted previously

(Figs. 8–2 and 8–8*B*) should help the pathologist distinguish cysts from other structures stained by methenamine-silver.[55] Nevertheless, a diagnosis should be based on the observation of clusters of cysts, not single structures that have the size and shape of cysts. Observation of clusters of cysts within the foamy material clinches the diagnosis.

Microbiologists and some pathologists prefer to use stains for sporozoites and trophozoites, especially the Giemsa and Wright's (Diff-Quik) stains. These take only minutes to perform and permit a rapid assessment of the adequacy of an induced sputum specimen (that is, presence of alveolar macrophages and only a few squamous cells).[22] Both the 2 to 8 μm free-living trophozoites and tiny (1 to 2 μm) intracystic sporozoites can be visualized in cytologic preparations with these stains. They are seen as clusters of organisms composing the foamy masses. Trophozoites have light blue or purple cytoplasm with dark blue, often eccentrically located nuclear material, and sporozoites have pale blue or violet cytoplasm and red nuclei.[139] Cysts are recognizable as round or oval structures with negatively stained walls and may have internal sporozoites (Fig. 8–9).[140]

A variety of fluorescence microscopy techniques are used to detect *P. carinii* in cytologic preparations. *Pneumocystis* fluoresces when stained by Papanicolaou's method and examined under ultraviolet light.[106,141,142] The orange G or eosin portions of the stain, or both, are believed responsible for this phenomenon.[141-143] This property is not specific, however, since it is shared by fungi. If cysts were not embedded in the familiar background of foamy material, it would be difficult to distinguish *Pneumocystis* from yeast forms such as *Blastomyces* and *Histoplasma*. Erythrocytes also fluoresce and could be confused with *Pneumocystis* in such preparations.[106] Cellufluor, a chemofluorescent optical brightening agent that nonspecifically binds to beta-linked polysaccharide polymers found in fungi and other organisms, stains cysts of *Pneumocystis* in BAL specimens.[144] Although details of cyst morphology such as the paired wall thickenings have been discerned by fluorescence microscopy with this stain, an inexperienced observer would have difficulty distinguishing *Pneumocystis* from fungal yeast forms.

Immunofluorescent staining methods using monoclonal antibodies to *Pneumocystis* are highly sensitive for the detection of the organism in cytologic specimens (Fig. 8–10) and

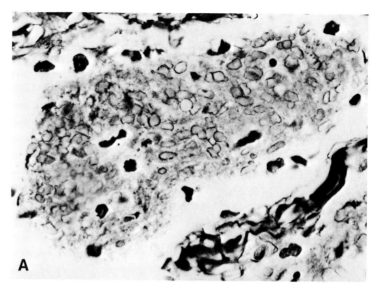

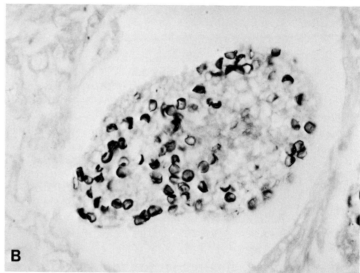

Figure 8–8. *A,* Biopsy specimen from patient with pulmonary hemorrhage overstained by methenamine-silver stain. Intraalveolar erythrocytes are outlined by silver and could mimic cysts of *Pneumocystis carinii.* Nuclei of inflammatory cells are also stained. *B,* Biopsy specimen from patient with *P. carinii* pneumonia stained by methenamine-silver. Focal capsular thickenings are readily apparent in many cysts. (*A* and *B,* ×250.)

increase the yield of organisms identified in induced sputum samples over that obtained by use of conventional histochemical stains.[23] Both indirect[23,145] and direct[146] methods have been described; the latter is less time consuming. The slightly greater sensitivity of immunofluorescence over conventional techniques may be offset by occasional false-positive readings resulting from extraneous fluorescence.[145,146] At this time immunofluorescence is not recommended for routine use but may have utility in evaluating specimens when conventional stains do not show large numbers of organisms.[1] Monoclonal antibodies have also been used for immunohistochemical identification of *Pneumocystis* in cytologic specimens[147] and formalin-fixed paraffin-embedded tissue.[148] These adapta-

tions would be too time consuming for routine application, but the latter was found to be particularly useful for identifying clinically occult extrapulmonary pneumocystosis in autopsy material. Molecular diagnostic techniques such as the Southern blot test or in situ hybridization that use specific labeled nucleic acid probes to detect *P. carinii* may find clinical application in the future.[47,106,149]

Cytomegalovirus

Epidemiology. Primary infection with CMV occurs either in childhood via sharing of respiratory secretions or in adulthood via sexual transmission, and the infection invariably becomes latent in the immunocompetent host.[1] From 50% to 95% of the adult popula-

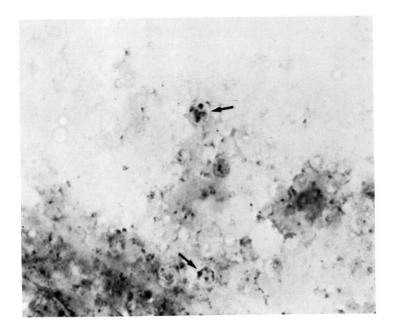

Figure 8–9. Smear of bronchoalveolar lavage sediment stained with Diff-Quik. Arrows denote cysts with negatively stained walls and intracystic bodies. Background contains numerous ill-defined trophozoites. (×250.)

tion and more than 95% of sexually active homosexual men have CMV infection.[1,150] Under the influence of HIV infection, latent CMV is often reactivated for a prolonged time, resulting in chronic persistent infection as evidenced by shedding of the virus in urine or semen.[1,151] Active CMV infection is common in patients with full-blown AIDS, and autopsy studies have demonstrated typical cytopathic CMV changes in approximately 70% to 90% of cases.[112,115,152-154] Moreover, disseminated CMV infection may be an important contributing cause of organ failure and

death.[112,155-157] Although the lung is commonly involved in CMV infections noted at autopsy, clinical evidence of a pathogenic role for the virus in AIDS-associated pneumonia is inconclusive.[151,158,159] In fact, no clinical syndrome that correlates with histopathologic evidence of CMV pneumonia in the absence of other etiologic agents has been defined in patients with AIDS.

Pathology. The histologic changes of CMV pneumonia in patients with AIDS are similar to those described in immunocompromised individuals without HIV infection. Any

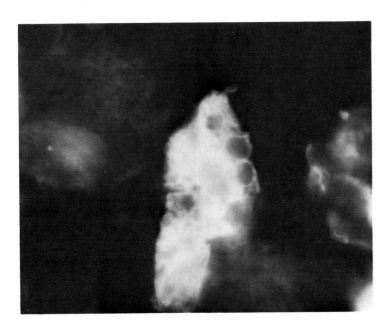

Figure 8–10. Smear of bronchoalveolar lavage sediment showing immunofluorescent staining of *Pneumocystis carinii* foam with monoclonal antibody to organism. (×250. Courtesy Dr. James Pullman.)

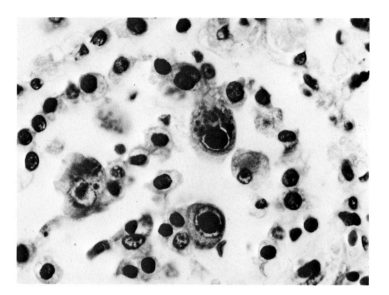

Figure 8–11. Cytomegalovirus pneumonia (diffuse type) with two typical cytomegalic cells containing "owl's eye" intranuclear inclusions. Upper cell also contains cytoplasmic inclusions. (Hematoxylin and eosin, ×250.)

of three patterns of lung involvement may be seen: diffuse (Figs. 8–11 and 8–12), necrotizing miliary lesions (Fig. 8–13), or rare cytomegalic cells.[160,161] The diffuse and rare cytomegalic cell patterns are typically associated with DAD.[161] The diffuse pattern is the most common, and the intensity of the infection, as gauged by the number of cytomegalic cells, varies from mild to severe.[18,162] Diagnostic cytomegalic cells in the lung are up to 40 μm in diameter and contain basophilic or eosinophilic intranuclear inclusions up to 17 μm that are separated from the nuclear membrane by a clear halo, imparting the classic owl's eye appearance to the nucleus (Fig. 8–11).[163] Small basophilic inclusions

may also be seen in the cytoplasm. Most cytomegalic cells are observed in alveolar spaces or lining alveolar walls and are thought to be alveolar macrophages and pneumocytes, respectively. Endothelial cells and bronchiolar epithelial cells may also exhibit CMV inclusions.[160,164,165]

When only a few diagnostic CMV cells are identified in lung tissue that shows DAD, the question is raised whether the viral infection is solely responsible for the profound pulmonary reaction. In this situation use of fluorescein-labeled monoclonal antibodies to CMV antigens[166] or CMV nucleic acid probes[167] (Fig. 8–12) typically reveals the virus in cells that do not have the classic ap-

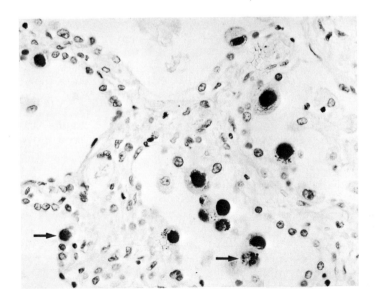

Figure 8–12. In situ DNA hybridization with biotinylated cytomegalovirus probe in patient with diffuse type of cytomegalovirus pneumonia. Probe (black in this photomicrograph) is present in nuclear and cytoplasmic inclusions. Most cells binding probe are typical cytomegalic cells. However, some cells *(arrows)* contain nuclear or cytoplasmic viral DNA but are not diagnostic cytomegalic cells. (Hematoxylin counterstain, ×100.)

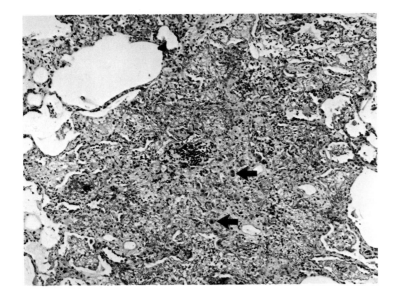

Figure 8–13. Miliary type of cytomegalovirus pneumonia. Necrotizing nodular lesion contains numerous cytomegalic cells *(arrows)*. (Hematoxylin and eosin, ×25.)

pearance of cytomegalic cells. In CMV pneumonia many cells that appear abnormal and suggestive but not diagnostic of CMV infection are probably the site of active infection after all. This evidence suggests that CMV may be the sole cause of DAD even when typical inclusion-bearing cells are rare. The pathogenesis of CMV pneumonia in AIDS is believed to involve direct damage to the lung caused by CMV replication.[158] Therefore, if only rare CMV-containing cells are identified, other infectious causes of DAD should be sought. In particular, CMV and *P. carinii* often coexist, and both cause DAD. If additional infectious agents cannot be identified, other conditions associated with DAD, such as oxygen intoxication and sepsis, should be considered.

Diagnosis. In the diagnosis of CMV pneumonia in AIDS patients, a distinction must be made between CMV infection and CMV disease (pneumonia). Moreover, if CMV pneumonia is present, its clinical significance must be ascertained before the initiation of potentially toxic, specific antiviral therapy. These are not easy questions to answer in this clinical setting.

The high correlation between isolation of CMV in cultures of BAL fluid and presence of CMV pneumonia in immunocompromised patients does not apply to AIDS patients.[28,158] Salivary glands are common sites of subclinical CMV infection in AIDS patients, and the virus may be found in cultures from respiratory secretions in the absence of morphologic confirmation of CMV pneumonia.[158,168] In

one study a third of patients who had CMV isolated from bronchoscopic specimens did not show histologic evidence of CMV pneumonitis at autopsy.[162] In the same study only half the patients with histologically proven CMV pneumonia at autopsy had positive cultures of bronchoscopy specimens within 2 months before their deaths. Thus both specificity and sensitivity of culture for the diagnosis of CMV pneumonia are suspect.

Most investigators believe that morphologic evidence of infected lung cells is necessary for the diagnosis of CMV pneumonia in AIDS patients.[151,158] Unfortunately, in these individuals routine histologic and cytologic identification of CMV infection in specimens obtained by all pulmonary procedures has a low diagnostic yield.[158] In a number of studies cytopathic changes were demonstrated cytologically in only 20% to 25% of culture-positive cases,[169-171] and classic cytomegalic cells are often sparse in lung biopsy specimens from AIDS patients.[41,158] Enlarged cells without typical nuclear or cytoplasmic inclusions but suggestive of CMV infection are often encountered in histologic and cytologic preparations. As noted previously, CMV can be diagnosed in such cells by immunohistochemical or immunofluorescence localization of viral antigens or identification of viral genome by in situ nucleic acid hybridization.[166,167,170,171] Detection of large numbers of CMV-infected cells (more than 0.5% of total) in BAL fluids stained with monoclonal antibodies has correlated with culture, histopathologic, and clinical evidence of CMV pneumonia.[158,172] Positive results of in situ hybridization must be interpreted carefully to avoid mistaking a latent infection for an active one because cloned DNA probes can detect as few as one or two viral genomes per cell; intact or replicating viruses are not required.[158,159] The number of positive cells, as well as correlation with viral cultures and the patient's clinical status, must also be considered in making a diagnosis of CMV pneumonia.

The clinical significance of CMV infection of the lung in AIDS patients has been difficult to assess. In contrast, the infection is a well-recognized cause of morbidity and mortality in organ transplant patients.[151,158,159] The main problem is that CMV in patients with AIDS usually coexists with other pulmonary pathogens, especially *P. carinii,* and the contribution of CMV to the pulmonary disease is difficult to isolate. Moreover, most patients with AIDS and pneumonia have a similar clinical course regardless of whether they have CMV in their lungs.[1,173,174] Despite the uncertain significance of CMV infection of the lung in most cases of AIDS-associated pneumonia, both clinical and autopsy studies have shown that occasionally CMV causes pulmonary disease in this setting.[162,175]

According to Murray and Mills,[1] criteria for a tentative clinical diagnosis of CMV pneumonia should include culture of CMV from the respiratory tract, identification of CMV inclusions in a BAL or lung biopsy specimen, absence of another pathogen, and progressive pneumonia. Response to specific antiviral therapy confirms the diagnosis. In Murray and Mills' experience less than 1% of patients with AIDS and pulmonary CMV infection fulfill these criteria.

Herpes Simplex Virus

Herpes simplex virus (HSV) is a well-recognized but unusual cause of lower respiratory tract infection in immunosuppressed patients, and only a few cases have been reported in patients with AIDS.[27] The infection is either localized to the lower respiratory tract or part of disseminated herpes. Localized infection is by far the more common and is characterized by necrotizing laryngotracheobronchitis (Fig. 8–14) or bronchopneumonia (Fig. 8–15), or both. Disseminated HSV infection produces miliary foci of necrosis throughout the lung, a pattern characteristic of hematogenous spread.[176-179] Herpetic laryngotracheobronchitis and bron-

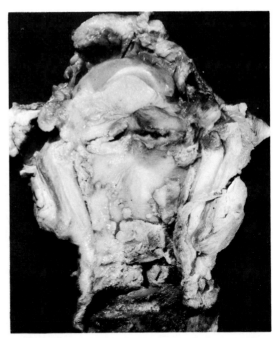

Figure 8–14. Herpetic lyaryngotracheitis. Punctate and confluent ulcers are covered by shaggy pseudomembrane.

chopneumonia probably represent reactivated latent HSV infection and are typically associated with immunosuppression and airway trauma caused by tracheal intubation.[180] Trauma facilitates HSV invasion of cells; furthermore, it leads to squamous metaplasia of the respiratory mucosa, and squamous epithelium is more susceptible to HSV infection than glandular epithelium.[176,181] Localized herpetic infection of the middle and lower respiratory tract usually occurs in hospitalized patients who require intubation for assisted ventilation. The infection begins in the larynx or trachea and either is self-limited or spreads by contiguity or aspiration down the tracheobronchial tree into the lungs.[177,178,181]

Herpetic lesions are characterized by extensive coagulation necrosis and karyorrhexis, which may be associated with a fibrinopurulent exudate (Fig. 8–15). A typical active lesion has central necrosis of infected tissue and characteristic cytopathic changes at the leading edge.[180] These changes include light-staining basophilic inclusion material, which gives the nucleus a ground-glass appearance, the classic Cowdry type A eosinophilic intranuclear inclusion surrounded by a clear halo (Fig. 8–15), multinucleated cells exhibiting nuclear molding,[180,182] and ballooning degeneration of the cytoplasm.[176] The last two

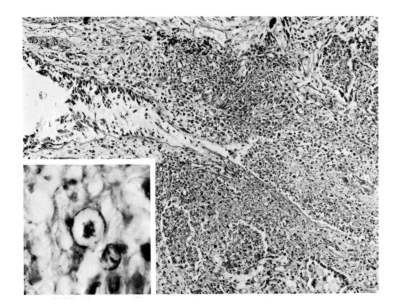

Figure 8–15. Herpetic broncho-pneumonia. Necrotizing process with marked karyorrhexis involves small airway and surrounding alveoli. *Inset,* Typical Cowdry type A intranuclear inclusion surrounded by clear halo. (Hematoxylin and eosin, ×25; inset ×250.)

changes typically occur in squamous mucosa and are seldom seen in the lung.

Herpetic tracheobronchitis and broncho-pneumonia in patients with AIDS are usually incidental findings at autopsy of individuals who required mechanical ventilation for another AIDS-related pulmonary disorder. Like CMV infection of the respiratory tract, HSV tracheobronchitis and pneumonia are difficult to diagnose during life. HSV is often isolated from oropharyngeal secretions and is a frequent contaminant of lower respiratory tract secretions.[1] Therefore culture of HSV from sputum or BAL fluid or identification of cytopathic changes of HSV infection in these materials does not establish the diagnosis of HSV pneumonia. Diagnosis requires histopathologic verification of the infection in respiratory tissue confirmed by isolation of the virus in culture, immunohistochemical identification of viral antigens in infected cells,[180,183,184] or detection of viral DNA by in situ hybridization. The most secure diagnosis is based on biopsy material obtained with direct bronchoscopic visualization of airway lesions.

Varicella-Zoster Virus

Varicella-zoster virus involves the lung as part of disseminated infection and is therefore easy to recognize. The infection has been described in patients with AIDS but is rare.[185] Pulmonary lesions of disseminated varicella-zoster infection are characterized by miliary foci of necrosis similar to the pattern of disseminated HSV and CMV infection.[17] The cytopathic changes are identical to those of HSV.

Miscellaneous Viruses

Other viruses that affect the lung, such as influenza, respiratory syncytial, and parainfluenza viruses, have been reported in HIV-infected patients and may be associated with more prolonged illness than in immunocompetent individuals.[1] The possible roles of Epstein-Barr virus (EBV) and HIV in HIV-related pulmonary disease are discussed in the section on lymphocytic interstitial pneumonitis.

Fungi

Patients with AIDS are predisposed to pulmonary fungal infections, especially those, such as cryptococcosis, histoplasmosis, and coccidioidomycosis, that require intact cellular immunity for their containment. In AIDS patients these fungal pneumonias are usually part of and overshadowed by disseminated infection. They occur in endemic and nonendemic areas, are most often caused by reactivation of latent infections, and often recur despite adequate therapy. Histologic features of these pneumonias include overwhelming numbers of organisms, which apparently multiply in macrophages that cannot kill them, and a poor granulomatous response.

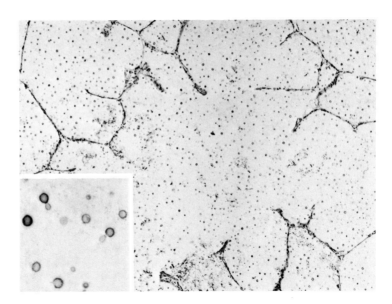

Figure 8–16. Cryptococcal bronchopneumonia with no inflammatory response. Yeasts fill alveolar spaces and appear to compress alveolar septa. Yeasts are widely separated from each other by thick capsules that are not stained by hematoxylin and eosin. *Inset,* Higher power magnification of yeasts showing two that are budding. Each bud is solitary and has narrow base. (Hematoxylin and eosin, ×25; inset ×100.)

Cryptococcus neoformans

Cryptococcus neoformans is the most common cause of fungal pneumonia in AIDS. It is a ubiquitous saprophytic yeast found in the feces of pigeons and other birds and in soil contaminated by their droppings.[186,187] The organisms are inhaled in airborne particles and lodge in the respiratory tract. Asymptomatic colonization of the tracheobronchial tree is common in both immunocompetent and immunocompromised individuals, with rates of cryptococcal isolation from sputum of at least 20% in most studies. When pulmonary infection occurs, it is usually self-limited in an immunocompetent host but occasionally leads to dissemination. In contrast, dissemination is a common sequel to pulmonary cryptococcosis in compromised hosts, especially those with AIDS. Cryptococcal pneumonia associated with HIV infection usually occurs in individuals who have meningoencephalitis or disseminated cryptococcosis. In less than 10% of patients with cryptococcosis and AIDS are the lungs the primary site of cryptococcal infection.[188]

Abnormal macrophage function related to T-cell deficiency is probably involved in the pathogenesis of cryptococcosis in AIDS, since unstimulated macrophages can phagocytose cryptococci but require stimulation by lymphokines secreted from activated T-cells to kill the intracellular organisms.[186,187] Cryptococci are unencapsulated in the environment, and the virulence of various strains depends partly on their ability to develop a thick polysaccharide capsule after deposition in the lungs.[1] Some AIDS patients have had infections caused by capsule-deficient cryptococci, which were found both in histologic sections and in primary cultures. Although some investigators believe that these organisms are pathogenic only in individuals with HIV-induced immunodeficiency, infections caused by capsule-deficient cryptococci were documented before the AIDS pandemic.[189-192] Diagnosis of pulmonary cryptococcosis requires isolation of the organism from sputum, BAL fluid, pleural fluid, or lung tissue.[1]

Pulmonary cryptococcosis has four basic morphologic patterns.[193]: (1) one or more peripheral granulomas with or without caseation, (2) a bronchopneumonia pattern with organisms in airways and adjacent alveoli associated with an inflammatory response that ranges from none (Fig. 8–16) to a diffuse intraalveolar granulomatous reaction (Fig. 8–17), (3) organisms in alveolar capillaries and interstitium with an inflammatory response ranging from nil to occasional interstitial granulomas (Fig. 8–18), and (4) a mixture of the bronchopneumonia and interstitial patterns with massive numbers of organisms and minimal inflammatory response. The interstitial and mixed patterns predominate in patients with AIDS.[190]

C. neoformans is an almost perfectly round monomorphic budding yeast that averages 4 to 7 μm in diameter with a range of 2 to 15 μm.[103,176] Budding forms are seen more frequently than with other fungi, and the buds tend to be single and have a narrow base (Fig. 8–16). The yeast is surrounded by a thick mu-

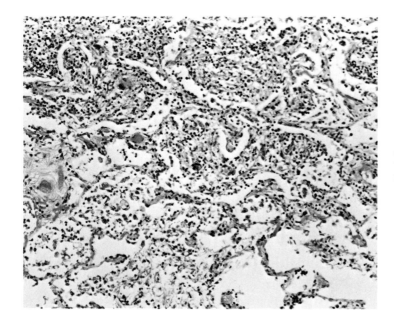

Figure 8–17. Cryptococcal bronchopneumonia with a diffuse intraalveolar granulomatous reaction. (Hematoxylin and eosin, ×25.)

copolysaccharide capsule that retracts in tissue sections, leaving a distinctive clear space 3 to 5 μm thick around each organism. This is best seen in intracellular organisms as a clear halo around the yeast. The organism stains moderately well with hematoxylin, appearing pale-blue or gray in hematoxylin and eosin preparations, and it is also stained with PAS and methenamine-silver stains. A diagnostic feature is the carminophilia of the mucopolysaccharide capsule, which stains bright red with Mayer's mucicarmine stain. This fea-

ture distinguishes *C. neoformans* from other budding yeasts such as *Histoplasma capsulatum* and *Blastomyces dermatitidis,* which are devoid of a mucopolysaccharide capsule.[176] In capsule-deficient cryptococcosis the organisms are in close contact with one another and could be confused with other yeasts. However, in most of these cases some carminophilic capsular material can be identified around a few yeasts and the distinction can be made.[194] The Fontana-Masson stain can also help make this distinction; *C. neoformans* stains positive

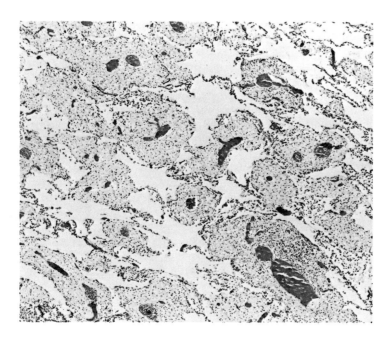

Figure 8–18. Interstitial form of cryptococcal pneumonia with histiocytes filling alveolar septa. (Hematoxylin and eosin, ×10.)

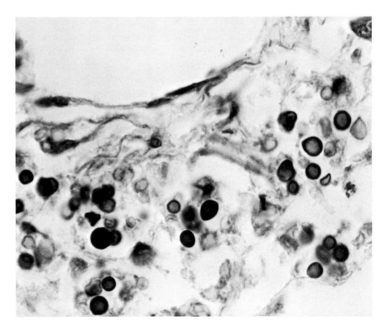

Figure 8–19. Cryptococci in alveolar wall (same patient as in Fig. 8–18) stained with Fontana-Masson stain. (×250.)

because it contains phenoloxidase and produces melanin-like pigment (Fig. 8–19), whereas the other yeasts are not stained.[195-197] If necessary, electron microscopy can be used to identify an attenuated mucopolysaccharide capsule.[194,197]

Histoplasma capsulatum

Histoplasma capsulatum is a dimorphic yeast that occurs as a yeast form at body temperature and a mycelial form in nature and thrives in soil contaminated with bird or bat droppings.[1] It is found in temperate regions throughout the world, and highly endemic areas in the United States include the Mississippi and Ohio river valleys. Spores liberated from the soil are inhaled and deposited in the lungs where they develop into yeasts, the parasitic form of the organism. In an immunocompetent host the primary pulmonary infection is inconsequential, but in immunosuppressed individuals it may lead to life-threatening disseminated histoplasmosis. Dissemination is the rule in HIV-infected patients, in whom both reactivation of latent infection and progression of newly acquired infection are believed to occur.[198]

Like cryptococcosis, disseminated histoplasmosis in patients with HIV infection is characterized by macrophages filled with multiplying fungi they cannot kill.[198] Granuloma formation is usually poor, although caseating and noncaseating granulomas have been described in persons with AIDS.[199] Chest roent-genograms of patients with pulmonary involvement most often show diffuse interstitial infiltrates; patterns consistent with granulomas are unusual.[198]

The *H. capsulatum* yeast form is ovoid and ranges from 1 to 5 μm in diameter with an average of 3 μm.[103] Budding may occur but is infrequent compared to *Cryptococcus*. Hematoxylin and eosin preparations stain the organism only when it is intracellular. Therefore hematoxylin and eosin is more likely to reveal the organism in a compromised host with disseminated infection than in an immunocompetent host who has well-formed granulomas in which organisms tend to be extracellular. Intracytoplasmic organisms appear as small oval yeasts with a central nucleus and clear zone between nucleus and cell wall, the latter representing an artifact of shrinkage of cytoplasm from the cell wall.[103]

A tentative diagnosis of disseminated histoplasmosis can be made on the basis of morphologic identification of yeasts consistent with the organism, but definitive diagnosis requires isolation of the organism by culture of bone marrow, blood, BAL fluid, or lung tissue[198] or by radioimmunoassay of *H. capsulatum* antigen in the urine or serum.[1]

Coccidioides immitis

Coccidioides immitis is another dimorphic soil fungus that typically produces self-limited disease in immunologically intact individuals and disseminated infection in patients with

HIV.[188,200] The fungus grows in the soil as a mycelium in semiarid regions of the Western Hemisphere (for example, the southwestern United States). Airborne arthrospores are deposited in small airways and alveoli where they are transformed into spherules, the parasitic phase.[1] In an immunologically competent host this eventually leads to granulomatous inflammation and containment of the infection. HIV-related coccidioidomycosis may result from reactivation of latent infection or progression of primary infection.[1] Pulmonary symptoms and signs and pathologic changes are more prominent in HIV-associated coccidioidomycosis than in histoplasmosis and are invariably associated with radiographic abnormalities, usually diffuse bilateral reticulonodular or nodular infiltrates.[1,188]

Diagnosis of coccidioidomycosis is based on morphologic identification of characteristic large, round, thick-walled, endosporulating spherules (Fig. 8–20) in cytologic or histologic material from the respiratory tract (sputum, BAL fluid, or transbronchial biopsy specimen) or by culture of the fungus from these specimens. Spherules measure 5 to 30 μm in diameter in the immature state and 30 to 100 μm in maturity and contain numerous 2 to 5 μm endospores. The spherules eventually rupture, liberating endospores to the surrounding tissue and leaving behind empty spherules in various stages of collapse. Spherules with their endospores stain with hematoxylin and are also well demonstrated with methenamine-silver. The inflammatory response to coccidioidomycosis in HIV-infected patients is similar to that in other immunocompromised hosts and ranges from suppurative (Fig. 8–20) to granulomatous.[200,201] However, patients with AIDS have a poorer granulomatous response and greater number of spherules in lung tissue.[200]

Other Fungi

Although mucocutaneous candidiasis is the most common HIV-associated opportunistic infection and often heralds the onset of AIDS, pulmonary candidiasis is uncommon in this setting.[188] HIV-associated *Candida* pneumonia is commonly a late complication of HIV infection, is associated with disseminated disease, and often coexists with other opportunistic infections or malignancies.[1] Diagnosis requires histologic identification of tissue invasion; culture alone is insufficient. Therefore antemortem diagnosis is uncommon, and most cases have been diagnosed only at autopsy.[112,115,202] Aspergillus is also not a significant HIV-related pulmonary pathogen but has been the etiologic agent in a number of respiratory infections in patients with AIDS.[115,153,188,202] Steroid therapy and neutropenia have been identified as risk factors for aspergillosis, as they are in immunosuppressed patients without HIV infection.[188,203] The histologic changes caused by HIV-related pulmonary candidiasis and invasive aspergillosis are generally similar to those in patients with other causes of immunodeficiency.

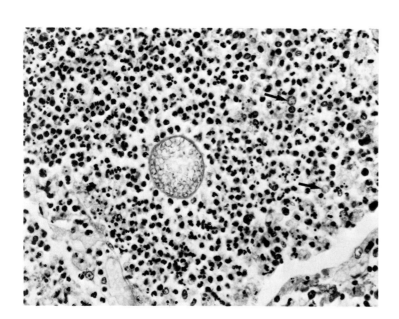

Figure 8–20. Fulminating suppurative pulmonary coccidioidomycosis. Spherule containing endospores is surrounded by neutrophilic exudate. Liberated endospores (arrows) are also enmeshed in exudate. (Hematoxylin and eosin, × 100.)

Bacteria

Mycobacterium avium Complex

Mycobacterium avium and *Mycobacterium intracellulare* are two closely related nonchromogenic mycobacteria that have been grouped together as *Mycobacterium avium* complex (MAC or MAI).[1] Although only 37 cases of disseminated MAC infection were reported before the AIDS epidemic,[204] MAC is the mycobacterium most commonly identified in AIDS patients and the most common cause of disseminated bacterial infection in this group.[205,206] Disseminated MAC infection has been diagnosed in approximately 5% of AIDS cases reported to the CDC,[207] but autopsy studies have revealed MAC infection in more than 50% of patients.[206] A declining prevalence of the infection with age suggests that it results from progressive recent infection instead of reactivation of latent infection.[1,207] Disseminated MAC typically occurs late in the course of HIV infection, and specific clinical features attributable to the organism are difficult to identify because other complications are present.[1]

MAC is ubiquitous in the environment, and the respiratory tract is a major portal of entry of aerosolized organisms. Person-to-person transmissions are uncommon. MAC typically causes lung disease resembling tuberculosis in elderly, presumably immunocompetent individuals with preexisting chronic lung disease.[208] MAC is frequently isolated from respiratory secretions in patients with AIDS, and in one large series 17% of patients were found to have MAC in cultures from specimens obtained by fiberoptic bronchoscopy.[27] In some of these cases recovery of the organism reflects only colonization, but in many instances further study reveals disseminated infection.[209] Disseminated MAC is associated with a variety of systemic symptoms and signs, but pulmonary symptoms are minimal.[205] Chest roentgenograms are nonspecific for MAC infection; they may be normal or show diffuse, localized, or nodular infiltrates, as well as hilar and mediastinal adenopathy. Cavitary disease is rare.[205]

Whereas MAC may elicit a necrotizing granulomatous inflammatory response in immunocompromised patients without AIDS, such a reaction is unusual in AIDS patients,[210] who usually have poorly formed granulomas.[154,211] This minimal inflammatory response to MAC has been associated with cell-mediated immunodeficiency.[212] The typical pathologic finding of pulmonary MAC infection in AIDS patients is that of focal interstitial collections of foamy or striated histiocytes that have pale blue cytoplasm when stained with hematoxylin and eosin (Fig. 8–21) and have been likened to Gaucher cells.[211,213] The striated pale blue histiocyte is characteristic of MAC infection in AIDS and should suggest the diagnosis. Confirmation is easily made if a mycobacterial stain shows the cells to be packed with rod-shaped

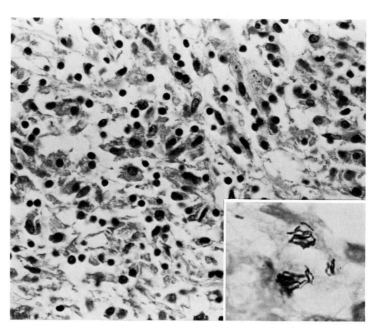

Figure 8–21. *Mycobacterium avium* complex in lung showing collection of histiocytes in interstitium. *Inset,* Acid-fast stain showing organisms within histiocytes. (Hematoxylin and eosin, ×100; inset ×250.)

acid-fast bacilli. The organisms are also stained with Giemsa, PAS, methenamine-silver, and Brown-Hopps stains.[211,213]

Abdominal involvement is the most clinically significant form of MAC infection in AIDS patients.[205] MAC involvement of the lung has little significance as a cause of respiratory disease in patients with AIDS, and cases in which respiratory symptoms are attributable to the organism are uncommon.[205] However, the observation of a few foamy histiocytes containing acid-fast bacilli in a respiratory specimen may be the first indication of disseminated infection with the organism. This is yet another example of the importance of routinely using special stains to evaluate specimens from HIV-infected individuals. Unfortunately, therapy has been ineffective in eradicating the infection in AIDS patients. Although MAC infection may cause significant morbidity in these patients, it is only rarely considered a cause of death.[205]

Mycobacterium tuberculosis

Tuberculosis has long been recognized as an opportunistic infection that is associated with impaired cell-mediated immunity.[214,215] In immunologically intact individuals infected with *Mycobacterium tuberculosis*, the likelihood of clinically apparent disease ever developing is approximately 10%.[214,215] People with impaired cellular immunity are at increased risk for tuberculosis, and generally the greater the degree of immunocompromise, the greater the risk. HIV-infected individuals constitute such a risk group. In fact, HIV infection is considered responsible for much of the excess (greater than predicted) cases of tuberculosis that have occurred since 1984 and for the increased tuberculosis case rate in 1986 after 33 years of successive decreases in the United States.[216] The greatest increases have occurred in large urban areas with the largest number of AIDS cases and in groups with the highest prevalence of HIV infection.

HIV-associated tuberculosis tends to occur in populations that have a high prevalence of preexisting tuberculous infection, including intravenous drug users, Haitians, and minorities.[215,217,218] This suggests that most new cases of tuberculosis in HIV-infected individuals, as in immunocompetent persons, arise from endogenous reactivation of old tuberculous infections.[217] However, progressive primary tuberculosis has been the predominant pattern of disease in some studies.[219,220] Tuberculosis characteristically occurs early in the course of HIV infection, usually preceding a diagnosis of AIDS.[215] This is in contrast to AIDS-defining infections such as pneumocystosis and disseminated MAC, which occur relatively late in the course of HIV infection when CD4 lymphocyte counts are low,[221] and is most likely a reflection of the greater pathogenicity of *M. tuberculosis* compared with these other agents.[217]

HIV-associated tuberculosis is noted for its atypical features. In general, the later tuberculosis occurs in the course of HIV infection (that is, the greater the impairment of cellular immunity), the more atypical are its features.[215] Typical pulmonary tuberculosis, with upper lobe involvement and cutaneous reactivity to tuberculin, may occur early in the course of HIV infection. In contrast, tuberculosis that develops late in HIV infection is characterized by a negative tuberculin skin test reaction and atypical roentgenographic findings, including intrathoracic adenopathy and lower lung zone or diffuse infiltrations without cavitation.[214,215] Dissemination to extrapulmonary sites frequently occurs, and involvement of the central nervous system, bone, pericardium, stomach, peritoneum, and scrotum has been described.[214,215]

The inflammatory response to *M. tuberculosis* depends on the degree of impairment of cell-mediated immunity. Granulomas may form early in the course of HIV infection, but classic granulomas are not seen in more advanced disease.[220] Postmortem examinations of AIDS patients who died of disseminated disease have revealed poorly formed granulomas with extensive caseation and numerous organisms.[115]

Some important differences between infections with *M. tuberculosis* and MAC in HIV-infected patients are worthy of reemphasis. Tuberculosis tends to occur earlier in the course of HIV infection and may be associated with typical caseating granulomas, whereas MAC infection develops later and is not characterized by granuloma formation. Thus observation of well-formed granulomas in an HIV-infected individual should raise a strong suspicion of tuberculosis. Unlike MAC infection in AIDS patients, which does not respond well to therapy, tuberculosis in this setting has a good response to antituberculous therapy.

Other Bacteria

Most pneumonias in AIDS patients are caused by nonbacterial opportunistic organisms known to produce disease in individuals with T-cell deficiencies. However, persons in all stages of HIV infection also have increased susceptibility to pneumonia caused by pyogenic bacteria.[12,188] This is largely due to functional defects in B-lymphocytes (impaired humoral immunity) and macrophages and neutrophils (abnormal phagocytic and bactericidal activity) associated with HIV infection.[12] In one autopsy study, more patients who died of AIDS (83%) had bacterial (nonmycobacterial) infection at some time during their illness than any other type of infection.[222]

The rate of community-acquired pneumonias is increased in HIV-infected individuals. These pneumonias tend to occur early in a patient's course, before an AIDS-defining illness has occurred. Most are caused by the encapsulated organisms *Streptococcus pneumoniae* and *Haemophilus influenzae*. They are readily diagnosed and respond to appropriate therapy, although bacteremia and recurrences are frequent sequellae.[12,188,223,224] In contrast, nosocomial pneumonias occur later in HIV infection, usually after AIDS has been diagnosed, and are often associated with other risk factors for bacterial infection such as drug-induced neutropenia and indwelling venous catheter. They tend to be unsuspected and inadequately treated, have a high fatality rate,[224] and are often diagnosed only at autopsy.[18,115,153,202,222] The majority are caused by *Pseudomonas aeruginosa*, *Klebsiella pneumoniae*, and *Staphylococcus aureus*. The histologic changes seen in HIV-associated nosocomial pneumonias are similar to those of acute necrotizing bacterial pneumonias in patients without HIV infection.

Other bacterial pathogens that have been documented as causes of pneumonia in AIDS patients include *Streptococcus* species other than *S. pneumoniae*, nonencapsulated *Haemophilus* species, *Branhamella catarrhalis*, *Legionella* species, *Salmonella* species, *Nocardia asteroides*, and *Mycoplasma pneumoniae*.[12,188,224]

Parasites

Toxoplasmosis is a relatively common infection in patients with AIDS, in whom it usually affects the central nervous system. Although lung involvement was identified at autopsy in 36% of cases in one study of toxoplasmosis in AIDS,[225] pulmonary toxoplasmosis is rarely diagnosed during life, either because it is clinically inapparent and overshadowed by the central nervous system infection or because organisms are sparse in lung tissue.[225,226] Toxoplasmosis is manifest in the lung as interstitial chronic inflammation or acute and chronic inflammation with areas of necrosis.[113,176,225-228] Cysts and trophozoites of *Toxoplasma gondii* are seen in alveolar lining cells and extracellularly. Although immunohistochemical staining of the organism has been useful in diagnosing central nervous system disease, in one study it was not as reliable in demonstrating pulmonary infection.[225]

Pulmonary cryptosporidiosis associated with intestinal infestation has been described in several patients with AIDS.[229-231] The organisms have been seen on the surface of bronchial epithelial cells (similar to their involvement of intestinal epithelium) or within alveolar exudates. Other pulmonary pathogens have also been present as a rule, so the contribution of cryptosporidiosis to the patient's respiratory disease is not clear. However, inflammation of the lamina propria and copious sputum production have been associated with cryptosporidial involvement of the airways.[231]

INTERSTITIAL PNEUMONIAS

Diffuse Alveolar Damage

Diffuse alveolar damage is the term used for a common nonspecific pattern of acute lung injury caused by a variety of biologic, chemical, and physical agents and associated with a large number of clinical conditions.[103] In particular, it is the lesion invariably seen in the adult respiratory distress syndrome from whatever cause.[103,232,233] DAD is also the most common histologic pattern of lung disease encountered in immunocompromised individuals with or without AIDS.[17,18,112]

DAD has two recognizable morphologic phases that are temporally related and merge imperceptibly, an acute exudative phase and an organizing or proliferative phase.[232-236] The exudative phase develops over 2 to 3 days and is characterized by interstitial edema and hyaline membranes lining the airspaces and respiratory bronchioles (Fig. 8–22).[232-234,236,237] Alveolar capillary congestion and interstitial hemorrhage are present in various degrees. The interstitium also contains scattered chronic inflammatory cells and neutrophils but the inflammation is usually not severe. Microthrombi and aggregates of neutrophils may be seen in some capillaries and small arteries.[232,236-238] Alveolar spaces contain variable amounts of proteinaceous fluid, erythrocytes, fibrin, and cell debris, as

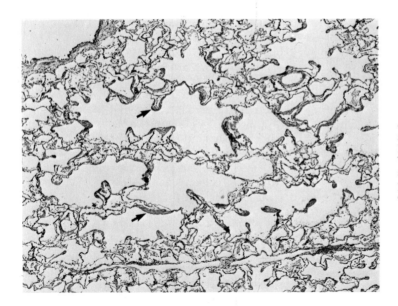

Figure 8–22. Exudative phase of diffuse alveolar damage showing hyaline membranes *(arrows)* lining dilated alveolar ducts and some alveoli. Widened (edematous) interlobular septum is evident in lower portion of photomicrograph. (Hematoxylin and eosin, × 10.)

well as small numbers of macrophages and acute and chronic inflammatory cells. At the ultrastructural level the alveolar epithelium may appear injured, necrotic, or even normal depending on the type and concentration of the etiologic agent. Typically destruction of type I alveolar cells is widespread, whereas type II cells appear to be more resistant to injury and show only minimal damage.[237-239] In places where the underlying epithelial basement membrane is exposed, sheetlike collections of alveolar exudate, including fragments of necrotic alveolar epithelial cells, adhere to the denuded alveolar surface, forming the hyaline membranes observed by light microscopy (Fig. 8–23).[237,238,240] Thus hyaline membranes serve as a convenient marker for alveolar epithelial necrosis.

The exudative phase of DAD may resolve within a few days or progress to a fibrosing organizing or proliferative phase within 7 to 10 days (Figs. 8–24 and 8–25).[103,232,237,238,241] Hyperplasia of alveolar lining cells is evident 3 days after the onset of DAD, and within 7 days the alveolar walls are repopulated by a layer of cuboidal epithelium (Fig. 8–24).[103,237] By electron microscopy these cells are similar to type II pneumocytes, which are believed to be the reserve cells of the alveolar epithelium.[103,237,239] This new

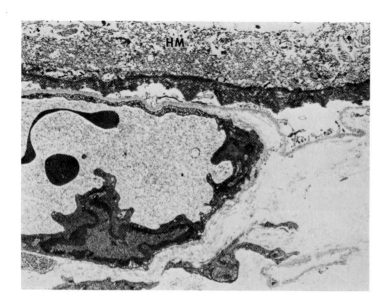

Figure 8–23. Electron micrograph of exudative diffuse alveolar damage. Hyaline membrane *(HM)* overlies epithelial basement membrane. Alveolar epithelium is destroyed, but capillary endothelium is intact. Hyaline membrane consists of cellular debris from necrotic alveolar epithelial cells (in upper portion of membrane) plus fibrillar material, presumably fibrin (in lower, more dense portion of membrane adjacent to epithelial basement membrane). Massive interstitial edema is evident to right of capillary. (× 13,600.) (From Nash G, Foley FD, Langlinais PC: Hum Pathol 5:149-160, 1974.)

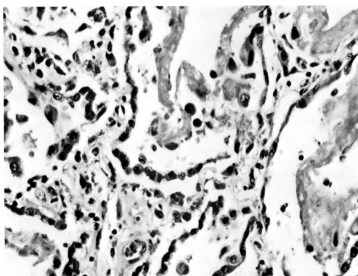

Figure 8–24. Transition from exudative phase to early proliferative phase of diffuse alveolar damage. Regenerating alveolar epithelium (strings of attached round or cuboidal cells lining alveoli) and residual hyaline membranes are evident. Interstitium is thickened and hypercellular. (Hematoxylin and eosin, ×100.)

epithelial layer can be transformed into type I cells in a few days or may persist.[242] Its presence increases the thickness of the air-blood membrane and probably diminishes gas exchange. Significant thickening of the interstitium results from a number of factors: an increase in extracellular matrix, including glycosaminoglycans (such as hyaluronic acid) and collagen[243,244]; persistent interstitial edema; an increased number of interstitial fibroblasts, myofibroblasts,[245,246] histiocytes, and chronic inflammatory cells; alveolar collapse with folding of portions of alveolar septa and permanent apposition of their walls (Fig. 8–26)[237,247,248]; and incorporation of intraal-

veolar exudates into alveolar septa.[247-250] Intraluminal organization also occurs in DAD, giving rise to obliterative fibrosis of lumens and intraluminal buds of connective tissue.[249]

At autopsy the gross appearance of DAD is distinctive and suggests the diagnosis. The lungs are heavy, airless, and firm and tend to be dark red in the exudative phase and pale gray in the organizing phase.[234] After fixation with formalin inflation, the cut surface is smooth and flat, interlobular septa are broadened, and the parenchyma has a homogeneous appearance of uniformly spaced pinpoint depressions, perhaps representing dilated small airways or alveolar ducts sur-

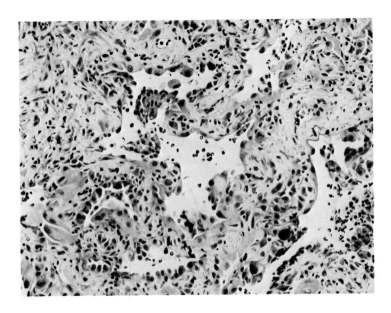

Figure 8–25. Well-developed proliferative phase of diffuse alveolar damage showing marked interstitial thickening with increased chronic inflammatory cells, fibroblasts, and extracellular matrix. The few remaining airspaces exhibit regenerated epithelium and absence of hyaline membranes. (Hematoxylin and eosin, ×50.)

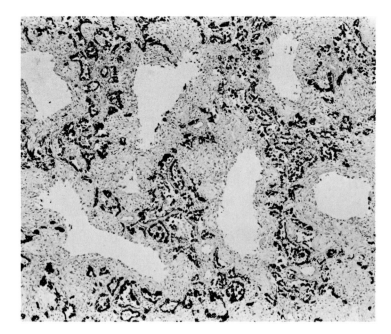

Figure 8–26. Proliferative phase of diffuse alveolar damage. Immunohistochemical stain for cytokeratin demonstrates regenerated alveolar epithelium and striking alveolar collapse. (×10.)

rounded by collapsed airspaces with thickened walls (Fig. 8–27).[237] A striking mucoid, slippery consistency is often present,[114] probably reflecting increased glycosaminoglycan levels. Since patients with DAD invariably require mechanical ventilation with high airway pressures because of decreased lung compliance, signs of barotrauma such as universal dilatation of the airways and interstitial emphysema are often evident.[114]

DAD is a common finding in the lungs of AIDS patients, especially at autopsy, in which it has been reported in more than 65% of cases.[18,112,251] The organizing phase of DAD

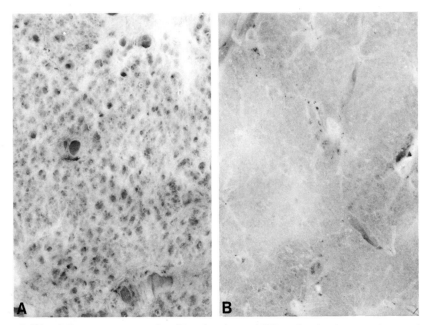

Figure 8–27. *A,* Gross appearance of proliferative phase of diffuse alveolar damage of approximately 3 weeks' duration. Formalin-inflated lung exhibits numerous pinpoint depressions, probably representing dilated small airways and alveolar ducts. *B,* Normal lung for comparison. (*A* and *B,* ×4.)

is most commonly observed, followed by mixed organizing-exudative and pure exudative patterns.[18,113,251,252] As previously noted, DAD is the most common pulmonary lesion encountered in immunocompromised patients without AIDS, in whom the condition is often idiopathic.[17] In contrast, in AIDS patients with DAD one or more potential etiologic agents (such as *P. carinii*) are usually identified (Table 8–4).[18] Even when an etiologic agent is not identified in lung tissue, patients often have a history of an infection caused by an agent known to elicit this pulmonary reaction.[252] The cause of organizing DAD in patients with AIDS is usually multifactorial, with some contribution from oxygen toxicity, a known cause of this injury pattern.[18,114,234]

Organizing DAD must be distinguished from chronic interstitial pneumonia with pulmonary fibrosis, even though the latter would be an unlikely finding in a patient with AIDS. Patients with DAD have extensive fibroblastic proliferation, relatively little collagen deposition, a great deal of hyaluronic acid in the interstitium, and much regenerative activity of the epithelium, whereas those with chronic interstitial pneumonia have more interstitial collagen and less fibroblastic activity, epithelial regeneration, and hyaluronic acid.[253]

The mortality rate of DAD in patients without AIDS is approximately 50% but varies considerably depending on the cause and severity.[103] Initially treatment of acute respiratory failure (DAD) caused by PCP in patients with AIDS yielded hospital survival rates of zero to 15%, but recent experience has improved the survival to approximately that of patients without AIDS who have DAD.[254] Severe organizing DAD with extensive alveolar collapse generally has a grim prognosis. However, recovery may occur at any stage,[255] and predicting the outcome from a lung biopsy in a given patient is hazardous, even when the underlying condition is AIDS.

Table 8–4. Common Causes of Diffuse Alveolar Damage in AIDS

Infectious agents
  Pneumocystis carinii
  Cytomegalovirus
Oxygen toxicity
Sepsis
Chemotherapeutic agents (bleomycin toxicity)

Nonspecific Interstitial Pneumonitis

An idiopathic nonspecific interstitial pneumonitis has been reported in lung biopsies of HIV-infected patients with and without AIDS. In one study 38% of patients with AIDS had transbronchial or open lung biopsies showing features of DAD, associated in some cases with interstitial lymphoid aggregates.[11] About one third of those patients had no known cause for the pulmonary changes. Clinical findings were indistinguishable from those in identifiable opportunistic infections, but the pneumonitis usually resolved without therapy. In another study 29% of transbronchial biopsies in AIDS patients revealed variable amounts of inflammatory cells within the interstitium or alveolar spaces with no etiologic agent identified.[256] Nevertheless, many of these patients improved without treatment. Ognibene et al.[257] found that approximately half of HIV-seropositive patients without clinical evidence of pneumonitis had transbronchial biopsies that showed nonspecific lymphoid interstitial infiltrates or lymphoid aggregates.

The preceding studies suggest that HIV infection is associated with an indolent inflammatory process in the lung that may be clinically evident or occult. Although many of these patients have lymphoid cells in the interstitium, a relationship to lymphoid interstitial pneumonitis has not been identified. Possibly the nonspecific pneumonitis reported in these studies is the histologic counterpart of a "lymphocytic alveolitis," composed of suppressor-cytotoxic cells (mainly the latter) noted in bronchoalveolar lavage specimens from individuals infected with HIV.[258-261] The cause of the lymphocyte expansion in the lung is unknown, but suggested etiologic agents include HIV, EBV, and cytomegalovirus; other possibilities include a response to therapeutic or illicit drugs.

Pulmonary Lymphoid Hyperplasia–Lymphoid Interstitial Pneumonitis Complex

A spectrum of pulmonary lymphoid infiltrates has been described with HIV infection, especially in children. These include pulmonary lymphoid hyperplasia (PLH), lymphoid interstitial pneumonitis (LIP), polyclonal polymorphic B-cell lymphoproliferative disorder (PBLD), and malignant lymphoma.[262] PBLD, an entity thought to be intermediate between benign and malignant lymphoid proliferation,[263] and malignant lymphoma in AIDS are discussed in Chapter 7.

Long before the AIDS pandemic, LIP was described as a diffuse infiltrate of predominantly mature lymphocytes, plasma cells, and reticuloendothelial cells in a lymphatic distribution around vessels and airways and in alveolar walls.[264,265] It typically occurs in adults and is rare in children who do not have AIDS.[266] LIP may be associated with other diseases such as Sjögren's syndrome, myasthenia gravis, and chronic active hepatitis. It is also associated with dysgammaglobulinemic states, frequently monoclonal gammopathies, and lymphomas have arisen in patients with these conditions.[267,268]

LIP is a common complication of AIDS in children and has been included in the CDC case definition of pediatric AIDS.[269-272] LIP has also been described in adults with AIDS, although its incidence in that population is low.[273-275] LIP in HIV infection is generally similar to that unassociated with AIDS and is characterized by diffuse infiltration of alveolar septa by mature lymphocytes, plasma cells with occasional Russell bodies, plasmacytoid lymphocytes, and immunoblasts.[262] Nodular aggregates of lymphoid cells and granuloma-like collections of pale mononuclear cells that may contain mutinucleated giant cells are sometimes encountered. Destruction of alveolar walls, vessels, or airways is not a feature of LIP, unlike lymphomatoid granulomatosis and bronchocentric granulomatosis.[262] Im-munohistochemical studies have demonstrated a mixed and polyclonal proliferation of both B- and T-cells.[262,275,276] Ruling out pneumocystosis is important before a pulmonary lymphoid infiltrate is designated LIP because, as previously noted, PCP may be associated with a marked lymphoid infiltrate with little or no characteristic alveolar foam.

PLH is characterized by lymphoid nodules in and around bronchi and bronchioles. The nodules may be large enough to see with the unassisted eye and often contain germinal centers with mature and immature lymphoid cells and plasma cells at the periphery.[262,277] PLH and LIP were initially regarded as separate entities, but considerable overlap was demonstrated so that now the lesions are designated the PLH-LIP complex (Fig. 8–28).[278]

The typical presentation of PLH-LIP complex is one of slowly progressive dyspnea and a chest roentgenogram showing bilateral interstitial or nodular infiltrates. In children the diagnosis is often suspected on the basis of clinical findings. The complex is distinguished from infectious pneumonia by the rapid course of the latter.[279] A biopsy is performed to confirm the diagnosis only when the patient's condition has deteriorated and steroid therapy is being considered.[280] LIP in adults cannot be distinguished clinically from other pulmonary diseases that affect HIV-infected individuals.[280]

The clinical course of LIP in children is variable. The typical course is a slowly pro-

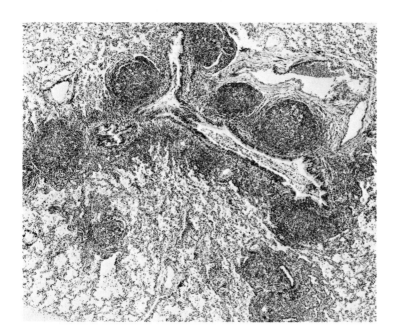

Figure 8–28. Lung biopsy specimen from child with pulmonary lymphoid hyperplasia–lymphoid interstitial pneumonitis complex characterized by lymphoid nodules around small airways and lymphoid cells infiltrating alveolar walls (Hematoxylin and eosin, × 10.)

gressive respiratory deterioration leading to respiratory failure, but spontaneous resolution may also occur.[277] In most children the condition remains stable without treatment or responds to steroid therapy for many years. In a few cases it progresses to a systemic lymphoproliferative disease, PBLD.[262]

The cause and pathogenesis of PLH-LIP associated with HIV infection are unknown, but a number of interesting theories have been offered.[262,280] One hypothesis suggests that it is an immunologic response to HIV infection in the lung. This is based on studies showing a significant presence of the virus in the lungs of patients with LIP and on the similarity of PLH-LIP to the lymphoid hyperplasia and infiltrates seen in sheep infected by ovine progressive pneumonia lentivirus, a subfamily of the retroviruses. However, the presence of HIV in the lungs has not been shown to be greater with LIP than without it. EBV replication in the lung has also been considered a cause of LIP. EBV DNA has been recovered from the lungs of children with LIP but not from HIV-infected children or adults without LIP. It has been suggested that LIP may consist of an infiltrate of EBV-infected cells and reactive lymphoid and mononuclear cells.[281] A third hypothesis, based on the finding that EBV-transformed B-cells are particularly susceptible to HIV infection,[282] suggests that the combination of EBV and HIV in the lung is responsible for PLH-LIP.

OTHER PULMONARY REACTIONS

A reaction resembling desquamative interstitial pneumonitis (DIP) and characterized by intraalveolar collections of alveolar macrophages, hyperplasia of alveolar lining cells, and a mild interstitial lymphoplasmacytic infiltrate has been described in a small number of children with AIDS. The DIP-like areas were near lesions of other pulmonary complications of AIDS and probably represent a nonspecific reaction rather than typical DIP.[262]

Secondary pulmonary alveolar proteinosis (PAP) has been reported in a few AIDS patients.[283] Unlike primary PAP, which has no identifiable cause, secondary PAP is associated with conditions that alter the immune system or with pulmonary infections. Since secondary PAP is caused by infections, such as CMV and mycobacterial infections, that occur in HIV-positive individuals, more cases will probably be encountered in the future.

MALIGNANT NEOPLASMS

Kaposi's Sarcoma

Involvement of the lung by Kaposi's sarcoma (KS) has been found in an average of 13% of AIDS patients at autopsy, and the incidence of KS at any site is approximately 50%.[202] In many of these patients pulmonary KS was implicated as a cause of death.[9,18,112,251,284,285]

The clinical presentation of pulmonary KS is similar to that of opportunistic pneumonias, with cough, dyspnea, and fever as the most common symptoms and signs.[284] Other symptoms are related to specific anatomic sites of tumor within the respiratory tract. Airway obstruction by tumor causes hoarseness, stridor, and wheezing from involvement of the vocal cords, trachea, and bronchi, respectively.[285] Hemoptysis resulting from endobronchial or parenchymal disease has also been described.[285] Most patients have hypoxemia, which may be severe enough to cause respiratory insufficiency and death.[9] Pulmonary KS usually follows cutaneous and lymph node involvement but occasionally is the main site of involvement when extrathoracic disease is minimal or not detectable.[9,286,287]

Pulmonary involvement as seen in open lung biopsies has a lymphatic-interstitial distribution, with KS infiltrating the pleura, bronchovascular sheaths, interlobular septa, and alveolar walls (Figs. 8–29 and 8–30).[18,288] This pattern is associated with diffuse interstitial or reticulonodular infiltrates on chest roentgenograms.[288,289] As the infiltrates expand, large tumor nodules develop and obliterate the underlying alveolar tissue. These are visualized roentgenographically as nodular densities.[289] The nodular pattern is the form usually seen at autopsy, and gross examination shows multiple hemorrhagic parenchymal nodules about 0.5 cm in diameter with occasional coalescence of the nodules to form large masses. Lesions of KS in the tracheobronchial tree are typically violaceous or cherry red, flat or raised plaques in the mucosa (Fig. 8–31), resembling the skin lesions.[36,284,285,287] Pleural involvement is common and is characterized by hemorrhagic plaques 0.3 to 1 cm in diameter.[285] The plaques are undoubtedly responsible for the serous or serosanguineous pleural effusions that occur in up to two thirds of patients.[280,284]

The histologic features of pulmonary KS are similar to those of the neoplasm in other tissues. The lesions generally have the ap-

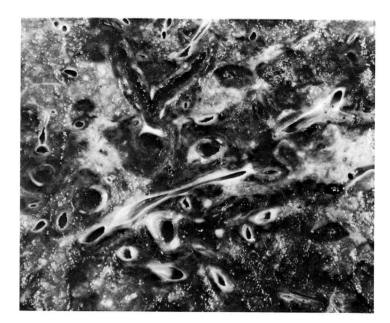

Figure 8–29. Kaposi's sarcoma involving bronchovascular sheaths (dark areas surrounding airways and vessels).

pearance of classic nodular KS of the skin and are highly cellular masses composed of spindle cells with hyperchromatic nuclei forming clefts that contain erythrocytes and deposits of hemosiderin (Fig. 8–30B).[288] Small, intracytoplasmic hyaline bodies can usually be identified in the spindle cells, and interspersed plasma cells are invariably present in such lesions.[288] A distinctive "polymorphous" or "early" form of KS,[288] analogous to inflammatory KS described in lymph nodes[290] and early patch or plaque lesions in the skin,[291] may be seen at the periphery of classic lesions or by itself and is characterized by fewer spindle cells, more chronic inflammatory cells, and nonspecific plump mesenchymal cells.[288] This form of the disease should not be mistaken for an organizing process such as the proliferative phase of DAD, organizing pneumonia, or bronchiolitis obliterans.[286,288] Careful evaluation is especially important with small biopsy specimens (such as transbronchial specimens) in which classic lesions may be sparse or absent. Identification of polymorphous KS in such a biopsy specimen from a patient known to have KS elsewhere should be sufficient for a diagnosis.[288]

Because of its patchy distribution, pulmonary KS is difficult to diagnose antemortem. Open lung biopsy has had the highest diagnostic yield,[251,288,292] but it is not 100% sensitive.[280] Although the diagnosis has been based on bronchial or transbronchial biopsies performed with fiberoptic bronchoscopy in many cases,[287,293,294] the small amounts of tissue obtained seldom permit identification of the characteristic architecture needed for histologic verification.[280] However, the presence of raised cherry red endobronchial lesions is considered characteristic enough to allow a presumptive diagnosis, and endobronchial KS is predictive of the concomitant presence of parenchymal KS.[36,280,285] Early reports suggested that bronchoscopic biopsy of KS was contraindicated because of a risk of hemorrhage owing to the tumor's vascular nature,[295,296] but excessive bleeding has not been encountered in subsequent studies.[280,287,294]

Complications of pulmonary KS may cause significant morbidity and mortality in AIDS patients. Involvement of the tracheobronchial tree by KS can cause life-threatening airway obstruction either directly or from hemorrhage.[284] Extensive parenchymal involvement or pleural effusions may cause respiratory failure. Parenchymal KS has been implicated as a cause of death in autopsy studies.[9,285] Although parenchymal hemorrhage is often noted to be associated with lesions of pulmonary KS at autopsy, clinically significant pulmonary hemorrhage is uncommon.[284]

Other Malignancies

Although the non-Hodgkin's lymphomas that occur with increased frequency in AIDS patients are characteristically extranodal neoplasms, the lung is usually not involved at the outset.[154,280] Lung involvement may occur as

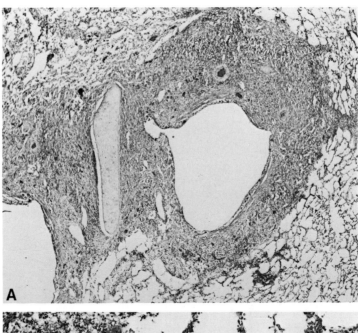

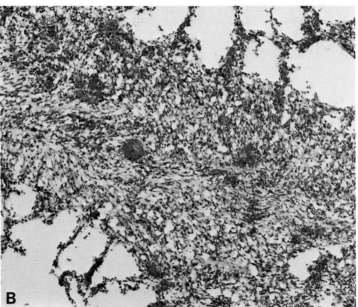

Figure 8–30. *A,* Kaposi's sarcoma involving bronchus. *B,* Spindle-cell infiltrate of Kaposi's sarcoma involving interlobular septum and adjacent alveolar walls. Erythrocytes are also evident among tumor cells. (Hematoxylin and eosin; *A,* × 10; *B,* × 50.)

part of disseminated disease; it is often not recognized clinically and is diagnosed only at autopsy.[297] Pulmonary involvement with HIV-related Hodgkin's disease occurs but is uncommon, and a few cases of AIDS-associated peripheral T-cell lymphoma-leukemia with pulmonary involvement have been reported.[280]

Neuroendocrine carcinomas of the lung have been reported in a few patients with AIDS,[298-300] but a relationship of lung cancer to HIV infection has not been identified.[280]

OTHER PULMONARY CONDITIONS

When evaluating a lung biopsy specimen from an HIV-positive individual, the pathologist should consider that the patient's pulmonary disease may not be directly related to immunosuppression or HIV infection. Examples of such unrelated conditions are talc granulomatosis in intravenous drug abusers and chemotherapeutic drug intoxication, especially with bleomycin.[280]

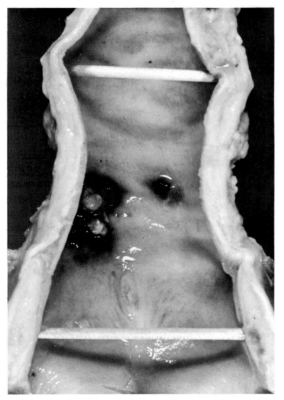

Figure 8–31. Kaposi's sarcoma involving trachea.

REFERENCES

1. Murray JF, Mills J: Pulmonary infectious complications of human immunodeficiency virus infection. Am Rev Respir Dis 141:1356-1372, 1582-1598, 1990.
2. Stover DE, White DA, Romano PA, et al: Spectrum of pulmonary diseases associated with the acquired immune deficiency syndrome. Am J Med 78:429-437, 1985.
3. Small PM, Hopewell PC: Respiratory system: A general approach. In Cohen PT, Sande MA, Volberding PA (eds): The AIDS Knowledge Base. Waltham, Mass, Medical Publishing Group, 1990.
4. Cohen BA, Pomeranz S, Rabinowitz JG, et al: Pulmonary complications of AIDS: Radiologic features. AJR 143:115-122, 1984.
5. Goodman PC, Gamsu G: Radiographic findings in the acquired immunodeficiency syndrome. Postgrad Radiol 7:3-15, 1987.
6. Golden JA, Sollitto RA: The radiology of pulmonary disease: Chest radiography, computed tomography, and gallium scanning. In White DA, Stover DE (eds): Pulmonary effects of AIDS. Clin Chest Med 9:481-495, 1988.
7. Small PM, Hopewell PC: Respiratory system: Radiographic findings. In Cohen PT, Sande MA, Volberding PA (eds): The AIDS Knowledge Base. Waltham, Mass, Medical Publishing Group, 1990.
8. Abd AG, Nieman DM, Ilowite JS, et al: Bilateral upper lobe *Pneumocystis carinii* pneumonia in a patient receiving inhaled pentamidine prophylaxis. Chest 94:329-331, 1988.
9. Ognibene FP, Steis RG, Macher AM, et al: Kaposi's sarcoma causing pulmonary infiltrates and respiratory failure in the acquired immunodeficiency syndrome. Ann Intern Med 102:471-475, 1985.
10. Morris JC, Rosen MJ, Marchevsky A, Teirstein AS: Lymphocytic interstitial pneumonia in patients at risk for the acquired immune deficiency syndrome. Chest 91:63-67, 1987.
11. Suffredini AF, Ognibene FP, Lack EE, et al: Nonspecific interstitial pneumonitis: A common cause of pulmonary disease in the acquired immunodeficiency syndrome. Ann Intern Med 107:7-13, 1987.
12. Chaisson RE: Bacterial pneumonia in patients with human immunodeficiency virus infection. Semin Respir Infect 4:133-138, 1989.
13. Suster B, Akerman M, Orenstein M, et al: Pulmonary manifestations of AIDS: Review of 106 episodes. Radiology 161:87-93, 1986.
14. Milligan SA, Stulbarg MS, Gamsu G, et al: *Pneumocystis carinii* pneumonia radiographically simulating tuberculosis. Am Rev Respir Dis 132:1124-1126, 1985.
15. Barrio JL, Sujarez M, Rodriguez JL, et al: *Pneumocystis carinii* pneumonia presenting as cavitating and noncavitating solitary pulmonary nodules in patients with the acquired immunodeficiency syndrome. Am Rev Respir Dis 134:1094-1096, 1986.
16. Scannell KA: Pneumothoraces and *Pneumocystis carinii* pneumonia in two AIDS patients receiving aerosolized pentamidine. Chest 97:479-480, 1990.
17. Nash G: Pathologic features of the lung in the immunocompromised host. Hum Pathol 13:841-858, 1982.
18. Nash G, Fligiel S: Pathologic features of the lung in the acquired immune deficiency syndrome (AIDS): An autopsy study of seventeen homosexual males. Am J Clin Pathol 81:6-12, 1984.
19. Walzer PD, Perl CP, Krogstad DJ, et al: *Pneumocystis carinii* pneumonia in the United States: Epidemiologic, diagnostic and clinical features. Ann Intern Med 80:83-93, 1974.
20. Bigby TD, Margolskee D, Curtis JL, et al: The usefulness of induced sputum in the diagnosis of *Pneumocystis carinii* pneumonia in patients with the acquired immunodeficiency syndrome. Am Rev Respir Dis 133:515-518, 1986.
21. Pitchenik AE, Ganjei P, Torres A, et al: Sputum examination for the diagnosis of *Pneumocystis carinii* pneumonia in the acquired immunodeficiency syndrome. Am Rev Respir Dis 133:226-229, 1986.
22. Ng VL, Gartner I, Weymouth LA, et al: The use of mucolysed induced sputum for the identification of pulmonary pathogens associated with human immunodeficiency virus infection. Arch Pathol Lab Med 113:488-493, 1989.
23. Kovacs JA, Ng VL, Masur H, et al: Diagnosis of *Pneumocystis carinii* pneumonia: Improved detection in sputum with use of monoclonal antibodies. N Engl J Med 318:589-93, 1988.
24. Del Rio C, Guarner J, Honig EG, et al: Sputum examination in the diagnosis of *Pneumocystis carinii* pneumonia in the acquired immunodeficiency syndrome. Arch Pathol Lab Med 112:1229-1232, 1988.

25. Small PM, Hopewell PC: Respiratory system: Techniques for definitive diagnosis. In Cohen PT, Sande MA, Volberding PA (eds): The AIDS Knowledge Base. Waltham, Mass, Medical Publishing Group, 1990.

26. Linder J, Radio SJ: Immunohistochemistry of *Pneumocystis carinii*. Semin Diagn Pathol 6:238-244, 1989.

27. Murray JF, Felton CH, Garay SM, et al: Pulmonary complications of the acquired immunodeficiency syndrome: Report of a National Heart, Lung, and Blood Institute Workshop. N Engl J Med 310:1682-1688, 1984.

28. Stover DE, Zaman MB, Hajdu SI, et al: Bronchoalveolar lavage in the diagnosis of diffuse pulmonary infiltrates in the immunosuppressed host. Ann Intern Med 101:1-7, 1984.

29. Hartman B, Koss M, Hui A, et al: *Pneumocystis carinii* pneumonia in the acquired immunodeficiency syndrome (AIDS): Diagnosis with bronchial brushings, biopsy, and bronchoalveolar lavage. Chest 87:603-607, 1985.

30. Broaddus C, Dake MD, Stulbarg MS, et al: Bronchoalveolar lavage and transbronchial biopsy for the diagnosis of pulmonary infections in the acquired immunodeficiency syndrome. Ann Intern Med 102:747-752, 1985.

31. Levine SJ, White DA: *Pneumocystis carinii*. Clin Chest Med 9:395-423, 1988.

32. Orenstein M, Webber CA, Heurich AE: Cytologic diagnosis of *Pneumocystis carinii* infection by bronchoalveolar lavage in acquired immune deficiency syndrome. Acta Cytol 29:727-731, 1985.

33. Luce JM, Clement MJ: Pulmonary diagnostic evaluation in patients suspected of having an HIV-related disease. Semin Respir Infect 4:93-101, 1989.

34. Caughey G, Wong H, Gamsu G, et al: Nonbronchoscopic bronchoalveolar lavage for the diagnosis for *Pneumocystis carinii* pneumonia in the acquired immunodeficiency syndrome. Chest 88:659-662, 1985.

35. Mann JM, Altus CS, Webber CA, et al: Nonbronchoscopic lung lavage for diagnosis of opportunistic infection in AIDS. Chest 9:319-322, 1987.

36. Murray JF, Garay SM, Hopewell PC, et al: Pulmonary complications of the acquired immunodeficiency syndrome: An update; Report of the Second National Heart, Lung and Blood Institute Workshop. Am Rev Respir Dis 135:504-509, 1987.

37. Centers for Disease Control: Acquired immunodeficiency syndrome (AIDS) update—United States. MMWR 32:309-311, 1983.

38. Centers for Disease Control: Update: Acquired immunodeficiency syndrome—United States. MMWR 34:245-248, 1985.

39. Masur H: New concepts in the therapy of infections in the acquired immunodeficiency syndrome. In Fauci AS (moderator): The acquired immunodeficiency syndrome: An update. Ann Intern Med 102:800-813, 1985.

40. Deleted.

41. Kovacs JA, Hiemenz JW, Macher AM, et al: *Pneumocystis carinii* pneumonia: A comparison between patients with the acquired immunodeficiency syndrome and patients with other immunodeficiencies. Ann Intern Med 100:663-671, 1984.

42. Centers for Disease Control: Guidelines for prophylaxis against *Pneumocystis carinii* pneumonia for persons infected with human immunodeficiency virus. MMWR 38:1-9, 1989.

43. Gutierrez Y: The biology of *Pneumocystis carinii*. Semin Diagn Pathol 6:203-211, 1989.

44. Barton EG Jr, Campbell WG Jr: *Pneumocystis carinii* in lungs of rats treated with cortisone acetate—ultrastructural observations related to the life cycle. Am J Pathol 54:209-236, 1969.

45. Vavra J, Kucera K: *Pneumocystis carinii* Delanoe, its ultrastructure and ultrastructural affinities. J Protozool 17:463-483, 1970.

46. Allegra CJ, Kovacs JA, Drake JC, et al: Activity of antifolates against *Pneumocystis carinii* dihydrofolate reductase and identification of a potent new agent. J Exp Med 165:926-931, 1987.

47. Edman JC, Kovacs JA, Masur H, et al: Ribosomal RNA sequence shows *Pneumocystis carinii* to be a member of the fungi. Nature 334:519-522, 1988.

48. Dutz W: *Pneumocystis carinii* pneumonia. Pathol Annu 5:309-341, 1970.

49. Kim HK, Hughes WT: Comparison of methods for identification of *Pneumocystis carinii* in pulmonary aspirates. Am J Clin Pathol 60:462-466, 1973.

50. Lanken PN, Minda M, Pietra GG, et al: Alveolar response to experimental *Pneumocystis carinii* pneumonia in the rat. Am J Pathol 99:561-588, 1980.

51. Henshaw NG, Carson JL, Collier AM: Ultrastructural observations of *Pneumocystis carinii* attachment to rat lung. J Infect Dis 151:181-186, 1985.

52. Yoneda K, Walzer PD: Attachment of *Pneumocystis carinii* to type 1 alveolar cells studied by freeze-fracture electron microscopy. Infect Immun 40:812-815, 1983.

53. Matsumoto Y, Yoshida Y: Sporogony in *Pneumocystis carinii:* Synaptonemal complexes and meiotic nuclear divisions observed in precysts. J Protozool 31:420-428, 1984.

54. Matsumoto Y, Yoshida Y: Advances in *Pneumocystis* biology. Parasitol Today 2:137-142, 1986.

55. Watts JC, Chandler FW: *Pneumocystis carinii* pneumonitis: The nature and diagnostic significance of the methenamine silver–positive "intracystic bodies." Am J Surg Pathol 9:744-751, 1985.

56. Ham EK, Greenberg SD, Reynolds RC, et al: Ultrastructure of *Pneumocystis carinii*. Exp Mol Pathol 14:362-372, 1971.

57. Price RA, Hughes WT: Histopathology of *Pneumocystis carinii* infestation and infection in malignant disease in childhood. Hum Pathol 5:737-752, 1974.

58. Walzer PD: Attachment of microbes to host cells: Relevance of *Pneumocystis carinii*. Lab Invest 54:589-592, 1986.

59. Singer C, Armstrong D, Rosen PP, et al: *Pneumocystis carinii* pneumonia: A cluster of 11 cases. Ann Intern Med 82:772-777, 1975.

60. Ruebush TK, Weinstein RA, Baehner RL, et al: An outbreak of *Pneumocystis* pneumonia in children with acute lymphocytic leukemia. Am J Dis Child 132:143-148, 1978.

61. Meuwissen JH, Tauber I, Leeuwenberg AD, et al: Parasitologic and serologic observations of infection with *Pneumocystis* in humans. J Infect Dis 136:43-49, 1977.

62. Pifer LL, Hughes WT, Stagno S, et al: *Pneumocystis carinii* infection: Evidence for high prevalence in

normal and immunosuppressed children. Pediatrics 61:35-41, 1978.

63. Sheldon WH: Subclinical *Pneumocystis* pneumonitis. Am J Dis Child 97:287-302, 1959.

64. Perera DR, Western KA, Johnson HD, et al: *Pneumocystis carinii* pneumonia in a hospital for children. JAMA 214:1074-1078, 1970.

65. Coleman DL, Luce JM, Wilber JC, et al: Antibody to the retrovirus associated with acquired immunodeficiency syndrome (AIDS): Presence in presumably healthy San Franciscans who died unexpectedly. Arch Intern Med 146:713-715, 1986.

66. Johnson JE, Anders GT, Hawkes CE, et al: Bronchoalveolar lavage findings in patients seropositive for the human immunodeficiency virus (HIV). Chest 97:1066-1071, 1990.

67. Frenkel JK, Good JT, Schultz JA: Latent *Pneumocystis* infection of rats, relapse, and chemotherapy. Lab Invest 15:1559-1577, 1966.

68. Masur H, Ognibene FP, Yarchoan R, et al: CD4 counts as predictors of opportunistic pneumonias in human immunodeficiency virus (HIV) infection. Ann Intern Med 111:223-231, 1989.

69. Phair J, Munoz A, Detels R, et al: The risk of *Pneumocystis carinii* pneumonia among men infected with human immunodeficiency virus type I. N Engl J Med 322:161-165, 1990.

70. Haverkos HW: Assessment of therapy for *Pneumocystis carinii* pneumonia: PCP therapy project group. Am J Med 76:501-508, 1984.

71. Engelberg LA, Lerner CW, Tapper ML: Clinical features of *Pneumocystis* pneumonia in the acquired immune deficiency syndrome. Am Rev Respir Dis 130:689-694, 1984.

72. Small CB, Harris CA, Friedland GH, et al: The treatment of *Pneumocystis carinii* pneumonia in the acquired immunodeficiency syndrome. Arch Intern Med 145:837-840, 1985.

73. Brenner M, Ognibene FP, Lack EE, et al: Prognostic factors and life expectancy of patients with acquired immunodeficiency syndrome and *Pneumocystis carinii* pneumonia. Am Rev Respir Dis 136:1199-1206, 1987.

74. Zaman MK, White DA: Serum lactate dehydrogenase levels and *Pneumocystis carinii* pneumonia: Diagnostic and prognostic significance. Am Rev Respir Dis 137:796-800, 1985.

75. Mason GR, Hashimoto CH, Dickman PS, et al: Prognostic implications of bronchoalveolar lavage neutrophilia in patients with *Pneumocystis carinii* pneumonia and AIDS. Am Rev Respir Dis 139:1336-1342, 1989.

76. Small PM, Goodman PC, Montgomery AB: Case 9-1989: AIDS and a cavitary pulmonary lesion [letter]. N Engl J Med 321:395, 1989.

77. Bleiweiss IJ, Jagirdar JS, Klein MJ, et al: Granulomatous *Pneumocystis carinii* pneumonia in three patients with the acquired immune deficiency syndrome. Chest 94:580-583, 1988.

78. Blumenfeld W, Basgoz N, Owen WF Jr, et al: Granulomatous pulmonary lesions in patients with the acquired immunodeficiency syndrome (AIDS) and *Pneumocystis carinii* infection. Ann Intern Med 15:505-507, 1988.

79. Liu YC, Tomashefski JF, Tomford JW, et al: Necrotizing *Pneumocystis carinii* vasculitis associated with lung necrosis and cavitation in a patient with acquired immunodeficiency syndrome. Arch Pathol Lab Med 113:494-497, 1989.

80. Beers MF, Sohn M, Swartz M: Recurrent pneumothorax in AIDS patients with *Pneumocystis* pneumonia: A clinicopathologic report of three cases and review of the literature. Chest 98:266-270, 1990.

81. Dyner TS, Lang W, Busch DF, et al: Intravascular and pleural involvement by *Pneumocystis carinii* in a patient with the acquired immunodeficiency syndrome (AIDS) [letter]. Ann Intern Med 111:94, 1989.

82. O'Doherty MJ, Thomas SH, Page CJ, et al: Does inhalation of pentamidine in the supine position increase deposition in the upper part of the lung? Chest 97:1343-1348, 1990.

83. LeGolvan DP, Heidelberger KP: Disseminated granulomatous *Pneumocystis carinii* pneumonia. Arch Pathol 95:344-348, 1973.

84. Barnett RN, Hull JG, Vortel V, et al: *Pneumocystis carinii* in lymph nodes and spleen. Arch Pathol 88:175-180, 1969.

85. Cote RJ, Rosenblum M, Telzak EE, et al: Disseminated *Pneumocystis carinii* infection causing extrapulmonary organ failure: Clinical, pathologic, and immunohistochemical analysis. Mod Pathol 3:25-30, 1990.

86. Unger PD, Rosenblum M, Krown SE: Disseminated *Pneumocystis carinii* infection in a patient with acquired immune deficiency syndrome. Hum Pathol 19:113-116, 1988.

87. Carter TR, Cooper PH, Petri WA Jr, et al: *Pneumocystis carinii* infection of the small intestine in a patient with acquired immune deficiency syndrome. Am J Clin Pathol 89:679-683, 1988.

88. Gallant JE, Enriquez RE, Cohen KL, et al: *Pneumocystis carinii* thyroiditis. Am J Med 84:303-306, 1988.

89. Poblete RB, Rodriguez K, Foust RT, et al: *Pneumocystis carinii* hepatitis in the acquired immunodeficiency syndrome (AIDS). Ann Intern Med 110:737-738, 1989.

90. Heyman MR, Rasmussen P: *Pneumocystis carinii* involvement of the bone marrow in acquired immunodeficiency syndrome. Am J Clin Pathol 87:780-783, 1987.

91. Gherman CR, Ward RR, Bassis ML: *Pneumocystis carinii* otitis media and mastoiditis as the initial manifestation of the acquired immunodeficiency syndrome. Am J Med 85:250-252, 1988.

92. Schinella RA, Breada SD, Hammerschlag PE: Otic infection due to *Pneumocystis carinii* in an apparently healthy man with antibody to the human immunodeficiency virus. Ann Intern Med 106:399-400, 1987.

93. Deleted.

94. Coulman CU, Greene I, Archibald RWR: Cutaneous pneumocystosis. Ann Intern Med 106:396-398, 1987.Deleted.

95. Montgomery AB, Debs RJ, Luce JM, et al: Aerosolized pentamidine as sole therapy for *Pneumocystis carinii* pneumonia in patients with acquired immunodeficiency syndrome. Lancet 2:480-483, 1987.

96. Raviglione MC, Mariuz P, Sugar J, et al: Extrapulmonary *Pneumocystis* infection [letter]. Ann Intern Med 111:339, 1989.

97. Fauci AS, Macher AM, Longo DL, et al: Acquired immunodeficiency syndrome: Epidemiologic, clinical, immunologic, and therapeutic considerations. Ann Intern Med 100:92-106, 1984.

98. Young LS: Clinical aspects of pneumocystosis in man: Epidemiology, clinical manifestations, diagnostic approaches, and sequelae. In Young LS (ed): *Pneumocystis carinii* Pneumonia. New York, Marcel Dekker, 1984, pp 139-174.

99. Burke BA, Good RA: *Pneumocystis carinii* infection. Medicine 52:23-51, 1973.

100. Richman DD, Zamvil L, Remington JS: Recurrent *Pneumocystis carinii* pneumonia in a child with hypogammaglobulinemia. Am J Dis Child 125:102-103, 1973.

101. Masur H, Jones TC: The interaction in vitro of *Pneumocystis carinii* with macrophages and L-cells. J Exp Med 147:157-170, 1978.

102. Weber WR, Askin FB, Dehner LP: Lung biopsy in *Pneumocystis carinii* pneumonia: A histopathologic study of typical and atypical features. Am J Clin Pathol 67:11-19, 1977.

103. Katzenstein AA, Askin FB: Surgical pathology of non-neoplastic lung disease. In Bennington JL (ed): Major Problems In Pathology, vol 13, ed 2. Philadelphia, Saunders, 1990.

104. Askin FB, Katzenstein ALA: *Pneumocystis* infection masquerading as diffuse alveolar damage: A potential source of diagnostic error. Chest 79:420-422, 1981.

105. Gal AA, Koss MN, Strigle S, et al: *Pneumocystis carinii* infection in the acquired immune deficiency syndrome. Semin Diagn Pathol 6:287-299, 1989.

106. Bedrossian CWM, Mason MR, Gupta PK: Rapid cytologic diagnosis of *Pneumocystis:* A comparison of effective techniques. Semin Diagn Pathol 6:245-261, 1989.

107. Luna MA, Cleary KR: Spectrum of pathologic manifestations of *Pneumocystis carinii* pneumonia in patients with neoplastic diseases. Semin Diagn Pathol 6:262-272, 1989.

108. Sterling RP, Bradley BB, Khalil KG, et al: Comparison of biopsy-proven *Pneumocystis carinii* pneumonia in acquired immune deficiency syndrome patients and renal allograft recipients. Ann Thorac Surg 38:494-499, 1984.

109. Limper AH, Offord KP, Smith TF, et al: Differences in lung parasite number and inflammation in patients with and without AIDS. Am Rev Respir Dis 140:1204-1209, 1989.

110. Shelhamer JH, Ognibene FP, Macher AM, et al: Persistence of *Pneumocystis carinii* in lung tissue of acquired immunodeficiency syndrome patients treated for *Pneumocystis* pneumonia. Am Rev Respir Dis 130:1161-1165, 1984.

111. DeLorenzo LJ, Maguire GP, Wormser GP, et al: Persistence of *Pneumocystis carinii* pneumonia in the acquired immunodeficiency syndrome: Evaluation of therapy by follow-up transbronchial lung biopsy. Chest 88:79-83, 1985.

112. Welch K, Finkbeiner W, Alpers CE, et al: Autopsy findings in the acquired immune deficiency syndrome. JAMA 252:1152-1159, 1984.

113. Marchevsky A, Rosen MJ, Chrystal G, et al: Pulmonary complications of the acquired immunodeficiency syndrome: A clinicopathologic study of 70 cases. Hum Pathol 16:659-670, 1985.

114. Saldana MJ, Mones JM, Martinez GR: The pathology of treated *Pneumocystis carinii* pneumonia. Semin Diagn Pathol 6:300-312, 1989.

115. Niedt GW, Schinella RA: Acquired immunodeficiency syndrome: Clinicopathologic study of 56 autopsies. Arch Pathol Lab Med 109:727-734, 1985.

116. Saldana MJ, Mones JM: Cavitation and other atypical manifestations of *Pneumocystis carinii* pneumonia. Semin Diagn Pathol 6:273-286, 1989.

117. Hartz JW, Geisinger KR, Scharyj M, et al: Granulomatous pneumocystosis presenting as a solitary pulmonary nodule. Arch Pathol Lab Med 109:466-469, 1985.

118. Bier S, Halton K, Krivisky B, et al: *Pneumocystis carinii* pneumonia presenting as a single pulmonary nodule. Pediatr Radiol 16:59-60, 1986.

119. Case records of the Massachusetts General Hospital (case 9-1989). N Engl J Med 320:582-587, 1989.

120. Lobenthal SW, Hajdu SI, Urmacher C: Cytologic findings in homosexual males with acquired immunodeficiency. Acta Cytol 27:597-604, 1983.

121. Rorat E, Garcia RL, Skolom J: Diagnosis of *Pneumocystis carinii* pneumonia by cytologic examination of bronchial washings. JAMA 254:1950-1951, 1985.

122. Greaves T, Strigle SM: The recognition of *Pneumocystis carinii* in routine Papanicolaou-stained smears. Acta Cytol 29:714-720, 1985.

123. Flint A, Beckwith AL, Naylor B: *Pneumocystis carinii* pneumonia: Cytologic manifestations and rapid diagnosis in routinely prepared Papanicolaou-stained preparations. Am J Med 81:1009-1011, 1986.

124. Stanley MW, Henry MJ, Iber C: Foamy alveolar casts: Diagnostic specificity for *Pneumocystis carinii* pneumonia in bronchoalveolar lavage fluid cytology. Diagn Cytopathol 4:112-115, 1988.

125. Walzer PD: Experimental models of *Pneumocystis carinii* infections. In Young LS (ed): *Pneumocystis carinii* Pneumonia. New York, Marcel Dekker, 1984.

126. Rosen PP, Martini N, Armstrong D: *Pneumocystis carinii* pneumonia: Diagnosis by lung biopsy. Am J Med 58:794-802, 1975.

127. Campbell WG: Ultrastructure of *Pneumocystis* in human lung: Life cycle in human pneumocystosis. Arch Pathol 93:312-324, 1972.

128. Hasleton PS, Curry A, Rankin EM: *Pneumocystis carinii* pneumonia: A light microscopical and ultrastructural study. J Clin Pathol 34:1138-1146, 1981.

129. Bedrossian CWM: Ultrastructure of *Pneumocystis carinii:* A review of internal and surface characteristics. Semin Diagn Pathol 6:212-237, 1989.

130. Michaelis LL, Leight GS Jr, Powell RD Jr, et al: *Pneumocystis carinii* pneumonia: The importance of early open lung biopsy. Ann Surg 183:301-306, 1976.

131. Grocott RG: A stain for fungi in tissue sections and smears using Gomori's methenamine-silver nitrate technic. Am J Clin Pathol 25:975-979, 1955.

132. Mahan CT, Sale GE: Rapid methenamine silver stain for *Pneumocystis* and fungi. Arch Pathol Lab Med 102:351-352, 1978.

133. Noble L: A simplified and reliable technique for the demonstration of *Pneumocystis carinii* in cytoprep smears. Histo-Logic 20:137-139, 1990.

134. Young RC, Bennet JE, Chu EW: Organisms mimicking *Pneumocystis carinii* [letter]. Lancet 2:1082-1083, 1976.

135. Reinhardt DJ, Kaplan W, Chandler FW: Morpho-

logic resemblance of zygomycete spores to *Pneumocystis carinii* cysts in tissue. Am Rev Respir Dis 115:170-172, 1977.

136. Schwarz J: Pathology of histoplasmosis. Pathol Annu 3:335-366, 1968.

137. Mark EJ: Lung biopsy interpretation. Baltimore, Williams & Wilkins, 1984, pp 37-40.

138. Dutz W, Burke BA: Cytologic diagnosis of *Pneumocystis carinii*. Natl Cancer Inst Monogr 43: 157-161, 1976.

139. Pintozzi RL, Blecka LJ, Nanos S: Morphologic identification of *Pneumocystis carinii*. Acta Cytol 23:35-39, 1979.

140. Blumenfeld W, Griffiss JM: *Pneumocystis carinii* in sputum: Comparable efficacy of screening stains and determination of cyst density. Arch Pathol Lab Med 112:816-820, 1988.

141. Ghali VS, Garcia RI, Skolom J: Fluorescence of *Pneumocystis carinii* in Papanicolaou stained smears. Hum Pathol 15:907-909, 1984.

142. Guarner J, Robey SS, Gupta PK: Cytologic detection of *Pneumocystis carinii*: A comparison of Papanicolaou and other histochemical stains. Diagn Cytopathol 2:133-137, 1986.

143. Gonzales MF, Brown RW, Bhathal PS: Fluorescence of fungi—not autofluorescence [letter]. Am J Clin Pathol 81:142, 1984.

144. Baselski VS, Robison MK, Pifer LW, et al: Rapid detection of *Pneumocystis carinii* in bronchoalveolar lavage samples by using Cellufluor staining. J Clin Microbiol 28:393-394, 1990.

145. Ng VL, Yajko DM, McPhaul LW, et al: Evaluation of an indirect fluorescent-antibody stain for detection of *Pneumocystis carinii* in respiratory specimens. J Clin Microbiol 28: 975-979, 1990.

146. Wolfson JS, Waldron MA, Luz SS: Blinded comparison of a direct immunofluorescent monoclonal antibody staining method and a Giemsa staining method for identification of *Pneumocystis carinii* in induced sputum and bronchoalveolar lavage specimens of patients infected with human immunodeficiency virus. J Clin Microbiol 28: 2136-2138, 1990.

147. Blumenfeld W, Kovacs JA: Use of a monoclonal antibody to detect *Pneumocystis carinii* in induced sputum and bronchoalveolar lavage fluid by immunoperoxidase staining. Arch Pathol Lab Med 112:1233-1236, 1988.

148. Radio SJ, Hansen S, Goldsmith J, et al: Immunohistochemistry of *Pneumocystis carinii* infection. Mod Pathol 3:462-468, 1990.

149. Tanabe K, Fuchimoto M, Egawa K, et al: Use of *Pneumocystis carinii* genomic DNA clones for DNA hybridization analysis of infected human lungs. J Infect Dis 157:593-596, 1988.

150. Mintz L, Drew WL, Miner RC, et al: Cytomegalovirus infections in homosexual men: An epidemiologic study. Ann Intern Med 99:326-329, 1983.

151. Jacobson MA, Mills J: Cytomegalovirus infection. Clin Chest Med 9:443-448, 1988.

152. Hui AN, Koss MN, Meyer PR: Necropsy findings in acquired immunodeficiency syndrome: A comparison of premortem diagnoses with postmortem findings. Hum Pathol 15:670-676, 1984.

153. Guarda LA, Luna MA, Smith JL, et al: Acquired immune deficiency syndrome: Postmortem findings. Am J Clin Pathol 81:549-557, 1984.

154. Reichert CM, Kelly VL, Macher AM: Pathologic features of AIDS. In DeVita VT Jr, Hellman S,

Rosenberg SA (eds): AIDS: Etiology, Diagnosis, Treatment and Prevention. Philadelphia, Lippincott, 1985.

155. Gold JWM: Clinical spectrum of infections in patients with HTLV-111-associated diseases. Cancer Res 45(suppl):4652s-4654s, 1985.

156. Macher AM, Reichert CM, Straus SE, et al: Death in the AIDS patient: Role of cytomegalovirus [letter]. N Engl J Med 309:1454, 1983.

157. Klatt EC, Shibata D: Cytomegalovirus infection in the acquired immunodeficiency syndrome. Arch Pathol Lab Med 112:540-544, 1988.

158. Wallace JM: Pulmonary infection in human immunodeficiency disease: Viral pulmonary infections. Semin Respir Infect 4:147-154, 1989.

159. Smith CB: Cytomegalovirus pneumonia: State of the art. Chest 95:182S-187S, 1989.

160. Beschorner WE, Hutchins GM, Burns WH, et al: Cytomegalovirus pneumonia in bone marrow transplant recipients: Miliary and diffuse patterns. Am Rev Respir Dis 122:107-114, 1980.

161. Craighead JE: Pulmonary cytomegalovirus infection in the adult. Am J Pathol 63:487-500, 1971.

162. Wallace JM, Hannah J: Cytomegalovirus pneumonitis in patients with AIDS: Findings in an autopsy series. Chest 92:198-203, 1987.

163. Lurie HI, Duma RJ: Opportunistic infections of the lungs. Hum Pathol 1:233, 1970.

164. Craighead JE: Cytomegalovirus pulmonary disease. Pathobiol Annu 5:197-220, 1975.

165. Shanley JD, Jordan MC: Viral pneumonia in the immunocompromised patient. Semin Respir Infect 1:193-201, 1986.

166. Hackman RC, Myerson D, Meyers JD, et al: Rapid diagnosis of cytomegaloviral pneumonia by tissue immunofluorescence with a murine monoclonal antibody. J Infect Dis 151:325-329, 1985.

167. Myerson D, Hackman RC, Meyers JD: Diagnosis of cytomegaloviral pneumonia by in situ hybridization. J Infect Dis 150:272-277, 1984.

168. Marder MZ, Barr CE, Mandel ID: Cytomegalovirus presence and salivary composition in acquired immunodeficiency syndrome. Oral Surg Oral Med Oral Pathol 60:372-376, 1985.

169. Cockerill FR: Diagnosing cytomegalovirus infection. Mayo Clin Proc 60:636-638, 1985.

170. Hilborne LH, Nieberg RK, Cheng L, et al: Direct in situ hybridization for rapid detection of cytomegalovirus in bronchoalveolar lavage. Am J Clin Pathol 87:766-769, 1987.

171. Paradis IL, Grgurich WF, Dummer JS, et al: Rapid detection of cytomegalovirus pneumonia from lung lavage cells. Am Rev Respir Dis 138: 697-702, 1988.

172. Emanuel D, Peppard J, Stover D, et al: Rapid immunodiagnosis of cytomegalovirus pneumonia by bronchoalveolar lavage using human and murine monoclonal antibodies. Ann Intern Med 104:476-481, 1986.

173. Miles PR, Baughman RP, Linnemann CC Jr: Cytomegalovirus in the bronchoalveolar lavage fluid of patients with AIDS. Chest 97:1072-1076, 1990.

174. Millar AB, Patou G, Miller RF, et al: Cytomegalovirus in the lungs of patients with AIDS: Respiratory pathogen or passenger? Am Rev Respir Dis 141:1474-1477, 1990.

175. Masur H, Lane HC, Palestine A, et al: Effect of 9-(1,3-dihydroxy-2-propoxymethyl) guanine on serious cytomegalovirus disease in eight immu-

nosuppressed homosexual men. Ann Intern Med 104:41-44, 1986.

176. Myerowitz RL: The pathology of opportunistic infections. New York, Raven Press, 1983.

177. Nash G, Foley FD: Herpetic infection of the middle and lower respiratory tract. Am J Clin Pathol 54:857-863, 1970.

178. Nash G: Necrotizing tracheobronchitis and bronchopneumonia consistent with herpetic infection. Hum Pathol 3:283-291, 1972.

179. Ramsey PG, Fife KH, Hackman RC, et al: Herpes simplex virus pneumonia: Clinical, virologic and pathologic features in 20 patients. Ann Intern Med 97:813-820, 1982.

180. Corey L, Spear PG: Infections with herpes simplex viruses. N Engl J Med 314:686-691, 749-757, 1986.

181. Graham BS, Snell JD Jr: Herpes simplex virus infection of the adult lower respiratory tract. Medicine 62:384-393, 1983.

182. Feiden W, Borchard F, Burrig KF, et al: Herpes oesophagitis: Light microscopical and immunohistochemical investigations. Virchows Arch [A] 404:167-176, 1984.

183. Kapur S, Patterson K, Chandra R: Detection of herpes simplex infection in cytologic smears. Arch Pathol Lab Med 109:464-465, 1985.

184. Bedrossian CWM, DeArce EAL, Bedrossian UK, et al: Herpetic tracheobronchitis detected at bronchoscopy: Cytologic diagnosis by the immunoperoxidase method. Diagn Cytopathol 1:292-299, 1985.

185. Cohen PR, Beltrani VP, Grossman ME: Disseminated herpes zoster in patients with human immunodeficiency virus infection. Am J Med 84:1076-1080, 1988.

186. Miller GPG: The immunology of cryptococcal disease. Semin Respir Infect 1:45-52, 1986.

187. Cairns MR, Durack DT: Fungal pneumonia in the immunocompromised host. Semin Respir Infect 1:166-185, 1986.

188. Fels AOS: Bacterial and fungal pneumonias. Clin Chest Med 9:449-457, 1988.

189. Bottone EJ, Toma M, Johansson BE, et al: Poorly encapsulated *Cryptococcus neoformans* from patients with AIDS. I. Preliminary observations. AIDS Res 2:211-218, 1986.

190. Gal AA, Koss MN, Hawkins J, et al: The pathology of pulmonary cryptococcal infections in the acquired immunodeficiency syndrome. Arch Pathol Lab Med 110:502-507, 1986.

191. Farmer SG, Komorowski RA: Histologic response to capsule-deficient *Cryptococcus neoformans*. Arch Pathol 96:383-387, 1973.

192. Kozel TR, Cazin J Jr: Nonencapsulated variant of *Cryptococcus neoformans*. Infect Immun 3:287-294, 1971.

193. McDonnell JM, Hutchins GM: Pulmonary cryptococcosis. Hum Pathol 16:121-128, 1985.

194. Watts JC, Chandler FW: Infection by capsule-deficient cryptococci [letter]. Arch Pathol Lab Med 111:688, 1987.

195. Shaw CE, Kapica L: Production of diagnostic pigment by phenoloxidase activity of *Cryptococcus neoformans*. Appl Microbiol 24:824-830, 1972.

196. Kwon-Chung KJ, Hill WB, Bennett JE: New special stain for histopathological diagnosis of cryptococcosis. J Clin Microbiol 13:383-387, 1981.

197. Ro JY, Lee SS, Ayala AG: Advantage of Fontana-Masson stain in capsule-deficient cryptococ-

cal infection. Arch Pathol Lab Med 111:53-57, 1987.

198. Johnson PC, Hamill RJ, Sarosi GA: Clinical review: Progressive disseminated histoplasmosis in the AIDS patient. Semin Respir Infect 4:139-146, 1989.

199. Wheat LJ, Slama TG, Zeckel ML: Histoplasmosis in the acquired immune deficiency syndrome. Am J Med 78:203-210, 1985.

200. Graham AR, Sobonya RE, Bronnimann DA, et al: Quantitative pathology of coccidioidomycosis in acquired immunodeficiency syndrome. Hum Pathol 19:800-806, 1988.

201. Prichard JG, Sorotzkin RA, James RE III: Cutaneous manifestations of disseminated coccidioidomycosis in the acquired immunodeficiency syndrome. Cutis 39:203-205, 1987.

202. Miller-Catchpole R, Variakojis D, Anastasi J, et al: The Chicago AIDS autopsy study: Opportunistic infections, neoplasms, and findings from selected organ systems with a comparison to national data. Mod Pathol 2:277-294, 1989.

203. Pervez NK, Kleinerman J, Kattan M, et al: Pseudomembranous necrotizing bronchial aspergillosis: A variant of invasive aspergillosis in a patient with hemophilia and acquired immune deficiency syndrome. Am Rev Respir Dis 131:961-963, 1985.

204. Horsburgh CR Jr, Mason UG, Farhi DC, Iseman MD: Disseminated infection with *Mycobacterium avium-intracellulare*. Medicine 64:36-48, 1985.

205. MacDonell KB, Glassroth J: *Mycobacterium avium* complex and other nontuberculous mycobacteria in patients with HIV infection. Semin Respir Infect 4:123-132, 1989.

206. Armstrong D, Gold JWM, Dryjanski J, et al: Treatment of infection in patients with acquired immune deficiency syndrome. Ann Intern Med 103:738-743, 1985.

207. Horsburgh CR Jr, Selik RM: The epidemiology of disseminated nontuberculous mycobacterial infection in the acquired immune deficiency syndrome (AIDS). Am Rev Respir Dis 139:4-7, 1989.

208. Wolinsky E: Nontuberculous mycobacteria and associated diseases. Am Rev Respir Dis 119:107-159, 1979.

209. Hawkins CC, Gold JWM, Whimbey E, et al: *Mycobacterium avium* complex infections in patients with the acquired immune deficiency syndrome. Ann Intern Med 105:184-188, 1986.

210. Farhi DC, Mason UG, Horsburgh CR Jr: Pathologic findings in disseminated *Mycobacterium avium-intracellulare* infection. Am J Clin Pathol 85:67-72, 1986.

211. Klatt EC, Jensen DF, Meyer PR: Pathology of *Mycobacterium avium-intracellulare* infection in acquired immunodeficiency syndrome. Hum Pathol 18:709-714, 1987.

212. Sohn CC, Schroff RW, Kliewer KE, et al: Disseminated *Mycobacterium avium-intracellulare* infection in homosexual men with acquired cell-mediated immunodeficiency: A histologic and immunologic study of two cases. Am J Clin Pathol 79:247-252, 1983.

213. Solis OG, Belmonte AH, Ramaswamy G, et al: Pseudogaucher cells in *Mycobacterium avium intracellulare* infections in acquired immune deficiency syndrome (AIDS). Am J Clin Pathol 85:233-235, 1986.

214. Rieder HL, Snider DE: Tuberculosis and the acquired immunodeficiency syndrome. Chest 90: 469-470, 1986.

215. Hopewell PC: Tuberculosis and human immunodeficiency virus infection. Semin Respir Infect 4:111-122, 1989.

216. Centers for Disease Control: Tuberculosis, final data—United States, 1986. MMWR 36:817-820, 1988.

217. Pitchenik AE, Fertel D, Bloch AB: Mycobacterial disease: Epidemiology, diagnosis, treatment and prevention. In White DA, Stover DE (eds): Pulmonary effects of AIDS. Clin Chest Med 9:425-441, 1988.

218. Handwerger S, Mildvan D, Senie R, et al: Tuberculosis and the acquired immunodeficiency syndrome at a New York City hospital: 1978-1985. Chest 91:176-180, 1987.

219. Pitchenik AE, Rubinson HA: The radiographic appearance of tuberculosis in patients with the acquired immune deficiency syndrome (AIDS) and pre-AIDS. Am Rev Respir Dis 131:393-396, 1985.

220. Sunderam G, McDonald RJ, Maniatis T, et al: Tuberculosis as a manifestation of the acquired immunodeficiency syndrome (AIDS). JAMA 256: 362-366, 1986.

221. Goedert JJ, Biggar RJ, Melbye M, et al: Effect of T4 count and cofactors on the incidence of AIDS in homosexual men infected with human immunodeficiency virus. JAMA 257: 331-334, 1987.

222. Nichols L, Balogh K, Silverman M: Bacterial infection in the acquired immune deficiency syndrome: Clinicopathologic correlations in a series of autopsy cases. Am J Clin Pathol 92:787-790, 1989.

223. Polsky B, Gold JWM, Whimbey E, et al: Bacterial pneumonia in patients with the acquired immunodeficiency syndrome. Ann Intern Med 104: 38-41, 1986.

224. Witt D, Craven DE, McCabe WR: Bacterial infections in adult patients with the acquired immune deficiency syndrome (AIDS) and AIDS-related complex. Am J Med 82:900-906, 1987.

225. Tschirhart D, Klatt EC: Disseminated toxoplasmosis in the acquired immunodeficiency syndrome. Arch Pathol Lab Med 112:1237-1241, 1988.

226. Catterall JR, Hofflin JM, Remington JS: Pulmonary toxoplasmosis. Am Rev Respir Dis 133: 704-705, 1986.

227. Mendelson MH, Finkel LJ, Meyers BR, et al: Pulmonary toxoplasmosis in AIDS. Scand J Infect Dis 19:703-706, 1987.

228. Tawney S, Masci J, Berger HW, et al: Pulmonary toxoplasmosis: An unusual nodular radiographic pattern in a patient with AIDS. Mt Sinai J Med 53:683-685, 1986.

229. Brady EM, Margolis ML, Korzeniowski OM: Pulmonary cryptosporidiosis in acquired immunodeficiency syndrome. JAMA 252:89-90, 1984.

230. Forgacs P, Tarshis A, Ma P, et al: Intestinal and bronchial cryptosporidiosis in an immunodeficient homosexual man. Ann Intern Med 99: 793-794, 1983.

231. Ma P, Villanueva TG, Kaufman D, et al: Respiratory cryptosporidiosis in the acquired immunodeficiency syndrome: Use of modified cold Kinyoun and Hemacolor stains for rapid diagnosis. JAMA 252:1298-1301, 1984.

232. Katzenstein AA, Bloor CM, Liebow AA: Diffuse alveolar damage: The role of oxygen, shock and related factors. Am J Pathol 85:209-228, 1976.

233. Pratt PC: Pathology of adult respiratory distress syndrome. In Thurlbeck WM, Abel MR (eds): The lung: Structure, function and disease. Baltimore, Williams & Wilkins, 1978.

234. Nash G, Blennerhassett JB, Pontoppidan H: Pulmonary lesions associated with oxygen therapy and artificial ventilation. N Engl J Med 276: 368-374, 1967.

235. Bachofen M, Weibel ER: Alterations of the gas exchange apparatus in adult respiratory insufficiency associated with septicemia. Am Rev Respir Dis 116:589-615, 1977.

236. Orell SR: Lung pathology in respiratory distress following shock in the adult. Acta Pathol Microbiol Scand [A] 79:65-76, 1971.

237. Bachofen M, Weibel ER: Structural alterations of lung parenchyma in the adult respiratory distress syndrome. Clin Chest Med 3:35-56, 1982.

238. Gould VE, Tosco R, Wheelis RF, et al: Oxygen pneumonitis in man: Ultrastructural observations on the development of alveolar lesions. Lab Invest 26:499-508, 1972.

239. Adamson IYR, Bowden DH: The type 2 cell as progenitor of alveolar epithelial regeneration: A cytodynamic study in mice after exposure to oxygen. Lab Invest 30:35-42, 1974.

240. Nash G, Foley FD, Langlinais PC: Pulmonary interstitial edema and hyaline membranes in adult burn patients: Electron microscopic observations. Hum Pathol 5:149-160, 1974.

241. Kapanci Y, Weibel ER, Kaplan HP, et al: Pathogenesis and reversibility of the pulmonary lesions of oxygen toxicity in monkeys. II. Ultrastructural and morphometric studies. Lab Invest 20:101-118, 1969.

242. Evans MJ, Cabral LJ, Stephens RJ, et al: Renewal of alveolar epithelium in the rat following exposure to NO$_2$. Am J Pathol 70:175-198, 1973.

243. Hallgren R, Samuelsson T, Laurent TC, et al: Accumulation of hyaluronan (hyaluronic acid) in the lung in adult respiratory distress syndrome. Am Rev Respir Dis 139:682-687, 1989.

244. Nettelbladt O, Bergh J, Schenholm M, et al: Accumulation of hyaluronic acid in the alveolar interstitial tissue in bleomycin-induced alveolitis. Am Rev Respir Dis 139:759-762, 1989.

245. Mitchell J, Woodcock-Mitchell J, Reynolds S, et al: α-Smooth muscle actin in parenchymal cells of bleomycin-injured rat lung. Lab Invest 60:643-650, 1989.

246. Adler KB, Low RB, Leslie KO, et al: Biology of disease: Contractile cells in normal and fibrotic lung. Lab Invest 60:473-485, 1989.

247. Katzenstein AA: Pathogenesis of "fibrosis" in interstitial pneumonia: An electron microscopic study. Hum Pathol 16:1015-1024, 1985.

248. Burkhardt A: Alveolitis and collapse in the pathogenesis of pulmonary fibrosis. Am Rev Respir Dis 140:513-524, 1989.

249. Basset F, Ferrans VJ, Soler P, et al: Intraluminal fibrosis in interstitial lung disorders. Am J Pathol 122:443-461, 1986.

250. Kuhn C III, Boldt J, King TE Jr, et al: An immunohistochemical study of architectural remodeling and connective tissue synthesis in pulmonary fibrosis. Am Rev Respir Dis 140:1693-1703, 1989.

251. Wallace JM, Hannah JB: Pulmonary disease at autopsy in patients with the acquired immunodeficiency syndrome. West J Med 149:167-171, 1988.

252. Ramaswamy G, Jagadha V, Tchertkoff V: Diffuse alveolar damage and interstitial fibrosis in acquired immunodeficiency syndrome patients without concurrent pulmonary infection. Arch Pathol Lab Med 109:408-412, 1985.

253. Katzenstein AA, Myers JL, Mazur MT: Acute interstitial pneumonia: A clinicopathologic, ultrastructural, and cell kinetic study. Am J Surg Pathol 10:256-267, 1986.

254. Wachter RM, Luce JM: Intensive care for patients with *Pneumocystis carinii* pneumonia and respiratory failure: Are we prepared for our new success? Chest 96:714-715, 1989.

255. Lamy M, Fallat RJ, Koeniger E, et al: Pathologic features and mechanisms of hypoxemia in adult respiratory distress syndrome. Am Rev Respir Dis 114:267-284, 1976.

256. Barrio JL, Harcup C, Baier HJ, Pitchenik AE: Value of repeat fiberoptic bronchoscopies and significance of nondiagnostic bronchoscopic results in patients with the acquired immunodeficiency syndrome. Am Rev Respir Dis 135:422-425, 1987.

257. Ognibene FP, Masur H, Rogers P, et al: Nonspecific interstitial pneumonitis without evidence of *Pneumocystis carinii* in asymptomatic patients infected with human immunodeficiency virus (HIV). Ann Intern Med 109:874-879, 1988.

258. Autran B, Mayaud CM, Raphael M, et al: Evidence for a cytotoxic T-lymphocyte alveolitis in human immunodeficiency virus–infected patients. AIDS 2:179-183, 1988.

259. Agostini C, Poletti V, Zambello R, et al: Phenotypical and functional analysis of bronchoalveolar lavage lymphocytes in patients with HIV infection. Am Rev Respir Dis 138:1609-1615, 1988.

260. Wallace JM, Barbers RG, Oishi JS, Prince H: Cellular and T-lymphocyte subpopulation profiles in bronchoalveolar lavage fluid from patients with acquired immunodeficiency syndrome and pneumonitis. Am Rev Respir Dis 130:786-790, 1984.

261. Young KR Jr, Rankin JA, Naegel GP, et al: Bronchoalveolar lavage cells and proteins in patients with the acquired immunodeficiency syndrome: An immunologic analysis. Ann Intern Med 103:522-533, 1985.

262. Joshi VV: Pathology of acquired immunodeficiency syndrome (AIDS) in children. In Joshi VV (ed): Pathology of AIDS and Other Manifestations of HIV Infection. Igaku-Shoin, New York, 1990, pp 239-269.

263. Joshi VV, Kauffman S, Oleske JM, et al: Polyclonal polymorphic B-cell lymphoproliferative disorder with prominent pulmonary involvement in children with acquired immune deficiency syndrome. Cancer 59:1455-1462, 1987.

264. Liebow AA: New concepts and entities in pulmonary disease. In Liebow AA, Smith DE (eds): The Lung. Baltimore, Williams & Wilkins, 1968, pp 332-365.

265. Liebow AA, Carrington CB: Diffuse pulmonary lymphoreticular infiltrations associated with dysproteinemia. Med Clin North Am 57:809-843, 1973.

266. O'Brodovich HM, Moser MM, Lu L: Familial lymphoid interstitial pneumonia: A long-term follow-up. Pediatrics 65:523-528, 1980.

267. Vath RR, Alexander CB, Fulmer JD: The lymphocytic infiltrative lung diseases. Clin Chest Med 3:619-634, 1982.

268. Kradin RL, Young RH, Kradin LA, et al: Immunoblastic lymphoma arising in chronic lymphoid hyperplasia of the pulmonary interstitium. Cancer 50:1339-1343, 1982.

269. Oleske J, Minnefor A, Cooper R Jr, et al: Immune deficiency syndrome in children. JAMA 249:2345-2349, 1983.

270. Scott GB, Buck BE, Leterman JG, et al: Acquired immunodeficiency syndrome in infants. N Engl J Med 310:76-81, 1984.

271. Joshi VV, Oleske JM, Minnefor AB, et al: Pathologic pulmonary findings in children with the acquired immunodeficiency syndrome: A study of ten cases. Hum Pathol 16:241-246, 1985.

272. Centers for Disease Control: Revision of the CDC surveillance case definition for acquired immunodeficiency syndrome. MMWR 36(suppl):3S-15S, 1987.

273. Solal-Celigny P, Couderc LJ, Herman D, et al: Lymphoid interstitial pneumonitis in acquired immunodeficiency syndrome–related complex. Am Rev Respir Dis 131:956-960, 1985.

274. Grieco MH, Chinoy-Acharya P: Lymphocytic interstitial pneumonia associated with the acquired immune deficiency syndrome. Am Rev Respir Dis 131:952-955, 1985.

275. Saldana MJ, Mones J, Buck BE: Lymphoid interstitial pneumonia in Haitian residents of Florida [abstract]. Chest 84:347, 1983.

276. Fackler JC, Nagel JE, Adler WH, et al: Epstein-Barr virus infection in a child with acquired immunodeficiency syndrome. Am J Dis Child 139:1000-1004, 1985.

277. Rubinstein A, Morecki R, Goldman H: Pulmonary disease in infants and children. In White DA, Stover DE (eds): Pulmonary effects of AIDS. Clin Chest Med 9:507-517, 1988.

278. Joshi VV, Oleske JM: Pulmonary lesions in children with the acquired immunodeficiency syndrome: A reappraisal based on data in additional cases and follow-up study of previously reported cases [letter]. Hum Pathol 17:641-642, 1986.

279. Rubinstein A, Morecki R, Silverman B, et al: Pulmonary disease in children with acquired immune deficiency syndrome and AIDS-related complex. J Pediatr 108:498-503, 1986.

280. White DA, Matthay FA: Noninfectious pulmonary complications of infection with the human immunodeficiency virus. Am Rev Respir Dis 140:1763-1787, 1989.

281. Andiman WA, Martin K, Rubinstein A, et al: Opportunistic lymphoproliferations associated with Epstein-Barr viral DNA in infants and children with AIDS. Lancet 2:1390-1393, 1985.

282. Montagnier L, Gruest J, Chamaret S, et al: Adaptation of lymphadenopathy associated virus (LAV) to replication in EBV-transformed B lymphoblastoid cell lines. Science 225:63-66, 1984.

283. Israel RH, Magnussen CR: Are AIDS patients at risk for pulmonary alveolar proteinosis? Chest 96:641-642, 1989.

284. Ognibene FP, Shelhamer JH: Kaposi's sarcoma. Clin Chest Med 9:459-465, 1988.

285. Meduri GU, Stover DE, Lee M, et al: Pulmonary Kaposi's sarcoma in the acquired immune defi-

ciency syndrome: Clinical, radiographic and pathologic manifestations. Am J Med 81:11-18, 1986.

286. Nash G, Fligiel S: Kaposi's sarcoma presenting as pulmonary disease in the acquired immunodeficiency syndrome: Diagnosis by lung biopsy. Hum Pathol 15:999-1001, 1984.

287. Fouret PJ, Touboul JL, Mayaud CM, et al: Pulmonary Kaposi's sarcoma in patients with acquired immune deficiency syndrome: A clinicopathological study. Thorax 42:262-268, 1987.

288. Purdy LJ, Colby TV, Yousem SA, Battifora H: Pulmonary Kaposi's sarcoma: Premortem histologic diagnosis. Am J Surg Pathol 10:301-311, 1986.

289. Sivit CJ, Schwartz AM, Rockoff SD: Kaposi's sarcoma of the lung in AIDS: Radiologic-pathologic analysis. Am J Radiol 148:25-28, 1987.

290. Moskowitz LB, Hensley GT, Gould EW, et al: Frequency and anatomic distribution of lymphadenopathic Kaposi's sarcoma in the acquired immunodeficiency syndrome: An autopsy series. Hum Pathol 16:447-456, 1985.

291. Gottlieb GJ, Ackerman AB: Kaposi's sarcoma: An extensively disseminated form in young homosexual men. Hum Pathol 13:882-892, 1982.

292. Garay SM, Belenko M, Fazzini E, Schinella R: Pulmonary manifestations of Kaposi's sarcoma. Chest 91:39-43, 1987.

293. Hanson PJV, Harcourt-Webster JN, Gazzard BG, Collins JV: Fibreoptic bronchoscopy in diagnosis of bronchopulmonary Kaposi's sarcoma. Thorax 42:269-271, 1987.

294. Hamm PG, Judson MA, Aranda CP: Diagnosis of pulmonary Kaposi's sarcoma with fiberoptic bronchoscopy and endobronchial biopsy: A report of five cases. Cancer 59:807-810, 1987.

295. Pitchenik AE, Fischl MA, Saldana MJ: Kaposi's sarcoma of the tracheobronchial tree: Clinical, bronchoscopic, and pathologic features. Chest 87:122-124, 1985.

296. Zibrak JD, Silvestri RC, Costello P, et al: Bronchoscopic and radiologic features of Kaposi's sarcoma involving the respiratory system. Chest 90:476-479, 1986.

297. Loureiro C, Gill PS, Meyer PR, et al: Autopsy findings in AIDS-related lymphoma. Cancer 62:735-739, 1988.

298. Moser RJ III, Tenholder MF, Ridenour R: Oat-cell-carcinoma in transfusion-associated acquired immunodeficiency syndrome [letter]. Ann Intern Med 103:478, 1985.

299. Nusbaum NJ: Metastatic small-cell carcinoma of the lung in a patient with AIDS [letter]. N Engl J Med 312:1706, 1985.

300. Weitberg AB, Mayer K, Miller ME, et al: Dysplastic carcinoid tumor and AIDS-related complex [letter]. N Engl J Med 314:1455, 1986.

9

GASTROINTESTINAL AND HEPATOBILIARY DISEASE

SHIRIN NASH

The gastrointestinal tract is a major target and site of entry for HIV. The presence of viral proteins has been documented by many studies demonstrating viral antigen in CD4 + T-lymphocytes in the lamina propria of the intestinal mucosa.[1-3] The possibility that HIV directly infects intestinal epithelial cells is supported by experiments in which human colorectal carcinoma cell lines are the only non-lymphoid cells that allow persistent infection and growth of HIV in a culture system.[4,5] However, no good evidence has shown that intestinal epithelium in vivo or in an experimental animal model can be infected by HIV.[2,6,7]

Primary HIV infection may be accompanied by gastrointestinal symptoms, such as diarrhea, nausea, and abdominal pain, associated with an acute mononucleosis syndrome[2,3] and occasionally odynophagia.[8] Recent studies indicate that these early symptoms may result from an HIV-induced enteropathy with minimal to mild inflammatory and atrophic changes in the small intestinal mucosa accompanied by a decrease in mucosal enzymes.[2,3,9,10] HIV may also be responsible for acute esophageal ulcers at the time of seroconversion. Retroviral-like particles have been identified by ultrastructural examination in esophageal ulcers in a group of homosexual men who had painful swallowing at the time of acute HIV infection.[8]

Venereally transmitted gastrointestinal infections are well recognized in homosexual men, and the spectrum of enteritis, colitis, and proctitis in this population has been referred to as the "gay bowel syndrome."[10,11] A study before the AIDS epidemic identified enteric pathogens in 80% of symptomatic and 39% of asymptomatic homosexual men.[11] *Neisseria gonorrhoeae*, herpes simplex virus (HSV), *Chlamydia trachomatis* (non–lymphogranuloma venereum serotypes), and *Treponema pallidum* were associated with proctitis. Most cases of colitis were associated with *Campylobacter, Shigella,* and *Entamoeba histolytica,* and enteritis was significantly associated with *Giardia lamblia*.[11] A more recent study of homosexual men with AIDS has shown that enteric disease in these patients is related to a different group of pathogens, most commonly cytomegalovirus (CMV), HSV, and *Cryptosporidium*.[12]

The gastrointestinal tract in AIDS patients reflects the immunologic deficits caused by HIV in peripheral blood and lymph nodes. Total numbers of T-lymphocytes in the small intestinal mucosa are significantly decreased in patients with AIDS and AIDS-related complex (ARC).[13] This decrease involves predominantly CD4 + T-lymphocytes, reversing the normal mucosal helper/suppressor T-lymphocyte ratios in the small intestine[13] and rectum.[14] The T-lymphocytes observed in the intestinal epithelium and lamina propria of patients with AIDS and ARC do not express the receptor for interleukin-2.[14] A significant decrease in immunoglobulin A (IgA) containing plasma cells has also been demonstrated in the small intestinal and rectal mucosa of patients with AIDS and ARC.[15] Clearly the opportunistic infections and neoplasms identified in patients with AIDS result directly from these specific deficits in intestinal immunity.

Although not as life threatening as respiratory or central nervous system disorders, gastrointestinal and liver involvement can produce significant symptoms and morbidity in AIDS patients. Intestinal disease has been diagnosed in 50% to 60% of AIDS patients in the United States and up to 100% of patients in Africa and Haiti.[16] The most common early symptoms are dysphagia and odynophagia or a prolonged watery diarrheal syndrome with loss of more than 10% of body weight over 2 to 3 months.[16] The infections and neoplasms discussed in the following paragraphs and outlined in Table 9–1 occur in patients who are immunosuppressed for a variety of reasons, but they have become much more prominent in the past 10 years in AIDS patients. Enteric infections in patients with AIDS may be due to bacteria, viruses, protozoa, parasites, or fungi. The infecting organisms are those generally present in the host's local environment. The disease is modified by behavioral patterns such as homosexuality and ultimately controlled by the components of the host's immune response.[17] Identification of the organism(s) responsible for the symptoms is important, particularly if therapy is available. Gastrointestinal and liver involvement in children with AIDS is similar to that in adults and is not discussed separately.[18]

GASTROINTESTINAL INFECTIONS IN AIDS

Vigorous diagnostic evaluation using multiple modalities has identified an intestinal pathogen in as much as 85% of patients with AIDS and diarrhea[19] suggesting that "AIDS-related enteropathy" probably occurs less often than was previously reported.[20] The majority of gastrointestinal biopsies, however, show only nonspecific inflammation as noted in 52% of biopsies performed at a New York hospital in 1985.[21] CMV was the most common infectious agent identified, especially in colonic biopsies, and *Candida* was the next, identified in 5 of 10 esophageal biopsies.[21] In another study of 22 AIDS patients (18 drug abusers and 4 homosexuals), 96% had weight loss and 55% had diarrhea. Gastrointestinal infections were identified in 45% of patients by microbiologic techniques, but histologic evidence of organisms was present in only

Table 9–1. Gastrointestinal, Hepatobiliary, and Pancreatic Disease in AIDS

Organ	Clinical Features	Pathologic Features	Etiology
Esophagus	Dysphagia/odynophagia/ retrosternal pain	Ulcers/esophagitis	HIV/HSV/CMV/ *Candida* sp.
Stomach	Hemorrhage/ obstruction	Ulcers/masses	Lymphoma/ Kaposi's sarcoma
Intestines	Abdominal pain/ hemorrhage/perforation	Ulcers with vasculitis	CMV
	Malabsorption/large volume watery diarrhea	Enteritis/enteropathy	MAI/Coccidiosis/HIV
Anorectum	Anorectal pain	Ulcers	HSV
Liver	Hepatomegaly/right upper quadrant pain/ jaundice	Acalculous cholecystitis/ sclerosing cholangitis	CMV or cryptosporidial biliary tract disease
	Hepatomegaly/increased alkaline phosphatase	Granulomas	MAI
	Hepatomegaly with increased bilirubin	Neoplasm	Lymphoma
Pancreas	Epigastric pain with increased serum amylase/lipase	Acute pancreatitis	Drugs/infections (CMV)

The most common presenting signs, symptoms, and associated causes are listed in this table. For less frequently seen infections and neoplasms, see text.

HSV, Herpes simplex virus; *CMV,* cytomegalovirus; *MAI,* Mycobacterium avium-intercellulare.

27%.[22] Gastrointestinal biopsies of patients with AIDS can show multiple opportunistic infections and possibly even contribute to the initial diagnosis of the disease (Fig. 9–1).

Cytomegalovirus Infection

The majority of CMV infections in normal adults are asymptomatic, and antibodies to the virus are present in 54% to 81% of people worldwide.[23-25] Gastrointestinal CMV infection in healthy adults is rare, although the virus may be an incidental finding at sites of proliferating granulation tissue in gastrointestinal ulcers.

CMV is the most commonly recognized opportunistic invader responsible for disease in patients immunosuppressed because of malignancy or chemotherapy, recipients of renal or bone marrow transplants, and patients with AIDS. The infection may be due to reactivation of the virus or may be acquired from exogenous sources such as blood transfusions or infected grafts from seropositive donors.[23-26] Serologic evidence of CMV infection is common in the male homosexual population; Drew et al. reported a 94% prevalence rate of positive CMV titers in homosexual men compared with 54% in heterosexual men at a venereal disease clinic.[27] CMV was initially thought to be responsible for the immune deficiency in AIDS patients, and numerous reports have identified it as the most often encountered infectious agent in biopsy and autopsy studies of patients with AIDS.[19,21,28] CMV was identified as the most common pathogen in AIDS patients undergoing emergency surgery in one study,[29] and CMV ileocolitis was the reason for emergency surgical intervention in 64% of patients in another.[30]

CMV infections of the gastrointestinal tract can be manifest as dysphagia, hematemesis, abdominal pain, ileus, diarrhea, melena, and occasionally intestinal pseudoobstruction.[31-36] Patients with AIDS and CMV appear incapacitated by fever, cramping abdominal pain, and copious watery diarrhea with 15 to 20 liquid stools per day.[32] The endoscopic appearances of CMV colitis have been recently described as multiple, submucosal, erythematous, violaceous lesions associated with discrete ulcers 5 mm to 2 cm in diameter.[32]

CMV ulcers may vary from small hemorrhagic erosions to larger more serpiginous ulcers with thicker heaped-up margins. In AIDS patients CMV ulcers occur most commonly in the esophagus and ileocolon and are superficial chronic ulcers or deep ulcers involving the entire muscularis propria and resulting in perforation in some cases.[32-36] CMV is a common cause of esophagitis in patients with

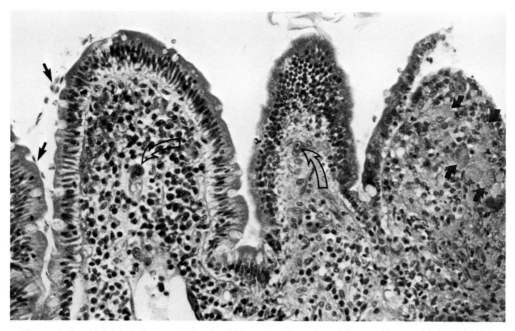

Figure 9–1. Multiple infections in duodenal biopsy specimen from 35-year-old man with AIDS include *Giardia (small arrows)*, cytomegalovirus *(open arrows)*, and foamy histiocytes *(curved arrows)*, which contained numerous bacilli on acid-fast stain (not shown). (Hematoxylin and eosin, × 100.)

AIDS. In one study the virus was identified in 28% of patients with esophageal ulcer or esophagitis resistant to antifungal therapy.[37]

The pathologist diagnoses CMV infection by noting large cells with single amphophilic intranuclear inclusions and multiple small basophilic intracytoplasmic inclusions. Viral inclusions are found most often in macrophages, fibroblasts, and endothelial cells and occasionally in glandular epithelial cells adjacent to ulcers. CMV infection may be identified as a focal active ileocolitis or within endothelial cells associated with fibrin thrombi in small capillaries with ulceration on a local ischemic basis (Fig. 9–2). Immunoperoxidase studies for CMV early antigen can help to identify infection in the absence of definite cytopathic inclusions,[37,38] but DNA in situ hybridization techniques do not appear to contribute to the diagnosis in difficult cases.[38,39] Diagnosing CMV infection has become particularly important with the availability of 9-(1,3-dihydroxy-2-propoxymethyl) guanine (ganciclovir), which produces clinical improvement and at least transient virologic response in some patients.[40]

Candida Infection

Candida species are commonly present as saprophytes in the gastrointestinal tract of healthy adults and have been cultured from 50% of mouth washings and 30% of fecal specimens from healthy individuals.[41] Candidiasis is the most commonly identified fungal infection in immunosuppressed patients. Severe

oral and esophageal candidiasis was originally described as a prominent feature of AIDS by Gottlieb et al.[43] in 1981. *Candida* esophagitis was subsequently included as a diagnostic criterion in the CDC definition of AIDS.

Although candidal infection can occur at multiple sites in the gastrointestinal tract, up to 45% of patients with AIDS have oral and esophageal involvement alone and systemic disease is rare. This lack of systemic disease is possibly related to the presence of intact neutrophil function in patients with AIDS, whereas systemic candidiasis is a major problem in severely neutropenic patients.[17] Symptoms include odynophagia, dysphagia, retrosternal pain, and gastrointestinal bleeding.[44] Double-contrast esophagograms may be useful in the diagnosis of *Candida* esophagitis, showing a ragged mucosal outline, ulcers, filling defects, and hypomotility, especially in cases of moderate to severe disease.[42] Until the recent recognition of *Candida* esophagitis as an important feature of AIDS, the diagnosis was rarely made during life. The most useful diagnostic modality is endoscopy with brushings and washings for smear, culture, and biopsy. Air-dried smears and wet mounts prepared with 10% potassium hydroxide are useful to distinguish the mycelial forms (pathogenic phase) from yeast forms (saprophytic phase), a distinction that cannot be made by culture. One study has shown that in patients with AIDS, oral candidiasis with esophageal symptoms is a marker of esophageal candidiasis, and endoscopy may not be necessary for the diagnosis in this clinical setting.[45]

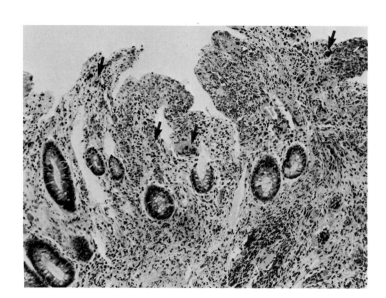

Figure 9–2. Cytomegalovirus (CMV) enteritis in 33-year-old man with AIDS. Ulcer of ileocecal valve is due to CMV vasculitis *(arrows)*. (Hematoxylin and eosin, ×100.)

Endoscopic appearances are characteristic early, with white 2 to 4 mm plaques on erythematous mucosa progressing to ulceration and later to a white pseudomembrane in severe disease.[42] Biopsies may show nonspecific inflammation indistinguishable from ulcers of reflux esophagitis; histologic diagnosis requires the presence of spores as well as hyphae admixed with viable tissues (not merely squamous debris), indicating pathogenic infection. *Candida* esophagitis in AIDS patients may have a prolonged course and be refractory to treatment.[44]

Mycobacterial Infection

The predominant mycobacterial organisms infecting patients with AIDS are the atypical mycobacteria *M. avium* and *M. intracellulare* (MAI), which are commonly found in soil, water, and plants and are carried by birds and farm animals.[46-48] Human infection is uncommon, and the organism has been considered a nonpathogen or occasionally opportunistic in humans.[48] The infection may be present as chronic pulmonary disease[47] or purely cutaneous involvement in nonimmunosuppressed adults[46] and as cervical adenopathy or rarely as disseminated disease in children.[47] It is rare even in patients with immunosuppression related to malignancy or chemotherapy. In one study of mycobacterial infections in patients with malignancies, only 10% were caused by MAI. Gastrointestinal involvement has not been identified in immunosuppressed patients without AIDS.[47,56]

In contrast, AIDS patients may have overwhelming MAI infections. In studies from Memorial Sloan-Kettering Cancer Center, 50% of AIDS patients had severe MAI infections at autopsy,[31] and in a study from the National Institutes of Health, 44% of patients had clinical evidence of MAI infection and 67% had MAI infection diagnosed at autopsy. MAI infection is now the most common disseminated bacterial infection in patients with AIDS and is probably a primary gastrointestinal infection acquired by ingestion of water.[49] In these patients MAI has been found in and grown from cultures of bone marrow, lymph nodes, lung, liver, brain, and gut and also grown from blood cultures.[50] AIDS patients have a high-grade persistent bacteremia with large numbers of acid-fast bacilli on direct stool smears.[31] Studies with a genetic probe have recently shown that the majority of AIDS patients are infected with *M. avium* rather than *M. intracellulare*.[51]

It is important to remember that AIDS patients die with rather than of MAI infection and that, although diagnosis is important for supportive and specific therapy, such treatment does not prolong life in these patients.[49] In one careful autopsy study of 12 patients with AIDS and MAI infection, only one death could be directly attributed to mycobacterial infection, which produced adrenal failure.[52] In most patients with AIDS and MAI infection the time course from diagnosis of infection to death is short (mean survival 4 months) and death is probably caused by profound immunodeficiency and infections with other pathogens.[49,52]

Original reports of the gross pathologic features of MAI infection of the gut were obtained from autopsy studies, which described a "new" lesion consisting of small yellow-white mucosal plaques seen on prominent folds in the small and large intestines (Fig. 9–3).[53] The gastrointestinal involvement is usually part of a disseminated process of systemic disease, but MAI involvement has also been reported as an inflammatory mass resembling Crohn's disease of the ileum.[54]

The pathologic findings by routine light microscopy are consistent and similar to those in Whipple's disease.[55] In the mucosa are collections of large foamy macrophages or striated histiocytes (pseudo-Gaucher cells) containing periodic acid–Schiff–positive diastase-resistant material. Unlike the organisms of Whipple's disease, MAI are acid-fast organisms when stained with Fite and Ziehl-Neelsen stains.[46] In biopsy specimens from the small intestine and colon, individual lesions may be small and focal, requiring serial sections or special stains when macrophage collections are scanty (Fig. 9–4). The malabsorption and resulting diarrhea most likely occur because the infiltrating macrophages produce villous distortion with loss of surface absorptive area.[46]

In attempts to distinguish MAI from Whipple's bacillus, indirect immunofluorescence patterns with bacterial grouping sera have shown strong reactivity with antisera to *Streptococcus* groups B and G in Whipple's disease and no reactivity with MAI, which appears to react with antisera to *Streptococcus* group D and *Salmonella*.[46] MAI can also be distinguished from Whipple's bacillus at the ultrastructural level. MAI organisms have been identified as intact rod-shaped bacilli with waxy, electron-lucent cell walls within macrophages.[55] Whipple's bacteria are 1.25 to

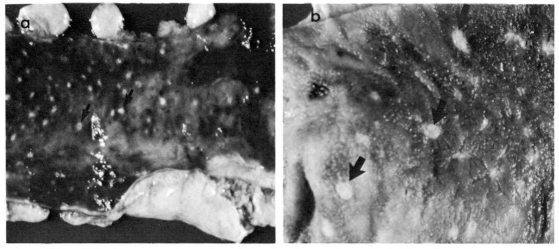

Figure 9–3. Autopsy specimen of small intestine from patient with AIDS. Yellow-white mucosal plaques *(arrows)* represent collections of mucosal macrophages caused by disseminated *Mycobacterium avium-intracellulare* infection. (*a,* Fresh specimen; *b,* formalin-fixed specimen.)

1.5 μm long and 0.25 μm wide, with a tubular, membranous central core, granular peripheral material, a double-layered capsule, and a brushed surface.[57]

Esophageal involvement by *Mycobacterium tuberculosis* has been recently described in six AIDS patients, five of whom had pulmonary tuberculosis and mediastinal adenopathy with esophageal fistulas to the mediastinum and bronchi.[58] Although mycobacterial involvement is important to recognize and treat in this clinical setting, localized MAI infection is unlikely to be responsible for transmural esophageal disease in AIDS patients.

Coccidiosis

Cryptosporidiosis. Cryptosporidia are intestinal protozoan parasites that can cause diarrhea in domestic and farm animals, reptiles, and birds.[59-62] Although cryptosporidiosis was initially described in mice in 1907,[63] human

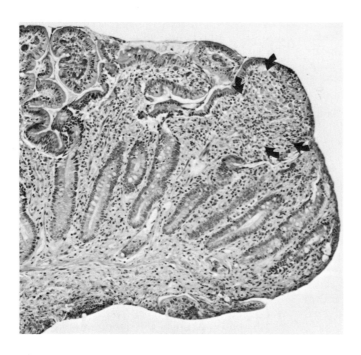

Figure 9–4. Biopsy specimen from small intestine of 36-year-old man with AIDS. Photomicrograph shows shortened blunted villi with focal aggregate of foamy macrophages *(arrows)* representing *Mycobacterium avium-intracellulare* infection identified only on deeper serial section of biopsy. (Hematoxylin and eosin, ×100.)

infection was considered rare until 1976 when sporadic case reports of diarrheal disease in immunocompromised patients were attributed to cryptosporidia.[64-66] Interest in this organism has been greatly stimulated by its role in causing an opportunistic infection with severe and often fatal consequences in AIDS patients. Within the last few years, however, improved methods for detecting this organism in stool have shown that cryptosporidia may be a common cause of diarrhea even in immunocompetent patients. A recent large outbreak of gastroenteritis in Georgia was attributed to contamination of public water supplies by *Cryptosporidium*.[67] The infection is reportedly more common in children, occurs more often in the summer months, and may be acquired either as a zoonosis (the organism is not species specific) or as a form of traveler's diarrhea along with *Giardia* from contaminated food or water.[59,60,68-74] Studies suggest that cryptosporidiosis commonly causes diarrhea in young children, with prevalence rates of 7% in developing countries and ranging from 6% to 54% in the United States.[75] Person-to-person transmission can occur, especially in confined environments and urban slums. Direct spread to laboratory personnel from animals and within the homosexual community has been reported.[76] An endoscopic study of nonimmunosuppressed adults with predominantly nondiarrheal symptoms identified cryptosporidial oocysts in 12.7%, suggesting a surprisingly high carrier rate.[77]

The clinical features of cryptospordiosis are less severe in immunocompetent patients than in patients with AIDS. The former may have nonbloody diarrhea accompanied by abdominal pain, fever, and nausea after an incubation period of approximately 8 days. The symptoms persist for 2 days to 2 weeks, followed by full recovery without any specific therapy and with the possible development of antibodies.[60,70] Numerous case reports and autopsy studies in AIDS patients emphasize the devastating illness associated with cryptosporidial infection in these patients, who have severe watery diarrhea, electrolyte imbalances, malabsorption, diffuse abdominal pain, and weight loss that persist for many months.[78-82] Chronic wasting diarrhea with stool volumes as great as 17 L per day has been reported in up to 11% of U.S. AIDS patients and in up to 46% of Haitian AIDS patients.[83] The pathogenesis of diarrhea in these patients is unknown. Its secretory nature suggests a possible enterotoxic mechanism, but damage to surface epithelium and enzymes may also contribute to malabsorption and diarrhea.[84]

Endoscopic examination in AIDS patients has identified small erosions on thickened folds with radiographic changes consistent with malabsorption.[78] The organisms were initially missed on biopsy specimens, but with increased awareness the spherical basophilic 2 to 4 µm organisms can be readily recognized in rows and clusters in the microvillus brush border of small intestinal villi on routine hematoxylin and eosin preparations (Fig. 9–5), although they are possibly better defined by Giemsa stain. Recent case studies have identi-

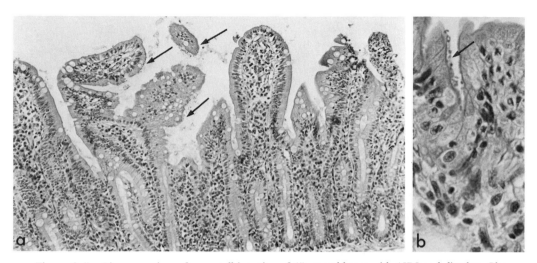

Figure 9–5. Biopsy specimen from small intestine of 45-year-old man with AIDS and diarrhea. Photomicrograph shows cryptosporidial organisms *(arrows)* focally present in microvillus brush border of villi. (Hematoxylin and eosin; *a*, ×100; *b*, ×400.)

fied organisms throughout the gastrointestinal tract and biliary tree and even in respiratory epithelium.[80] On air-dried smears the organisms appear to contain cytoplasmic vacuoles, which are more prominent than in paraffin-embedded tissues. Cryptosporidia may be seen free in the intestinal lumen and until recently were thought to remain extracellular. Mucosal abnormalities are minimal, with mild to moderate villus blunting and a decrease in villus/crypt ratio to 2:1 or 1:1. The epithelial cells show mild damage with shortening and vacuolation. The lamina propria contains a mild lymphoplasmacytic infiltrate with scattered polymorphonuclear leukocytes. The ultrastructural features of *Cryptosporidium* species were described first by Vetterling[85] and later by many other authors to consist of an asexual and sexual life cycle of trophozoites, schizonts, macrogametes, and microgametes.[64-66,78-81] Oocysts, the infectious form produced by the fertilization of macrogametes by microgametes, are not often seen in biopsy specimens. The controversy over the presence of intracytoplasmic organisms has been resolved by the elegant ultrastructural studies of Marcial and Madara,[86] who found cryptosporidial organisms in the apex of absorptive cells and also deep in the cytoplasm of M cells overlying intestinal lymphoid follicles (Fig. 9–6). Cryptosporidia were also noted in macrophages subjacent to M cells, which suggests that although cryptosporidial antigens can be sampled by intestinal immune cells, immunodeficient patients may not be able to mount an appropriate response. No therapy is effective for cryptosporidiosis in AIDS patients, and the mortality rate is greater than 70%.[87]

Until the recent interest in *Cryptosporidium*, simple methods for its identification in stool specimens were not available. Initial diagnosis in patients with AIDS was based on examination of biopsy tissue. In the past 5 years several authors have compared and improved on available methods of stool examination.[88,89] Although stool concentration techniques may be necessary for immunocompetent patients who do not shed numerous oocysts, modified Ziehl-Neelsen carbolfuchsin or modified Kinyoun acid-fast staining of smears of unconcentrated formalin-preserved or fresh stool specimens is safe, quick, and efficient.[76,90] By these methods the oocysts in fecal smears appear as round, densely stained red bodies in a green background. They have a thick wall with up to four inner sporozoites, an eccentric dot, and vacuoles. Other useful stains are auramine-carbolfuchsin and Giemsa stains. Sheather's flotation technique with phase-contrast microscopy is a useful concentration technique for screening specimens.[88-91] If a stool examination shows no abnormalities, it should be repeated, especially in AIDS patients, since the parasites may be excreted intermittently.

Isosporiasis. Before the AIDS epidemic, human coccidiosis was reportedly caused more

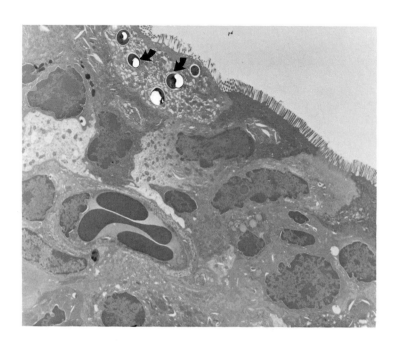

Figure 9–6. Electron micrograph of cryptosporidial organisms *(arrows)* within cytoplasm of intestinal M cells from ileum of spontaneously infested guinea pig. (Approximately ×6000. Courtesy Dr. James L. Madara, Brigham & Women's Hospital, Boston.)

often by *Isospora* than by *Cryptosporidium*. Isosporiasis appears to be widespread among vertebrates, but sporadic cases of human infection in immunocompetent patients, acquired by ingestion of infective sporulated oocysts, have been regularly reported over the past 40 years, especially in Central and South America.[83,92] In immunocompetent patients the illness has an acute onset with fever, malaise, diarrhea, abdominal pain, and weight loss. It is usually self-limited with full recovery in a few days or months, although occasionally malabsorption and a prolonged illness occur.[92] Organisms causing diarrheal disease include *I. belli, I. hominis,* and *I. natalensis.*[50] Although diarrheal disease from *I. belli* infection occurs in less than 0.2% of AIDS cases reported to the Centers for Disease Control, a recent report from Haiti has documented isosporiasis in 15% of patients with AIDS.[83] Chronic watery diarrhea and crampy abdominal pain of greater than 2 months' duration with weight loss and nausea are similar to the symptoms of cryptosporidiosis, but *Isospora* can be eradicated by oral administration of trimethoprim-sulfamethoxazole even in recurrent cases.[83] Therefore identification of the organism in biopsy specimens is important.

The pathologic features of isosporiasis have been well described by Trier et al.[92] and more recently by Restrepo et al.[93] The small intestinal mucosa shows moderate villous abnormality with mild damage to epithelial cells. The lamina propria may have increased numbers of eosinophils and neutrophils. The organisms released from sporulated oocysts can be seen in all stages of the life cycle in parasitophorous vacuoles in villous epithelial cells, which may appear undamaged (Fig. 9–7). The simplest method for diagnosis is stool examination for oocysts by staining stool smears with modified Kinyoun acid-fast stain. Oocysts of *I. belli* stain red and can be distinguished from cryptosporidia by their large size (20 to 30 μm by 10 to 20 μm), oval shape, and two intracystic sporoblasts.[83]

Microsporidiosis. The microsporidium *Enterocytozoon bieneusi* was recently described as a cause of diarrhea in 10 patients with AIDS.[94] The parasites have been identified within enterocytes in the small intestine. Although identification by light microscopy may be difficult, spores can be identified with Gram's stain and the proliferative phase can be recognized with Giemsa stains of air-dried smears of duodenal and jejunal biopsy mate-

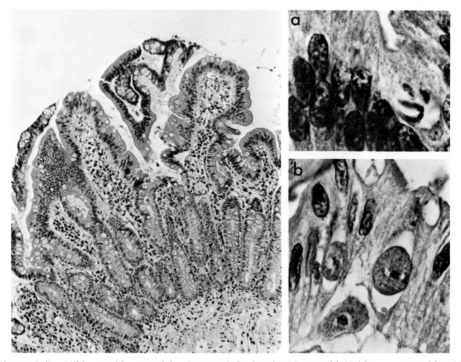

Figure 9–7. Mild enteritis caused by *Isospora* infection in 33-year-old Haitian woman with AIDS, diarrhea, and malabsorption. (Hematoxylin and eosin, × 100.) Intracellular organisms are present in intestinal surface epithelium. *a,* Merozoites. *b,* Schizonts or gametocytes. (Hematoxylin and eosin, × 1000.)

rial. When stained with Giemsa stain the parasites (2 to 9 μm in diameter) exhibit hyaline pale-blue cytoplasm with one to many reddish purple nuclei. In a recent study of 67 patients with AIDS or ARC and chronic diarrhea, in whom no other pathogens could be identified, electron microscopy revealed *E. bieneusi* in 22 biopsies from 20 patients. Parasites and spores were noted by light microscopy of semithin plastic sections and in retrospect could be identified by light microscopy of standard hematoxylin and eosin–stained, paraffin-embedded sections. The key to identification of the organisms is to search for them in biopsy specimens from the small intestine, which show villus damage with atrophy and necrosis of surface epithelial cells. The organisms are intracellular in a supranuclear location with lightly stained oval parasites, containing prominent clefts, and densely stained clusters of spores.[95] Another microsporidium, *Encephalitozoon cuniculi*, has been reported to cause peritonitis in a patient with AIDS.[96] Whether these organisms are natural parasites in humans or represent an opportunistic zoonosis is not yet known.[94]

Herpes Simplex Infection

Viral esophagitis is found in approximately one third of patients with AIDS, and in 11% of these the cause is herpes simplex virus (HSV) as a single pathogen or in a mixed infection with CMV and *Candida* species.[97] HSV esophagitis can be accurately identified at endoscopy only in the early stages when vesicles or small (1 to 3 mm) punched-out ulcers are present in otherwise normal mucosa. The ulcers enlarge later and become confluent with a diffuse erosive esophagitis in the lower third of the esophagus. The inflammatory changes end abruptly at the gastroesophageal junction. Biopsy specimens from the ulcer bed may show nonspecific inflammation and diagnostic inclusions, or multinucleated cells with "ground-glass" nuclei may be present only in intact squamous epithelium at the edges of the ulcer. It is likely that more cases of HSV esophagitis could be identified with immunoperoxidase or in situ hybridization techniques.

HSV proctitis is probably the most common cause of nongonococcal proctitis in sexually active male homosexuals and was identified in 23% of such patients in one study.[98] Perianal and anal vesicular and ulcerative lesions combined with mucosal friability and ulcers within 10 cm of the anal verge suggest the correct diagnosis. Anorectal biopsy specimens show extensive ulceration with acute inflammation,

multinucleated cells, and cells with classic intranuclear inclusions. The attack in immunocompetent patients is usually self-limited and may last from 7 to 44 days, but latency and recurrent infection may occur.[16] Although proctitis may be caused by HSV-1 or HSV-2, symptomatic proctitis is usually due to a first infection with HSV-2.[99] Siegal et al.[99] described severe enlarging mucocutaneous ulcers in the perianal and oral regions of patients with AIDS. In one study HSV was isolated from 35 patients with AIDS, 26 of whom had severe perianal ulcers that were chronic, large (up to 20 cm), and unresponsive to therapy.[31] Pathologists should remember that proctitis in AIDS patients may be due to multiple pathogens such as HSV and CMV (Fig. 9–8).

MISCELLANEOUS GASTROINTESTINAL DISEASE IN AIDS

Infections by nonmycobacterial organisms may be the most common infections in patients with AIDS.[100] Salmonellosis has an incidence up to 20 times higher in these patients and is associated with bacteremia in 40% of cases.[101] Recurrent infections with *Salmonella*, *Campylobacter*, and *Shigella* are common, even after effective therapy.[102] The incidence of *Helicobacter pylori* gastritis in patients with AIDS is controversial, with some reports suggesting a higher and others a lower incidence than in the general population.[102]

Recent studies have described the ultrastructural findings in the gut in AIDS. Dobbins and Weinstein[103] found tubuloreticular structures (modified endoplasmic reticulum) in endothelial cells and in intraepithelial lymphocytes and mononuclear cells in the lamina propria of intestinal and rectal mucosa. These authors also identified tube- and ring-shaped forms (cytoplasmic tubules formed by fusion of endoplasmic reticulum membranes with dense material between) in lamina propria lymphocytes of three of six patients. None of these features is specific, nor can they be used as diagnostic markers for AIDS. Weber and Dobbins[104] demonstrated an increase in intraepithelial lymphocytes that appear "activated" in intestinal biopsies from patients with AIDS, but they were unable to find histologic evidence of immune-mediated gastrointestinal injury. However, reports of increased numbers of apoptotic bodies in the rectal crypts of AIDS patients may represent an immunologically mediated HIV enteropathy.[3,105]

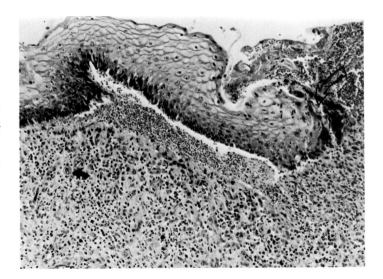

Figure 9–8. HIV-positive man with anal ulcer. Herpes simplex virus is in squamous epithelium at edge of ulcer *(open arrow)*, and cytomegalovirus is in granulation tissue in ulcer bed *(closed arrow)*. (Hematoxylin and eosin, × 100.)

GASTROINTESTINAL NEOPLASMS IN AIDS

The gastrointestinal tract is involved in 32% of patients with AIDS and neoplasia. Kaposi's sarcoma (KS) and high-grade lymphomas are the most common neoplasms in AIDS, with gastrointestinal involvement in 32% and 24% of patients, respectively. KS is most commonly identified in the oropharynx, and lymphomas are noted most often in the stomach and intestines. Other reported neoplasms are uncommon but include squamous carcinoma of the esophagus.[106] The neoplasms in AIDS patients probably represent virally induced tumors arising in a background of reduced immune surveillance.[107]

Kaposi's Sarcoma

Visceral involvement by lesions of nonepidemic KS has been known since Kaposi originally described the disease in 1872.[108-110] This form of KS is associated with a 10% incidence of visceral involvement,[50] and postmortem studies have shown the gastrointestinal tract to be the most frequently involved site.[108,109] Whereas KS comprises 0.6% of all cancers in the general population, the incidence of KS in immunosuppressed organ transplant patients is 3.2%.[111] KS in these patients appears to develop between 8 and 43 months after transplantation, and the most effective therapy for KS in this clinical setting is the cessation of immunosuppression.[111,112]

Since 1979 KS has emerged as the most common malignant neoplasm in patients with AIDS, affecting one third to one half of patients (Fig. 9–9).[21,113] In the United States KS is reported to be 20,000 times more common in AIDS patients than in the general population, with the majority of cases occurring in homosexual and bisexual males.[114] In this group of patients the incidence dropped from a high of 79% in 1981 to 25% in 1989.[115] Although the causative agent is not yet known, KS appears to be related to a cofactor that exists in patients who acquire the disease by sexual transmission.[114,115]

In the majority of cases epidemic KS is an aggressive disease with an unusual distribution on skin surfaces and rapid involvement of oral mucosa, lymph nodes, and viscera.[116-118] In one series of 183 patients with AIDS and KS, 70% had tumors in the skin, 47% had nodal involvement, and 37% and 33%, respectively, had upper and lower gastrointestinal tract involvement.[117] In a study from the University of San Francisco, 40% of patients with KS had morphologically visible lesions recognized with either upper endoscopy or sigmoidoscopy. There is no apparent correlation between the presence of gastrointestinal neoplasms and skin, nodal, or oral involvement.[108] However, Saltz et al.[119] in their study of 19 patients found that 71% with advanced cutaneous disease and 75% with oral mucosal lesions had gastrointestinal tumors. In three patients gastrointestinal KS before involvement of other sites has been described.[109] Gastrointestinal tumors are asymptomatic in most patients, although massive gastrointestinal bleeding, obstruction, and perforation with peritonitis have occasionally been reported in both the nonepidemic and epidemic forms of the disease.[120,121] The mortal-

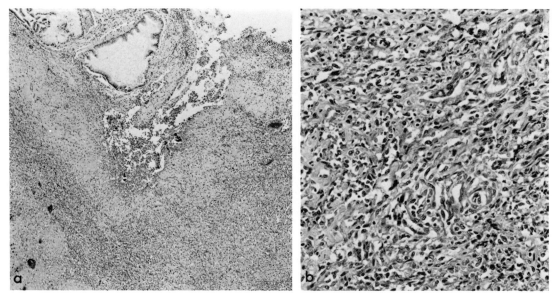

Figure 9–9. Gastric antropyloric ulcer identified at autopsy in 28-year-old man with AIDS. Photomicrograph shows Kaposi's sarcoma at base of ulcer. (Hematoxylin and eosin; *a*, ×25; *b*, ×100.)

ity rate is reportedly higher in patients with gastrointestinal involvement, although death is not directly attributable to the neoplasm.[108]

Radiographic techniques are not helpful in the diagnosis except when neoplastic masses are present as intraluminal filling defects.[108,109] Since the onset of the AIDS epidemic, several authors have described the endoscopic appearance of gastrointestinal KS. Lesions may range from maculopapular reticulated purple spots 1 to 2 mm in diameter to multiple or solitary polypoid lesions up to 3 cm with central umbilication.[108,109,120,121] Occasionally with massive involvement the endoscopist sees serpiginous ulcers covered by a fibrinous membrane. Because of the submucosal nature of the tumor nodules and the superficial biopsies, a positive histologic diagnosis was obtained in only 15% to 23% of patients with endoscopically visible lesions.[108,119] Sigmoidoscopy gave a better yield (36%) than upper endoscopy (13%).[108]

The pathologic findings in KS of the gastrointestinal tract are similar to those in skin and any other site, with a proliferation of thin, irregular vascular channels associated with spindle cells in the earlier, less diagnostic stage, followed by an infiltrate composed of nodules of atypical spindle cells with entrapped red blood cells, mononuclear cells, and siderophages. Vascular channels and cords of neoplastic cells, some with intracytoplasmic eosinophilic globules, dissect between collagen bundles. Mitoses are generally sparse,

and atypia of endothelial cells may be mild. The neoplastic infiltrate separates and destroys intestinal crypts and extends from the submucosa luminally into the mucosa and peripherally into muscularis propria and possibly into subserosal tissues.[116,120,122] There are apparently no histologic differences between the nonepidemic forms of KS and the tumors in AIDS patients, but a recent ultrastructural study demonstrated necrosis of individual endothelial cells in some patients with KS and AIDS but not in the classic variant.[116]

Lymphomas

An increased incidence of high-grade B-cell lymphomas and an aggressive form of Hodgkin's disease have been reported in patients with or at risk for AIDS.[123,124] These neoplasms appear to be equally distributed among homosexual male patients and intravenous drug users.[106] In 90 homosexuals with non-Hodgkin's lymphoma, all but two had extranodal disease involving the central nervous system, bone marrow, bowel, and mucocutaneous sites.[123] In this study 17% of patients had bowel involvement, four other patients had intraoral tumors, and three patients had anorectal tumors. It is well known that lymphomas of high-grade malignancy can develop in extranodal sites in immunosuppressed transplant patients[125,126] and may follow the development of KS by several months.[123,127] In a series from the University of Southern California, in 61 patients with AIDS-related lymphomas, 26% had initial gastrointestinal involvement and half of these had rectal involvement.[128] Primary anorectal lymphoma is an unusual presentation reported recently in six other patients with AIDS.[129,130] Esophageal lymphoma was seen in four patients with AIDS at one institution within 9 months.[131] In contrast to KS, gastrointestinal lymphomas usually are large bulky neoplasms and often are symptomatic, with bleeding or obstruction.[132] Diagnosis can often be established with endoscopic techniques.

The lymphomas are composed of large or undifferentiated cells of B-cell phenotype. Possibly the loss of immune surveillance produced by HIV infection allows the development of B-cell lymphomas potentiated by reactivation of Epstein-Barr virus (EBV) in these patients. Despite aggressive therapy the prognosis is poor.[107,133]

Anorectal Squamous Carcinoma

Recent epidemiologic and pathologic studies have demonstrated an increase in anal squamous carcinoma and its precursor, atypical lesions, in young homosexual men.[134-138] Several of these studies have also demonstrated an association between anal dysplasia-carcinoma and serum antibody to HIV.[135,138] Human papilloma virus (HPV) has been identified in these neoplasms by cytologic[138] and immunohistochemical techniques, and HPV mRNA has been detected in 12 of 18 anal carcinomas, suggesting that this may be a sexually transmitted disease.[139] Despite these data it is not yet apparent that anorectal carcinomas arise in patients with AIDS more often than in otherwise healthy homosexual males, and the diagnosis of anorectal carcinoma does not establish a diagnosis of AIDS in an HIV-positive individual.[132]

HEPATOBILIARY AND PANCREATIC INVOLVEMENT IN AIDS

Hepatomegaly and liver function abnormalities are common in AIDS patients. In several large studies of patients from centers where AIDS has been reported since the start of the epidemic, hepatomegaly and mild elevations in transaminase and alkaline phosphatase levels have been noted in approximately 70% of patients. This is not surprising,

since the predominant groups affected by the epidemic are homosexual men and intravenous drug abusers who are constantly exposed to hepatotropic viruses, hepatotoxic drugs, and alcohol.[140-145] Although the liver is rarely normal on biopsy or at autopsy, pathologic findings are poorly correlated with abnormal biochemical findings, no hepatic pathologic findings are characteristic of AIDS, and liver involvement does not contribute to death.

The most commonly identified pathologic changes are nonspecific, with periportal or centrilobular steatosis, sinusoidal dilatations, and portal mononuclear infiltrates noted in 30% to 60% of biopsies and autopsies.[140-145] As in the gastrointestinal tract, recent studies have identified HIV p24 protein in 40% to 80% of liver biopsies performed in patients with AIDS or ARC. The viral antigens are present in Kupffer cells, histiocytes in granulomas, sinusoidal lining cells, and rare hepatocytes.[146,147] This suggests that some of the nonspecific histologic changes present, especially the peliotic lesions and the sinusoidal dilatations, may be related to the presence of the virus in sinusoidal macrophages and endothelial cells.[148]

Exposure to hepatitis B virus (HBV) is noted in 80% to 90% of homosexual men and intravenous drug abusers, and 15% of the latter have also been exposed to hepatitis D virus.[140-145] In homosexual men, anal intercourse allows the acquisition of both HBV and HIV, but the former appears to be transmitted eight times more efficiently.[149] HIV infection increases the risk of becoming a carrier of HBV and allows the reactivation of any underlying HBV or HDV infection, although the inflammatory response to the replicating viruses is greatly reduced in these immunodeficient patients. Studies of homosexual men with AIDS do not show any greater incidence of chronic active hepatitis or cirrhosis (10%) than in the general population because HBV is usually acquired and eliminated before the onset of HIV infection.[140,141,143] In a study predominantly of drug abusers in New York, the incidence of cirrhosis was 23%, related not to viral hepatitis but to alcohol abuse.[144] EBV and HSV hepatitis are rare in patients with AIDS as shown by a recent in situ hybridization study in which these viruses were identified in hepatocyte nuclei in four of 37 cases studied.[150]

Specific infections in AIDS patients can involve the liver as part of a disseminated process and have been noted in approximately one third of cases in most studies.[140-145] Not surprisingly, the organisms most commonly identified in the liver at biopsy or autopsy are MAI (30% to 50%) and CMV (40%). MAI is most often associated with a granulomatous response composed of large lobular and portal aggregates of foamy macrophages (Fig. 9–10a), occasionally ill-defined granulomas, or well-formed granulomas (Fig. 9–10b). In a patient population environmentally exposed to *M. tuberculosis*, this is the most common organism identified in hepatic granulomas, as in a group of Haitian patients with AIDS studied at the University of Miami.[142] Hepatic granulomas in AIDS may also be due to fungi such as

Histoplasma capsulatum (Fig. 9–10c) and *Cryptococcus neoformans*, parasites, and occasionally drugs.[141] Microsporidian hepatitis and *Pneumocystis* hepatitis (Fig. 9–10d) secondary to dissemination following successful aerosolized pentamidine prophylaxis have also been reported.[151,152]

Liver involvement has been reported in 5% to 40% of patients with generalized CMV.[140-145] CMV inclusions may be primarily sinusoidal in endothelial cells but may also be found in hepatocytes and bile duct epithelium. CMV may be present without associated necrosis or inflammation or as acute or

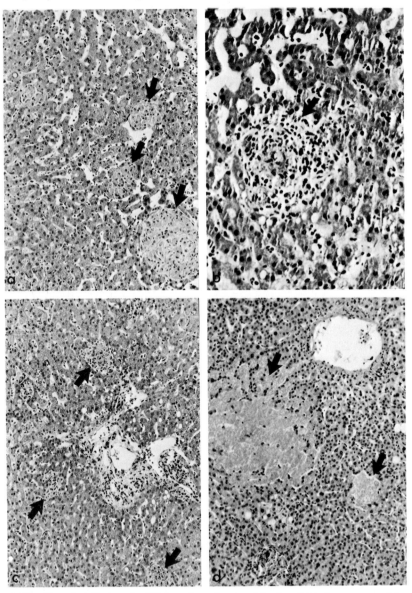

Figure 9–10. Hepatic infections in AIDS. *a,* Granulomas of "striated" histiocytes caused by disseminated *Mycobacterium avium-intracellulare* (MAI). *b,* Well-formed granuloma caused by MAI. *c,* Granulomas of disseminated histoplasmosis. *d,* Foamy exudate of *Pneumocystis carinii* infection. (*a, c,* and *d,* ×100; *b,* ×400. Slide *d* Courtesy Dr. Urmilla Khettry, New England Deaconess Hospital, Boston.)

granulomatous hepatitis. CMV DNA has been identified in 92% of liver biopsies of AIDS patients without associated necroinflammatory activity; CMV may be present as a latent infection.[150]

KS may involve the liver in the presence of disseminated disease of the skin and other viscera. It has been identified at autopsy in 14% to 18% of cases but is rarely seen in biopsies.[140-145] The neoplasm originates in hilar, capsular, and portal areas and can spread into sinusoids, simulating fibrosis. Extensive involvement of the hilum and compression of main bile ducts occasionally leads to cholestasis and ascending cholangitis.[28] High-grade B-cell lymphomas have also been reported in the liver, usually as part of disseminated disease but occasionally as a primary hepatic neoplasm.[145] Diagnosis during life is rare but may be suggested by markedly elevated bilirubin levels as well as radiologic findings. Response to chemotherapy can be dramatic but is almost inevitably associated with relapse and death.[145]

Acalculous cholecystitis and cholangitis with obstruction have recently been reported in patients with AIDS.[153-156] Symptoms include biliary colic, fever, and jaundice. In 75% of these patients, radiologic techniques including endoscopic retrograde cholangiopancreatography reveal dilated intrahepatic and extrahepatic bile ducts with strictures suggestive of sclerosing cholangitis with or without papillary stenosis.[153] Endoscopic sphincterotomy relieves symptoms in most patients.

The pathologic features on biopsy or cholecystectomy include acute or chronic inflammation with edema responsible for acalculous cholecystitis and benign strictures of the distal common bile duct. Cryptosporidial organisms or CMV is most often detected in association with the inflammatory reaction in reported cases, although bacteria and *Candida albicans* have also been isolated.[155–157] Biliary tract abnormalities have been reported in 10% of patients with cryptosporidiosis.[75] In patients with generalized CMV infection, cholestatic changes have been reported in one third and sclerosing cholangitis or papillary stenosis in 3% to 11%.[154] Although these reactions may be entirely inflammatory, immunologic mechanisms may also play a role. In this context, HLA class II antigens have been identified on bile duct epithelium in five of 10 patients with AIDS and may be involved in immune-mediated mechanisms of bile duct injury.[158,159]

The role of liver biopsy in patients with AIDS is controversial. Most hepatologists at centers having a large experience with this disease have found that the yield of a positive diagnosis on liver biopsy is about 25%, the same diagnostic yield as in non-AIDS patients with pyrexia of unknown origin. Liver biopsy is recommended only for patients with fever and liver function abnormalities that persist after withdrawal of hepatotoxic medications.[141,153] Liver biopsy may be useful in patients with elevated alkaline phosphatase levels and no radiologic evidence of biliary tract abnormalities. Such biopsies may provide the first diagnosis of an infection (MAI) or neoplasm (lymphoma) and may influence therapy.[160,161] Diagnostic yield can be maximized when tissue is sent for culture, held for possible ultrastructural or immunohistochemical study, and stained for specific organisms even when appearances are "normal" in routine hematoxylin-eosin stains.

Pancreatic involvement has recently been documented both clinically and at autopsy in 22% to 65% of AIDS patients. Approximately half the patients with AIDS are found to have pancreatic involvement at postmortem examination. In about 40% of these, specific infections and neoplasms are identified, and in the remainder findings are nonspecific.[162] In data combined from several large studies the most significant finding was opportunistic infections, particularly CMV, MAI, and *C. neoformans* in 24% of cases.[162,163] Most of these were generalized infections, and pancreatic involvement was clinically inapparent. Other lesions were nonspecific and probably not responsible for symptoms. Pancreatitis in AIDS patients may also be related to therapeutic agents such as trimethoprimsulfamethoxazole and pentamidine,[162] both of which are used for the treatment of *P. carinii* pneumonia, and the new purine analog 2',3'-dideoxyinosine,[164] a therapeutic agent that suppresses the replication of HIV.

CONCLUSION

With the increasing number of patients infected by HIV throughout the world, the surgical pathologist must assume an important role in the accurate diagnosis of tissue specimens from these patients. When the pathologist is confronted with a gastrointestinal or liver specimen from an HIV-positive patient, the following may be helpful:

1. History is important. HIV-positive patients often belong to high-risk groups predisposed to certain health hazards that may be

responsible for the signs, symptoms, and associated pathologic changes. Homosexual male patients are prone to infections by a number of venereally transmitted organisms that can cause gay bowel disease. These organisms should be identified and distinguished from those responsible for AIDS. Intravenous drug abusers are exposed to the effects of hepatotoxic drugs and sometimes alcohol, which may be responsible for disease in these patients rather than specific AIDS-related infections and neoplasms.

2. Opportunistic infections in HIV-positive patients are caused by organisms not commonly seen in ordinary pathology practice, and these may be associated with unusual patterns of reaction, such as acalculous cholecystitis caused by CMV and cryptosporidia. Accurate diagnosis requires an awareness of these infections, bearing in mind that patients are infected by organisms normally present in their environment; hence *M. tuberculosis* and *Isospora* infections are identified primarily in Haitian and African patients. Examination of several levels through the biopsy specimen may be necessary to ensure that focal involvement is not missed, and special stains may be required, particularly for the identification of acid-fast bacteria and fungi. Most important is the accurate diagnosis of treatable infections such as CMV, HSV, *M. tuberculosis, Candida,* and *Isospora.*

3. Special and expensive techniques in pathology, such as electron microscopy for microsporidial infections, have only a small place in routine diagnosis. Immunohistochemical studies for viral antigens may prove useful in ulcers without easily recognizable cytopathic changes, since viral infections such as CMV and HSV can now be treated. The usual special techniques are required for the diagnosis of lymphomas.

4. HIV-positive patients may exhibit gastrointestinal and hepatic symptoms unrelated to HIV infection but caused by such conditions as peptic esophagitis, duodenal ulcer disease, and inflammatory bowel disease. The correct diagnosis is vital for appropriate management.

REFERENCES

1. Sierra-Madero J, Yen-Lieberman B, Proffit MR, et al: Enhanced replication of the human immunodeficiency virus (HIV) in intestinal mucosal cells as compared to peripheral blood cells. Gastroenterology 98:A474, 1990.
2. Ullrich R, Zeitz M, Heise W, et al: Small intestinal structure and function in patients infected with human immunodeficiency virus (HIV): Evidence for HIV-induced enteropathy. Ann Intern Med 111:15-21, 1989.
3. Reka S, Kotler DP: An inflammatory bowel disease associated with HIV infection. Gastroenterology 98:A472, 1990.
4. Adachi A, Koenig S, Gendelman HE, et al: Productive, persistent infection of human colorectal cell lines with human immunodeficiency virus. J Virol 61:209-213, 1987.
5. Ramirez A, Suarez-McKee M, Luna J, et al: Propagation of human immunodeficiency virus (HIV) in human colon cancer (HCC) cells. Gastroenterology 98:A664, 1990.
6. Nelson JA, Wiley CA, Reynolds-Kohler C, et al: Human immunodeficiency virus detected in bowel epithelium from patients with gastrointestinal symptoms. Lancet 1:259-262, 1988.
7. Winter HS, Fox CH, Hendren RB, et al: An animal model for the study of human intestinal epithelial infection with HIV. Gastroenterology 98: A480, 1990.
8. Rabeneck L, Popovic M, Gartner S, et al: Acute HIV infection presenting with painful swallowing and esophageal ulcers. JAMA 263:2318-2322, 1990.
9. Batman PA, Miller AR, Forster SM, et al: Jejunal enteropathy associated with human immunodeficiency virus infection: Quantitative histology. J Clin Pathol 42(3):275-281, 1989.
10. Smith PD, Janoff EN: Infectious diarrhea in human immunodeficiency virus infection. Gastroenterol Clin North Am 17:587-598, 1988.
11. Quinn TC, Stamm WE, Goodell SE, et al: The polymicrobial origin of intestinal infections in homosexual men. N Engl J Med 309:576-582, 1983.
12. Laughon BE, Druckman DA, Vernon A, et al: Prevalence of enteric pathogens in homosexual men with and without acquired immunodeficiency syndrome. Gastroenterology 94:984-993, 1988.
13. Rodgers VD, Fassett R, Kagnoff MF: Abnormalities in intestinal mucosal T cells in homosexual populations including those with the lymphadenopathy syndrome and acquired immunodeficiency syndrome. Gastroenterology 90:552-558, 1986.
14. Ellakany S, Whiteside TL, Schade RR, et al: Analysis of intestinal lymphocyte subpopulations in patients with acquired immunodeficiency syndrome (AIDS) and AIDS-related complex. Am J Clin Pathol 87:356-364, 1987.
15. Kotler DP, Scholes JV: Altered intestinal plasma cell immunoglobulins in the acquired immunodeficiency syndrome. Gastroenterology 86:1144, 1987.
16. Quinn TC, Bender BS, Bartlett JG: New developments in infectious diarrhea. Dis Mon 32:231, 1986.
17. Janoff EN, Smith PD: Perspectives on gastrointestinal infections in AIDS. Gastroenterol Clin North Am 17:451-463, 1988.
18. McLoughlin LC, Nord KS, Joshi VV, et al: Severe gastrointestinal involvement in children with the

acquired immunodeficiency syndrome. J Pediatr Gastroenterol Nutr 6:517-524, 1987.

19. Smith PD, Lane HC, Gill VJ, et al: Intestinal infections in patients with the acquired immunodeficiency syndrome: Etiology and response to therapy. Ann Intern Med 108:328-333, 1988.

20. Kotler DP, Gaetz HP, Lange M, et al: Enteropathy associated with the acquired immunodeficiency syndrome. Ann Intern Med 101:421-428, 1984.

21. Rotterdam H, Sommers SC: Alimentary tract biopsy lesions in the acquired immune deficiency syndrome. Pathology 17:181-192, 1985.

22. Dworkin B, Wormser GP, Rosenthal WS, et al: Gastrointestinal manifestations of the acquired immunodeficiency syndrome: A review of 22 cases. Am J Gastroenterol 80:774-778, 1985.

23. Rosen PP: Cytomegalovirus infection in cancer patients. Pathol Annu 13:175-208, 1978.

24. Betts RF: Syndromes of cytomegalovirus infection. Adv Intern Med 26:447-466, 1980.

25. Betts RF, Hanshaw JB: Cytomegalovirus (CMV) in the compromised host(s). Annu Rev Med 28:103-110, 1977.

26. Nankervis GA, Kumar ML: Diseases produced by cytomegaloviruses. Med Clin North Am 62:1021-1035, 1978.

27. Drew WL, Mintz L, Miner RC, et al: Prevalence of cytomegalovirus infection in homosexual men. J Infect Dis 143:188-192, 1981.

28. Niedt GW, Schinella RA: Acquired immunodeficiency syndrome: Clinicopathologic study of 56 autopsies. Arch Pathol Lab Med 109:727-734, 1985.

29. Wilson SE, Robinson G, Williams RA, et al: Acquired immune deficiency syndrome (AIDS): Indications for abdominal surgery, pathology, and outcome. Ann Surg 210(4):428-433, 1989.

30. Wexner SD, Smithy WB, Trillo C, et al: Emergency colectomy for cytomegalovirus ileocolitis in patients with the acquired immune deficiency syndrome. Dis Colon Rectum 31(10):755-761, 1988.

31. Gold JWM, Armstrong D: Infectious complications of the acquired immune deficiency syndrome. Ann NY Acad Sci 437:383-393, 1984.

32. Meiselman MS, Cello JP, Margaretten W: Cytomegalovirus colitis: Report of the clinical, endoscopic, and pathologic findings in two patients with the acquired immune deficiency syndrome. Gastroenterology 88:171-175, 1985.

33. Clive DM, Stoff JS: Intestinal pseudoobstruction related to cytomegalovirus infection of myenteric plexus [letter]. N Engl J Med 311:196-197, 1984.

34. Frank D, Raicht RF: Intestinal perforation associated with cytomegalovirus infection in patients with acquired immune deficiency syndrome. Am J Gastroenterol 79:201-205, 1984.

35. Knapp AB, Horst DA, Eliopoulos G, et al: Widespread cytomegalovirus gastroenterocolitis in a patient with acquired immunodeficiency syndrome. Gastroenterology 85:1399-1402, 1983.

36. St. Onge G, Bezahler GH: Giant esophageal ulcer associated with cytomegalovirus. Gastroenterology 83:127-130, 1982.

37. Theise ND, Rotterdam H, Dieterich D: CMV esophagitis in AIDS: Diagnosis by endoscopic biopsy. Gastroenterology 96:A509, 1989.

38. Robey SS, Gage WR, Kuhajda FP: Comparison of immunoperoxidase and in situ hybridization techniques in the diagnosis of cytomegalovirus colitis. Am J Clin Pathol 89:666-671, 1988.

39. Clayton F, Klein EB, Kotler DP: Correlation of in situ hybridization with histology and viral culture in patients with acquired immunodeficiency syndrome with cytomegalovirus colitis. Arch Pathol Lab Med 113:1124-1126, 1989.

40. Chachoua A, Dieterich D, Krasinski K, et al: 9-(1,3-Dihydroxy-2-propoxymethyl) guanine (ganciclovir) in the treatment of cytomegalovirus gastrointestinal disease with the acquired immunodeficiency syndrome. Ann Intern Med 107:133-137, 1987.

41. Marples MJ, DiMenna ME: The incidence of *Candida albicans* in Dunedin, New Zealand. J Pathol Bacteriol 64:497-500, 1952.

42. Kodsi BE, Wickremesinghe PC, Kozinn PJ, et al: *Candida* esophagitis. Gastroenterology 71:715-719, 1976.

43. Gottlieb MS, Schroff R, Schanker HM, et al: *Pneumocystis carinii* pneumonia and mucosal candidiasis in previously healthy homosexual men: Evidence of a new acquired cellular immunodeficiency. N Engl J Med 305:1425-1431, 1981.

44. Gottlieb MS, Groopman JE, Weinstein WM, et al: The acquired immunodeficiency syndrome. Ann Intern Med 99:208-220, 1983.

45. Tavitian A, Raufman JP, Rosenthal L: Oral candidiasis as a marker for esophageal candidiasis in the acquired immunodeficiency syndrome. Ann Intern Med 104:54-55, 1986.

46. Roth RI, Owen RL, Keren DF, et al: Intestinal infection with *Mycobacterium avium* in acquired immune deficiency syndrome (AIDS): Histological and clinical comparison with Whipple's disease. Dig Dis Sci 30:497-504, 1985.

47. Zakowski P, Fligiel S, Berlin OGW, et al: Disseminated *Mycobacterium avium-intracellulare* infection in homosexual men dying of acquired immunodeficiency. JAMA 248:2980-2982, 1982.

48. Sohn CC, Schroff RW, Kliewer KE, et al: Disseminated *Mycobacterium avium-intracellulare* infection in homosexual men with acquired cell-mediated immunodeficiency: A histologic and immunologic study of two cases. Am J Clin Pathol 79:247-252, 1983.

49. Chaisson RE, Hopewell PC: Mycobacteria and AIDS mortality. Am Rev Respir Dis 139:1-3, 1989.

50. Fauci AS, Macher AM, Longo DL, et al: Acquired immunodeficiency syndrome: Epidemiologic, clinical, immunologic and therapeutic considerations. Ann Intern Med 100:92-106, 1984.

51. Guthertz LS, Damsker B, Bottone EJ, et al: *Mycobacterium avium* and *Mycobacterium intracellulare* infections in patients with and without AIDS. J Infect Dis 160(6):1037-1041, 1989.

52. Klatt EC, Jensen DF, Meyer PR: Pathology of *Mycobacterium avium-intracellulare* in acquired immunodeficiency syndrome. Hum Pathol 18:709-714, 1987.

53. Strom RL, Gruninger RP: AIDS with *Mycobacterium avium-intracellulare* lesions resembling those of Whipple's disease [letter]. N Engl J Med 309:1323-1324, 1983.

54. Schneebaum CW, Novick DM, Chabon AB, et al: Terminal ileitis associated with *Mycobacterium*

avium-intracellulare infection in a homosexual male with acquired immune deficiency syndrome. Gastroenterology 92:1127-1132, 1987.

55. Gillin JS, Urmacher C, West R, et al: Disseminated *Mycobacterium avium-intracellulare* infection in acquired immunodeficiency syndrome mimicking Whipple's disease. Gastroenterology 85:1187-1191, 1983.

56. Farhi DC, Mason UG, Horsburgh CR: Pathologic findings in disseminated *Mycobacterium avium-intracellulare* infection: A report of 11 cases. Am J Clin Pathol 85:67-72, 1986.

57. Morningstar WA: Whipple's disease: An example of the value of the electron microscope in diagnosis, follow-up and correlation of a pathologic process. Hum Pathol 6:443-454, 1975.

58. deSilva R, Stoopjack PM, Raufman JP: Esophageal fistulas associated with mycobacterial infection in patients at risk for AIDS. Radiology 175:449-453, 1990.

59. Jokipii L, Pohjola S, Jokipii AMM: Cryptosporidiosis associated with traveling and giardiasis. Gastroenterology 89:838-842, 1985.

60. Wolfson JS, Richter JM, Waldron MA, et al: Cryptosporidiosis in immunocompetent patients. N Engl J Med 312:1278-1282, 1985.

61. Reese NC, Current WL, Ernest JV, Bailey WS: Cryptosporidiosis of man and calf: A case report and results of experimental infections in mice and rats. Am J Trop Med Hyg 31:226-229, 1982.

62. Current WL, Reese NC, Ernst JV, et al: Human cryptosporidiosis in immunocompetent and immunodeficient persons: Studies of an outbreak and experimental transmission. N Engl J Med 308:1252-1257, 1983.

63. Tyzzer EE: A sporozoan found in peptic glands of the common mouse. Proc Soc Exp Biol Med 5:12-13, 1907.

64. Weisburger WR, Hutcheon DF, Yardley JH, et al: Cryptosporidiosis in an immunosuppressed renal transplant recipient with IgA deficiency. Am J Clin Pathol 72:473-478, 1979.

65. Nime FA, Burek JD, Page DL, et al: Acute enterocolitis in a human being infected with the protozoan *Cryptosporidium*. Gastroenterology 70:592-598, 1976.

66. Lasser KH, Lewin KJ, Ryning FW: Cryptosporidial enteritis in a patient with congenital hypogammaglobulinemia. Hum Pathol 10:234-240, 1979.

67. Hayes EB, Matte TD, O'Brien TR: Large community outbreak of cryptosporidiosis due to contamination of a filtered public water supply. N Engl J Med 320:1372-1376, 1989.

68. Hart CA, Baxby D: Cryptosporidiosis in immunocompetent patients [letter]. N Engl J Med 313:1018, 1985.

69. Arnaud-Battandier F, Naciri M, Maurage C: Cryptosporidiosis in immunocompetent patients [letter]. N Engl J Med 313:1019, 1985.

70. Bossen AN, Britt EM: Cryptosporidiosis in immunocompetent patients [letter]. N Engl J Med 313:1019, 1985.

71. Jokipii AMM, Hemila M, Jokipii L: Prospective study of acquisition of *Cryptosporidium, Giardia lamblia* and gastrointestinal illness. Lancet 2:487-489, 1985.

72. Tzipori S, Smith M, Birch C, et al: Cryptosporidiosis in hospital patients with gastroenteritis. Am J Trop Med Hyg 32:931-934, 1983.

73. Soave R, Ma P: Cryptosporidiosis: Traveler's diarrhea in two families. Arch Intern Med 145:70-72, 1985.

74. Jokipii L, Pohjola S, Jokipii AMM: *Cryptosporidium*: A frequent finding in patients with gastrointestinal symptoms. Lancet 2:358-361, 1983.

75. Soave R, Armstrong D: *Cryptosporidium* and cryptosporidiosis. Rev Infect Dis 8:1012-1023, 1986.

76. Current WL: Human cryptosporidiosis [letter]. N Engl J Med 309:1326-1327, 1983.

77. Roberts MG, Green PH, Ma J, et al: Prevalence of cryptosporidiosis in patients undergoing endoscopy: Evidence for an asymptomatic carrier state. Am J Med 87:537-539, 1989.

78. Lefkowitch JH, Krumholz S, Feng-Chen KC, et al: Cryptosporidiosis of the human small intestine: A light and electron microscopic study. Hum Pathol 15:746-752, 1984.

79. Chiampi NP, Sundberg RD, Klompus JP, et al: Cryptosporidial enteritis and *Pneumocystis* pneumonia in a homosexual man. Hum Pathol 14:734-737, 1983.

80. Guarda LA, Stein SA, Cleary KA, Ordonez NGL: Human cryptosporidiosis in the acquired immune deficiency syndrome. Arch Pathol Lab Med 107:562-566, 1983.

81. Weinstein L, Edelstein SM, Madara JL, et al: Intestinal cryptosporidiosis complicated by disseminated cytomegalovirus infection. Gastroenterology 81:584-591, 1981.

82. Modigliani R, Bories C, LeCharpentier Y, et al: Diarrhoea and malabsorption in acquired immune deficiency syndrome: A study of four cases with special emphasis on opportunistic protozoan infestation. Gut 26:179-187, 1985.

83. DeHovitz JA, Pape JW, Boncy M, et al: Clinical manifestations and therapy of *Isospora belli* infection in patients with the acquired immunodeficiency syndrome. N Engl J Med 315:87-90, 1986.

84. Casemore DP, Sands RL, Curry A: *Cryptosporidium* species a "new" human pathogen. J Clin Pathol 38:1321-1336, 1985.

85. Vetterling JM, Takeuchi A, Madden PA: Ultrastructure of *Cryptosporidium wrairi* from the guinea pig. J Protozool 18:248-260, 1971.

86. Marcial MA, Madara JL: *Cryptosporidium*: Cellular localization, structural analysis of absorptive cell-parasite membrane-membrane interactions in guinea pigs, and suggestion of protozoan transport by M cells. Gastroenterology 90:583-594, 1986.

87. Pitlik SD, Fainstein V, Garza D, et al: Human cryptosporidiosis: Spectrum of disease; Report of six cases and review of the literature. Arch Intern Med 143:2269-2275, 1983.

88. Ma P, Soave R: Three-step stool examination for cryptosporidiosis in 10 homosexual men with protracted watery diarrhea. J Infect 147:824-828, 1983.

89. Garcia LS, Bruckner DA, Brewer TC, Shimizu RY: Techniques for the recovery and identification of *Cryptosporidium* oocysts from stool specimens. J Clin Microbiol 18:185-190, 1983.

90. Henriksen SA, Pohlenz JFL: Staining of cryptosporidia by a modified Ziehl-Neelsen technique. Acta Vet Scand 22:594-596, 1981.

91. Nicholas G, Thom BT: Screening for *Cryptosporidium* in stools [letter]. Lancet 1:735, 1984.

92. Trier JS, Moxey PC, Schimmel EM, et al: Chronic

intestinal coccidiosis in man: Intestinal morphology and response to treatment. Gastroenterology 66:923-935, 1974.

93. Restrepo C, Macher AM, Radany EH: Disseminated extraintestinal isosporiasis in a patient with acquired immune deficiency syndrome. Am J Clin Pathol 87:536-542, 1987.

94. Rijpstra AC, Canning EU, Van Ketel RJ, et al: Use of light microscopy to diagnose small intestinal microsporidiosis in patients with AIDS. J Infect Dis 157:827-831, 1988.

95. Orenstein JM, Chiang J, Steinberg W, et al: Intestinal microsporidiosis as a cause of diarrhea in human immunodeficiency virus-infected patients: A report of 20 cases. Hum Pathol 21: 475-481, 1990.

96. Zender HO, Arrigoni E, Eckert J, et al: A case of *Encephalitozoon cuniculi* peritonitis in a patient with AIDS. Am J Clin Pathol 92:352-356, 1989.

97. Bonacini M, Laine L, Martin SE: Viral esophagitis in patients with AIDS. Gastroenterology 96:A50, 1989.

98. Goodell SE, Quinn TC, Mkrtichian E, et al: Herpes simplex virus proctitis in homosexual men: Clinical, sigmoidoscopic and histopathologic features. N Engl J Med 308:868-871, 1983.

99. Siegal FP, Lopez C, Hammer GS, et al: Severe acquired immunodeficiency in male homosexuals, manifested by chronic perianal ulcerative herpes simplex lesions. N Engl J Med 305:1439-1444, 1981.

100. Nichols L, Balogh K, Silverman M: Bacterial infections in the acquired immune deficiency syndrome. Am J Clin Pathol 92:787-790, 1989.

101. Chaisson RE: Infections due to encapsulated bacteria, *Salmonella, Shigella,* and *Campylobacter.* Infect Dis Clin North Am 2(2):475-484, 1988.

102. Kotler DP: Intestinal and hepatic manifestations of AIDS. Adv Intern Med 34:43-72, 1989.

103. Dobbins WO, Weinstein WM: Electron microscopy of the intestine and rectum in acquired immunodeficiency syndrome. Gastroenterology 88:739-749, 1985.

104. Weber JR, Dobbins WO: The intestinal and rectal epithelial lymphocyte in AIDS: An electron-microscopic study. Am J Surg Pathol 10:627-639, 1986.

105. Kotler DP, Weaver SC, Terzakis JA: Ultrastructural features of epithelial cell degeneration in rectal crypts of patients with AIDS. Am J Surg Pathol 10:531-538, 1986.

106. Danzig J, Brandt LJ, Reinus JF, et al: GI malignant neoplasms in patients with AIDS. Gastroenterology 98:A444, 1990.

107. Purtilo DT: Opportunistic cancers in patients with immunodeficiency syndromes. Arch Pathol Lab Med 111:1123-1129, 1987.

108. Friedman SL, Wright TL, Altman DF: Gastrointestinal Kaposi's sarcoma in patients with acquired immunodeficiency syndrome: Endoscopic and autopsy findings. Gastroenterology 89:102-108, 1985.

109. Altman DF: Kaposi's sarcoma: Gastrointestinal manifestations. Front Radiat Ther Oncol 19:123-125, 1985.

110. Digiovanna JJ, Safai B: Kaposi's sarcoma: Retrospective study of 90 cases with particular emphasis on the familial occurrence, ethnic background

and prevalence of other diseases. Am J Med 71: 779-782, 1981.

111. Penn I: Kaposi's sarcoma in organ transplant recipients. Transplantation 27:8-11, 1979.

112. Stribling J, Weitzner S, Smith GV: Kaposi's sarcoma in renal allograft recipients. Cancer 42: 442-446, 1978.

113. Weller IVD: AIDS and the gut. Scand J Gastroenterol 114(suppl):77-89, 1985.

114. Beral V, Peterman TA, Berkelman RL, et al: Kaposi's sarcoma among persons with AIDS: A sexually transmitted infection? Lancet 335(8682): 123-128, 1990.

115. Lifson AR, Darrow WW, Hessol NA, et al: Kaposi's sarcoma in a cohort of homosexual and bisexual men. Am J Epidemiol 131(2):221-231, 1990.

116. McNutt NS, Fletcher V, Conant MA: Early lesions of Kaposi's sarcoma in homosexual men: An ultrastructural comparison with other vascular proliferations in skin. Am J Pathol 111:62-77, 1983.

117. Safai B, Sarngadharan MG, Koziner B, et al: Spectrum of Kaposi's sarcoma in the epidemic of AIDS. Cancer Res 45(suppl):4646-4648, 1985.

118. Leslie W, Templeton A, Braun D: Kaposi's sarcoma in the acquired immune deficiency syndrome. Med Pediatr Oncol 12:336-342, 1984.

119. Saltz RK, Kurtz RC, Lightdale CJ, et al: Kaposi's sarcoma: Gastrointestinal involvement correlation with skin findings and immunologic function. Dig Dis Sci 29:817-823, 1984.

120. Ell C, Matek W, Gramatzki M, et al: Endoscopic findings in a case of Kaposi's sarcoma with involvement of the large and small bowel. Endoscopy 17:161-164, 1985.

121. Bernal A, del Junco GW, Gibson SR: Endoscopic and pathologic features of gastrointestinal Kaposi's sarcoma: A report of four cases in patients with the acquired immune deficiency syndrome. Gastrointest Endosc 31:74-77, 1985.

122. Blumfeld W, Egbert BM, Sagebiel RW: Differential diagnosis of Kaposi's sarcoma. Arch Pathol Lab Med 109:123-127, 1985.

123. Ziegler JL, Beckstead JA, Volberding PA, et al: Non-Hodgkin's lymphoma in 90 homosexual men: Relation to generalized lymphadenopathy and the acquired immunodeficiency syndrome. N Engl J Med 311:565-570, 1984.

124. Unger PD, Strauchen JA: Hodgkin's disease in AIDS complex patients: Report of four cases and tissue immunologic marker studies. Cancer 58:821-825, 1986.

125. Louie S, Daoust PR, Schwartz RS: Immunodeficiency and the pathogenesis of non-Hodgkin's lymphoma. Semin Oncol 7:267-284, 1980.

126. Hanto DW, Frizzera G, Purtilo DT, et al: Clinical spectrum of lymphoproliferative disorders in renal transplant recipients and evidence for the role of Epstein-Barr virus. Cancer Res 41: 4253-4261, 1981.

127. Safai B, Miké V, Giraldo G, et al: Association of Kaposi's sarcoma with second primary malignancies: Possible etiopathogenic implications. Cancer 45:1472-1479, 1980.

128. Levine AM, Gill PS, Muggia F: Malignancies in the acquired immunodeficiency syndrome. Curr Probl Cancer 11:209-255, 1987.

129. Lee MH, Waxman M, Gillooley JF: Primary malignant lymphoma of the anorectum in homosexual men. Dis Colon Rectum 29:413-416, 1986.

130. Ioachim HL, Weinstein MA, Robbins RD, et al: Primary anorectal lymphoma: A new manifestation of AIDS. Cancer 60:1449-1453, 1987.

131. Bernal A, del Junco GW: Endoscopic and pathologic features of esophageal lymphoma: A report of four cases in patients with acquired immune deficiency syndrome. Gastrointest Endosc 32: 96-99, 1986.

132. Friedman SL: Gastrointestinal and hepatobiliary neoplasms in AIDS. Gastroenterol Clin North Am 17:465-486, 1988.

133. Groopman JE, Sullivan JL, Mulder C, et al: Pathogenesis of B-cell lymphoma in a patient with AIDS. Blood 67:612-615, 1986.

134. Cooper HS, Patchefsky AJ, Marks G: Cloacogenic carcinoma of the anorectum in homosexual men: An observation of four cases. Dis Colon Rectum 27:325-330, 1984.

135. Frazer IH, Medley G, Crapper RM, et al: Association between anorectal dysplasia, human papilloma virus and human immunodeficiency virus infection in homosexual men. Lancet 2:657-660, 1986.

136. Nash G, Allen W, Nash S: Atypical lesions of the anal mucosa in homosexual men. JAMA 256:873-876, 1986.

137. Daling JR, Weiss NS, Hislop TG, et al: Sexual practices, sexually transmitted diseases and the incidence of anal cancer. N Engl J Med 317: 973-977, 1987.

138. Croxson T, Chabon AB, Rorat E, et al: Intraepithelial carcinoma of the anus in homosexual men. Dis Colon Rectum 27:325-330, 1984.

139. Gal AA, Saul SH, Stoler MH: In situ hybridization analysis of human papillomavirus in anal squamous cell carcinoma. Mod Pathol 2:439-443, 1989.

140. Palmer M, Braly LF, Schaffner F: The liver in acquired immune deficiency disease. Semin Liver Dis 7:192-202, 1987.

141. Lebovics E, Dworkin BM, Heier SK, et al: The hepatobiliary manifestations of human immunodeficiency virus infection. Am J Gastroenterol 83:1-7, 1988.

142. Gordon SC, Reddy KR, Gould EE, et al: The spectrum of liver disease in the acquired immunodeficiency syndrome. J Hepatol 2:475-484, 1986.

143. Glasgow BJ, Anders K, Layfield LJ, et al: Clinical and pathologic findings of the liver in the acquired immune deficiency syndrome (AIDS). Am J Clin Pathol 83:582-588, 1985.

144. Dworkin BM, Stahl RE, Giardina MA, et al: The liver in acquired immune deficiency syndrome: Emphasis on patients with intravenous drug abuse. Am J Gastroenterol 82:231-236, 1987.

145. Schneiderman DJ, Arenson DM, Cello JP, et al: Hepatic disease in patients with the acquired immune deficiency syndrome (AIDS). Hepatology 7:925-930, 1987.

146. Housset C, Boucher O, Girard PM, et al: Immunohistochemical evidence for human immunodeficiency virus-1 infection of the liver Kupffer cells. Hum Pathol 21:404-408, 1990.

147. Hoda S, Gerber MA: Immunohistochemical studies of human immunodeficiency virus type 1 (HIV-1)

148. Scoazec JY, Marche C, Girard PM, et al: Peliosis hepatis and sinusoidal dilatation during infection by the human immunodeficiency virus (HIV). Am J Pathol 131:38-47, 1988.

149. Kingsley LA, Rinaldo CR, Lyter DW: Sexual transmission efficiency of hepatitis B virus and human immunodeficiency virus among homosexual men. JAMA 264:230-234, 1990.

150. Li XM, Jeffers LJ, Reddy KR, et al: Viral infections of liver in AIDS patients evaluated by in situ hybridization. Gastroenterology 98:A459, 1990.

151. Terada S, Reddy KR, Jeffers LJ, et al: Microsporidian hepatitis in the acquired immunodeficiency syndrome. Ann Intern Med 107:61-62, 1987.

152. Hagopian WA, Huseby JS: *Pneumocystis* hepatitis and choroiditis despite successful aerosolized pentamidine pulmonary prophylaxis. Chest 96: 949-951, 1989.

153. Schneiderman DJ: Hepatobiliary abnormalities of AIDS. Gastroenterol Clin North Am 17:615-630, 1988.

154. Jacobson MA, Cello JP, Sande MA: Cholestasis and disseminated cytomegalovirus disease in patients with the acquired immunodeficiency syndrome. Am J Med 84:218-224, 1987.

155. Schneiderman DJ, Cello JP, Laing FC: Papillary stenosis and sclerosing cholangitis in the acquired immunodeficiency syndrome. Ann Intern Med 106:546-549, 1987.

156. Margulis SJ, Honig CL, Soave R, et al: Biliary tract obstruction in the acquired immunodeficiency syndrome. Ann Intern Med 105:207-210, 1986.

157. Roulot D, Valla D, Brun-Vezinet F, et al: Cholangitis in the acquired immunodeficiency syndrome: Report of two cases and review of the literature. Gut 28:1653-1660, 1987.

158. Viteri AL, Greene JF: Bile duct abnormalities in the acquired immune deficiency syndrome. Gastroenterology 92:2014-2018, 1987.

159. Sieratzki J, Thung SN, Gerber MA, et al: Major histocompatibility antigen expression in the liver in acquired immunodeficiency syndrome. Arch Pathol Lab Med 111:1045-1049, 1987.

160. Prego V, Glatt AE, Roy V, et al: Liver biopsy is the most rapid method for detecting occult mycobacterial infection in patients infected with the human immunodeficiency virus (HIV). Gastroenterology 96:A399, 1989.

161. Theise ND, Rotterdam H, Dieterich D: The role of liver biopsy in AIDS. Gastroenterology 96:A668, 1989.

162. Schwartz MS, Brandt LJ: The spectrum of pancreatic disorders in patients with the acquired immune deficiency syndrome. Am J Gastroenterol 84:459-462, 1989.

163. Dowell SF, Moore GW, Hutchins GM: The spectrum of pancreatic pathology in patients with AIDS. Mod Pathol 3:49-53, 1990.

164. Lambert JS, Seidlin M, Reichman RC, et al: 2',3'-Dideoxyinosine (ddI) in patients with the acquired immunodeficiency syndrome or AIDS-related complex:. A phase 1 trial. N Engl J Med 322:1333-1340, 1990.

in liver tissues of patients with AIDS [abstract]. Am J Clin Pathol 93:452, 1985.

10

CARDIOVASCULAR SYSTEM

MICHAEL C. FISHBEIN AND JIAN-HUA QIAO

Cardiac abnormalities are found at autopsy in two thirds of patients with AIDS,[1] and more than 150 reports of cardiac complications in AIDS patients have been published. Yet the majority of AIDS patients die of noncardiac causes. As control of noncardiac infectious and neoplastic complications improves and survival time of AIDS patients lengthens, more cardiac complications are emerging. Based on reported morbidity rates of 6% to 7% and mortality rates of 1% to 6%, Anderson and Virmani[2] have estimated that during the next few years clinical heart disease will develop in between 2860 and 5032 AIDS patients in the United States. As many as 3465 AIDS patients may die of cardiac complications each year. In this chapter we review the cardiac lesions observed in AIDS and discuss their clinical significance (Table 10–1).

PERICARDIUM

Neoplasms

Two neoplasms associated with AIDS may involve the pericardial tissues: Kaposi's sarcoma and lymphoma. Kaposi's sarcoma most often involves the visceral pericardium with multifocal infiltrates in the epicardial adipose tissue. These neoplastic nodules are often perivascular and closely associated with the adventitia of muscular arteries (Fig. 10–1). The adventitia of the aorta and main pulmonary artery may be involved. In one patient reported by Cammarosano and Lewis[3] the sarcoma had infiltrated a branch of the left

Table 10–1. Cardiac Lesions in AIDS

I. Pericardial lesions
  A. Neoplasms
    1. Kaposi's sarcoma
    2. Lymphoma
  B. Pericarditis
    1. Infective
      a. Common bacteria
      b. *Mycobacterium avium* or *M. tuberculosis*
      c. Actinomycetales (*Nocardia asteroides*)
      d. Fungi
      e. Viruses
    2. Nonspecific
  C. Pericardial effusion
    1. Heart failure
    2. Nonspecific
II. Myocardial lesions
  A. Neoplasms
    1. Kaposi's sarcoma
    2. Lymphoma
  B. Myocarditis
    1. Infective
      a. Viruses: HIV(?), cytomegalovirus, and others
      b. Bacteria
      c. Fungi
      d. Protozoa: *Toxoplasma gondii*
    2. Nonspecific: inflammation with or without necrosis
      a. Infectious
      b. Autoimmune
      c. Toxic
  C. Myocardial necrosis without inflammation
    1. Catecholamines
    2. Toxins
    3. Vascular lesions: arteriopathy, arteritis, thromboemboli
  D. Dilated cardiomyopathy
III. Endocardial lesions
  A. Nonbacterial thrombotic endocarditis
  B. Infective endocarditis
    1. Bacteria
    2. Fungi

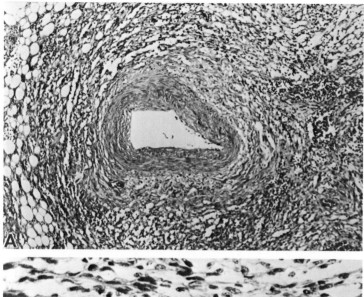

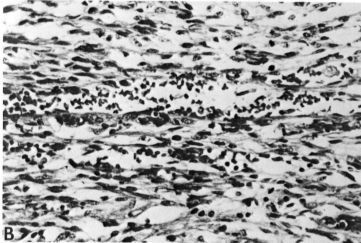

Figure 10–1. Kaposi's sarcoma in epicardial adipose tissue. *A,* Perivascular localization. *B,* Characteristic erythrocyte-filled vascular spaces with intervening spindle cells. (Hematoxylin and eosin; *A,* ×40; *B,* ×160.)

anterior descending coronary artery. When Kaposi's sarcoma involves the epicardial tissues, the neoplasm is usually widely disseminated. Myocardial neoplasm is often present. Although cardiac involvement is rarely detected by clinical assessment, we have seen one patient with clinical and pathologic evidence of constrictive pericardial disease resulting from Kaposi's sarcoma (Fig. 10–1). Tamponade has been observed infrequently.[2] The greatest frequency of pericardial Kaposi's sarcoma reported is the series of Silver et al.,[4] who found it in 28% of cases (5 of 18).

Malignant lymphomas in AIDS are primarily high-grade, B-cell proliferations, histologically of Burkitt or immunoblastic cell types.[5] They may involve the pericardium as distinct nodules or diffuse infiltrates. As with other neoplasms involving the pericardium, clinical manifestations may or may not be present.

The findings are nonspecific and often limited to asymptomatic pericardial effusions, which may be hemorrhagic.

Pericarditis

The pericardium is the most common site of cardiac infection in AIDS, with reports of fungal, bacterial, and viral pathogens.[2] Opportunistic organisms such as *Mycobacterium avium-intracellulare,*[6] *Cryptococcus neoformans,* and Actinomycetales *(Nocardia asteroides),*[7] as well as more common bacteria and viruses, have been grown on cultures of pericardial fluid. Although one might expect *Mycobacterium tuberculosis* to be a common pathogen in AIDS patients, pericardial involvement is relatively infrequent and occurs in patients with disseminated tuberculosis.[8,9]

Pericardial Effusion

Much more common than neoplasm or infection of the pericardium is a nonspecific pericardial effusion, which may be accompanied by inflammation. Pericardial effusions detected by echocardiography have been reported in as much as 40% of adult AIDS patients[10]; in larger series of adults and children they have been found in an average of 25% to 30% of cases studied.[11-13] Among asymptomatic adults with HIV, 25% have echocardiographic evidence of pericardial effusion. In a large autopsy series of 115 cases, Lewis[14] reported a 59% frequency in patients with other cardiac lesions and an overall frequency of 30% of cases. Most of these patients had cultures negative for organisms and no evidence of neoplasm. Pericardial effusion is seen in patients with chronic lung disease and dilatation of the right side of the heart, so is often assumed to be related to right-sided heart failure. Pericardial effusion with tamponade, constrictive pericarditis, or both has been implicated as the cause of death in 9.5% of AIDS patients thought to have died of cardiac causes.[2]

MYOCARDIUM

Neoplasms

Although Kaposi's sarcoma most often involves the pericardial layer of the heart, myocardial involvement also occurs with extensive myocardial infiltration manifest clinically as cardiomegaly, sinus tachycardia, and a "gallop rhythm." The data reported suggest that AIDS patients with cardiac Kaposi's sarcoma are more likely to have clinical manifestations of pericardial disease than myocardial disease.

Malignant lymphoma is one of the more common neoplasms to metastasize to the heart[15] in patients with and without HIV-related diseases. Primary lymphomas of the heart are rare, comprising approximately 5% of primary cardiac neoplasms. There are few cases of purported primary cardiac lymphomas in AIDS patients.[16,17]

Most neoplasms of the heart are clinically inapparent. The most common abnormality is sinus tachycardia, which is too nonspecific to be of diagnostic value, especially in AIDS patients who may be tachycardic secondary to infection. Pericardial effusion and heart failure are also nonspecific. The sudden appearance of heart block is less common but strongly suggests cardiac involvement by neoplasm.

Myocarditis and Myocardial Necrosis Without Inflammation

Almost any agent that can cause disseminated infection in AIDS patients may involve the myocardium. Clinical evidence of cardiac disease is usually overshadowed by manifestations of involvement of other organs, primarily the brain or lungs. Opportunistic organisms, such as *Toxoplasma gondii* and *Cryptococcus neoformans*, which rarely cause myocarditis in immunocompetent hosts, are common pathogens in AIDS myocarditis (Fig. 10–2). Common viruses, such as Coxsackie B and cytomegalovirus (CMV) with inclusions, have also been reported.[18,19] The absence of the characteristic inclusions may not rule out CMV infection, since in situ hybridization studies suggest that some infected cells do not have them. The interpretation of these findings is complicated by the fact that CMV may be present without necessarily being the cause of pathologic changes which are present.

Far more common in AIDS than infectious myocarditis is nonspecific lymphocytic myocarditis, which is present in more than 40% of autopsy cases in some series (Fig. 10–3).[20] In 80% of patients with lymphocytic myocarditis, however, no etiologic agent is identified. If both necrosis and inflammation are present, often *T. gondii* infection can be proved. An intriguing, unanswered question is whether HIV directly infects myocardial fibers and causes myocardial injury. HIV, its protein components, or both have been demonstrated by culture, in situ hybridization, and Southern blot test in hearts of AIDS patients with and without cardiac abnormalities. Initially, studies found evidence of HIV only in inflammatory cells. HIV-1 DNA has been identified in three hearts of patients with AIDS by Southern blot techniques.[21] More recently, HIV proteins, p17, p24, and gp 120/160 have been detected by monoclonal antibodies in myocardial fibers from nine patients.[1] Six of these patients died of cardiac complications. All nine had large amounts of protein. Establishing a causal relationship between the presence of viral proteins and myocardial dysfunction is obviously complex and remains under investigation.

Sometimes myocardial necrosis without inflammation is observed in the hearts of

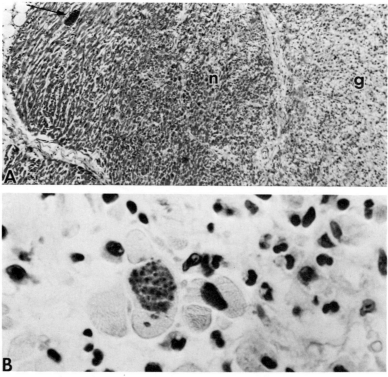

Figure 10–2. *Toxoplasma gondii* myocarditis. *A,* Broad zones of granulation tissue *(g)* and necrosis *(n),* with a cyst containing bradyzoites *(arrow)* in adjacent normal myocardium. *B,* In another patient, cyst surrounded by inflammatory cell infiltrate. (Hematoxylin and eosin; *A,* ×16, *B,* ×256.)

AIDS patients. The differential diagnosis includes infection in a lymphopenic host, "catecholamine-induced" necrosis in a stressed individual,[22] toxic injury caused by a drug,[23] specific vascular lesions, or generalized hypotension or hypoxia leading to myocardial necrosis. Solving this conundrum requires detailed knowledge of the patient's clinical history and familiarity with drugs to which the patient may have been exposed. Agents currently used in the treatment of AIDS are not known to cause myocardial necrosis. Doxorubicin (Adriamycin), which has been used to treat Kaposi's sarcoma, and the immunosuppressive agent cyclophosphamide (Cytoxan) may cause myocardial injury and cardiomyopathy. Cocaine abuse, common in our society and among AIDS patients, can lead to cardiomyopathy with myocardial necrosis.[23] As new drugs are developed and tested in AIDS patients, possible injury to the heart and other organs will have to be considered. For example, in three AIDS patients with Kaposi's sarcoma, reversible cardiac dysfunction was related to interferon alfa therapy.[24]

Cardiomyopathy

Cardiomegaly is a common autopsy finding in AIDS patients. Right-sided dilatation is expected, since many patients die with pulmonary hypertension secondary to parenchymal disease. Biventricular or four-chamber dilatation without histologic abnormalities is known to occur with sepsis and perhaps accompanies chronic hypoxia of the myocardium.

In addition to these nonspecific findings, a dilated cardiomyopathy seems to be associated with HIV-related disease.[25] Himelman et al.[26] documented left ventricular dilatation and hypokinesia by echocardiography in 8 of 70 AIDS patients studied. Accumulated data indicate that approximately 25% of AIDS patients have otherwise unexplained myocardial dysfunction.[25-31] Dilated cardiomyopathy has also been observed in congenital AIDS.[30,31] Cardiomyopathy usually becomes manifest late in the course of AIDS; accordingly, evidence of myocardial dysfunction has ominous implications, with 50% of adult patients dying within 6 months.[26]

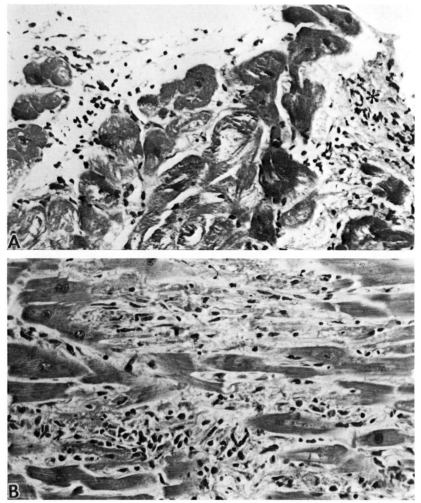

Figure 10–3. Nonspecific myocarditis in AIDS. *A,* Nonspecific lymphocytic myocarditis with fibrosis *(asterisk). B,* Nonspecific myocarditis with myocardial necrosis. (Hematoxylin and eosin, × 160.)

AIDS-related dilated cardiomyopathy is clinically and pathologically similar to other idiopathic forms.[2] Patients show evidence of heart failure, arrhythmias, or both. At autopsy the heart weight may be increased; the degree of dilatation varies. Histologic findings include hypertrophy and atrophy of myocardial fibers, myocytolysis, and interstitial and replacement fibrosis of varying severity. A minority of patients with the clinical diagnosis of idiopathic dilated cardiomyopathy have nonspecific myocarditis or some identifiable pathogen in the heart. Dilated cardiomyopathy is reported to be the cause of death in as much as one third of AIDS patients dying of heart disease.[2] Cardiac dysfunction is also common in the pediatric population with AIDS. Stewart et al.[30] reported decreased left ventricular function detected by echocardiography in 20% of patients studied (8 of 40). Two had frank dilated cardiomyopathy at autopsy. Lipshultz et al.[31] studied 31 pediatric AIDS patients prospectively with two-dimensional echocardiography and found diminished contractility in 26%, including four patients with symptomatic dilated cardiomyopathy. Four patients had high-grade atrial or ventricular ectopy as well. In the preceding studies some patients had autopsy evidence of myocarditis.

Proposed pathogenetic mechanisms for dilated cardiomyopathy in AIDS patients include viral disease, autoimmune disease (possibly postviral), drugs, or nutritional deficits such as vitamin or selenium deficiency. None of these has been established as the cause.

ENDOCARDIUM

Nonbacterial Thrombotic Endocarditis

Nonbacterial thrombotic endocarditis (NBTE), or marantic endocarditis, associated with wasting diseases, malignancies, and hypercoagulable states, is the endocardial lesion most common in AIDS patients. Although all four cardiac valves may be involved, right-sided lesions are reportedly more common, perhaps related to indwelling catheters.[2] In non-AIDS patients, left-sided lesions are more common.[32] As in other disorders, the lesions are small, friable, easily detachable valvular vegetations composed primarily of platelets and fibrin, with few erythrocytes and leukocytes present. Although characterized as nondestructive, these lesions do organize, with granulation tissue proliferation and fibrosis in the underlying valve leaflet (Fig. 10–4). Echocardiographic recognition of even small vegetations is possible,[33] but relatively few lesions have been detected during life. Embolization occurs, and death has been attributed to systemic thromboembolism from NBTE in three AIDS patients.[2]

Infective Endocarditis

AIDS patients have multiple risk factors for infective endocarditis. Some AIDS patients are known users of injectable illicit drugs. Many, when hospitalized, have indwelling catheters. AIDS patients commonly have multiple infections that can lead to sepsis and seeding of heart valves. Underlying NBTE, with endothelial injury, may predispose patients to an infected vegetation. Last

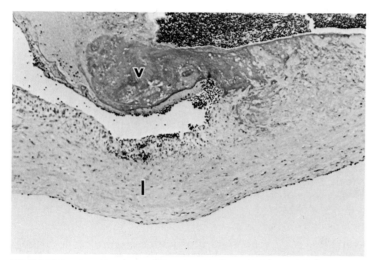

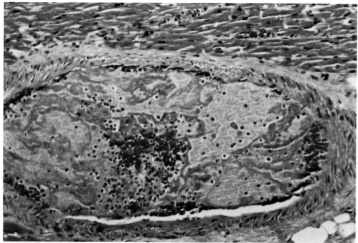

Figure 10–4. Nonbacterial thrombotic endocarditis. *A*, Mitral valve leaflet *(l)* with organizing bland vegetation *(v)*. *B*, Intramyocardial arterial embolus. (Hematoxylin and eosin; *A*, ×40; *B*, ×64.)

and most important, by definition all AIDS patients are immunosuppressed. Thus it is surprising that infectious endocarditis has not been a more prominent finding in AIDS. There are reports of healed lesions, which could be of bacterial or nonbacterial origin, and one case report of pulmonary *Aspergillus fumigatus* infection with mitral valve endocarditis, myocardial abscesses, and cerebral embolization.[34] Clinical features of endocarditis in AIDS patients are similar to those in other patients, except perhaps for involvement of a greater variety of more unusual organisms because of profound immunosuppression in AIDS patients.

VASCULAR LESIONS

Most vascular lesions occurring in AIDS have been in children and have been described as arteriopathy, with or without aneurysm formation, a fibrocalcific lesion, and thrombosis of the coronary arteries.[35-37] Arteritis or periarteritis may be present.[37] Calabrese et al.[36] reviewed 14 cases of arteritis in AIDS patients. Most of these were angiocentric lymphoid proliferations. Vascular involvement was greater in peripheral muscle than in viscera. The pathogenesis of vascular inflammation and destruction is unknown. Direct HIV infection seems unlikely. Autoimmune mechanisms, infection (mycotic aneurysm), and drug effects are more plausible etiologic agents. Besides therapeutic agents, illicit drugs such as cocaine can cause coronary arteritis with thrombosis.[23]

OTHER LESIONS

AIDS patients may have non-AIDS-related cardiovascular disease. We have seen two apparently well HIV-positive patients die suddenly. One, a 31-year-old man with a strong family history of coronary artery disease and hypercholesterolemia, died of acute thrombotic occlusion of a severely atherosclerotic coronary artery. The second, a 35-year-old man with no stigmata of Marfan's disease, died of cardiac tamponade secondary to an aortic dissection with rupture into the pericardial sac. He had cystic medial necrosis of the aorta. Active rheumatic heart disease with Aschoff nodules has been reported in one AIDS patient.[38] As the AIDS epidemic expands, more patients with coexisting unrelated diseases will appear.

CLINICAL SYNDROMES OF CARDIAC INVOLVEMENT IN AIDS

Knowing the spectrum of diseases that can affect the heart in AIDS is useful in pathologic evaluation of specimens from HIV-positive patients.

Pericarditis, Tamponade, and Constriction

In some series, pericardial disease is the most common cardiac problem in AIDS patients.[39] Patients with pericardial disease may have neoplasm (Kaposi's sarcoma or lymphoma), infection, nonspecific pericarditis, or simple effusion. If pericardiocentesis is performed, fluid should be cultured for organisms and sent for cytologic examination. The fluid should be stained with an India ink preparation if *Cryptococcus* infection is suspected. If the patient has lymphocytosis, lymphocyte marker studies of the fluid may yield the diagnosis of lymphoma. If the pericarditis is nonspecific or right-sided heart failure causes effusion, studies of the fluid show no abnormalities; this is usually the case.

Myocardial Dysfunction

Subclinical (detected by echocardiography) or clinical (manifest as heart failure) myocardial dysfunction may be related to a variety of disorders. Myocardial dysfunction secondary to coronary artery disease, valvular disease, or congenital malformations should be ruled out by clinical studies. A myocardial biopsy may detect infiltrative neoplastic or infectious diseases.[40] Lymphoma and lymphocytic myocarditis are easily confused, but lymphocyte marker studies should help to differentiate them. The infections most likely to be apparent on biopsy are *T. gondii* and CMV. The most common finding, however, is lymphocytic myocarditis unaccompanied by necrosis of myocytes. Degenerative changes, such as vacuolization or necrosis without inflammation, should suggest drug-related injury to the myocardium. If the patient has dilated cardiomyopathy, nonspecific hypertrophy, atrophy, or fibrosis may be present. If the heart failure is secondary to sepsis or pulmonary disease (cor pulmonale), the myocardial biopsy findings are normal.

Endocarditis

The symptoms and signs of infective endocarditis in AIDS patients are similar to those in non-AIDS patients. NBTE is rarely diagnosed clinically, although two-dimensional echocardiography has made this feasible.[33] Stroke, myocardial infarction, or some other thromboembolic event may be the first, and perhaps a fatal, manifestation of NBTE.

Arrhythmias and Conduction Abnormalities

An AIDS patient with arrhythmias may have pericardial, myocardial, endocardial, or no anatomic cardiac disease. The nature of the arrhythmia and other clinical findings are crucial in unraveling the pathogenesis of the arrhythmia. In AIDS patients who have ventricular tachycardia or have undergone sudden death, idiopathic myocarditis, infectious myocarditis (*T. gondii* and *M. tuberculosis*), and cardiac lymphoma have been found.[2] Bharati et al.[37] performed detailed postmortem histologic studies of the conduction system and hearts of six pediatric AIDS patients born to intravenous drug addicts. All hearts had degenerative vascular changes, including fibrosis, calcification, or intimal or medial proliferation. Perivascular lymphocytic infiltrates were also present. The conduction system sections showed angiitis, myocarditis, or fragmentation of the bundle of His with fibrosis. In only one had electrocardiography shown an abnormal, left hemiblock. Conduction problems may be related to inflammatory or neoplastic infiltrates. Electromechanical dissociation is classically associated with cardiac tamponade. If arrhythmias have no anatomic cause, they may be due to generalized hypoxia, electrolyte imbalance, or sepsis.

CONCLUSION

The number of AIDS patients with cardiac abnormalities at autopsy greatly exceeds the number with significant cardiac disease during life. However, as the AIDS epidemic progresses and other complications are better controlled, cardiovascular disorders may assume importance in a greater percentage of patients. In addition, AIDS may provide the opportunity to gain insights into the pathogenesis of little-understood cardiac diseases such as lymphocytic myocarditis and dilated cardiomyopathy.

REFERENCES

1. Cotton P: AIDS giving rise to cardiac problems. JAMA 263:2149, 1990.
2. Anderson DW, Virmani R: Emerging patterns of heart disease in human immunodeficiency virus infection. Hum Pathol 21:253-259, 1990.
3. Cammarosano C, Lewis W: Cardiac lesions in acquired immune deficiency syndrome (AIDS). J Am Coll Cardiol 5:703-706, 1985.
4. Silver MA, Macher AM, Reichert CM, et al: Cardiac involvement by Kaposi's sarcoma in acquired immune deficiency syndrome. Am J Cardiol 53:983-985, 1984.
5. Ziegler J, Beckstead J, Volberding P, et al: Non-Hodgkin's lymphoma in 90 homosexual men: Relation to generalized lymphadenopathy in the acquired immunodeficiency syndrome. N Engl J Med 311:565-570, 1984.
6. Woods GL, Goldsmith JC: Fatal pericarditis due to *Mycobacterium avium-intracellulare* in acquired immunodeficiency syndrome. Chest 95:1355-1357, 1989.
7. Holtz HA, Lavery DP, Kapila R: *Actinomycetales* infection in the acquired immunodeficiency syndrome. Ann Intern Med 102:203-205, 1985.
8. Sunderam G, McDonald RJ, Maniatis T, et al: Tuberculosis as a manifestation of the acquired immunodeficiency syndrome (AIDS). JAMA 256:362-366, 1986.
9. Dalli E, Quesadda A, Juan G, et al: Tuberculous pericarditis as the first manifestation of acquired immunodeficiency syndrome. Am Heart J 114:905-906, 1987.
10. Fink L, Reichek N, Sutton M: Cardiac abnormalities in acquired immune deficiency syndrome. Am J Cardiol 54:1161-1163, 1984.
11. Reilly JM, Cunnion RE, Anderson DW: Frequency of myocarditis, left ventricular dysfunction and ventricular tachycardia in the acquired immunodeficiency syndrome. Am J Cardiol 62:789-793, 1988.
12. Hecht S, Berger M, Tosh A, Croxson S: Unsuspected cardiac abnormalities in the acquired immune deficiency syndrome. Chest 96:805-808, 1989.
13. Corolla S, Mutinelli M, Moroni M, et al: Echocardiography detects myocardial damage in AIDS: Prospective study in 102 patients. Eur Heart J 9:887-892, 1988.
14. Lewis W: AIDS: Cardiac findings from 115 autopsies. Prog Cardiovasc Dis 32:207-215, 1989.
15. Roberts WC, Glancy DL, DeVita VT Jr: Heart in malignant lymphoma (Hodgkin's disease, lymphosarcoma, reticulum cell sarcoma and mycosis fungoides): A study of 196 autopsy cases. Am J Cardiol 22:85-107, 1968.
16. Constatino A, West TE, Gupta M, Loghmanee F: Primary cardiac lymphoma in a patient with acquired immune deficiency syndrome. Cancer 60:2801-2805, 1987.
17. Guarner J, Brynes RK, Wing CC, et al: Primary non-Hodgkin's lymphoma of the heart in two patients with the acquired immunodeficiency syndrome. Arch Pathol Lab Med 111:254-256, 1987.

18. Wink KI, Schmitz H: Cytomegalovirus myocarditis. Am Heart J 100:667-672, 1980.

19. Wilson R, Morris T, Rossel R Jr: Cytomegalovirus myocarditis. Br Heart J 34:856-858, 1982.

20. Anderson D, Virmani R, Reilly J, et al: Prevalent myocarditis at necropsy in the acquired immunodeficiency syndrome. J Am Coll Cardiol 11:792-799, 1988.

21. Flomenbaum M, Soeiro R, Udem SA, et al: Proliferative membranopathy and human immundeficiency virus in AIDS hearts. J AIDS 2:129-135, 1989.

22. Cebelin MS, Hirsch CS: Human stress cardiomyopathy: Myocardial lesions in victims of homicidal assaults without internal injuries. Hum Pathol 11:123-132, 1980.

23. Chokshi SK, Moore R, Pandian NG, Isner JM: Reversible cardiomyopathy associated with cocaine intoxication. Ann Intern Med 111:1039-1040, 1989.

24. Deyton LR, Walker RE, Kovacs JA, et al: Reversible cardiac dysfunction associated with interferon alfa therapy in AIDS patients with Kaposi's sarcoma. N Engl J Med 321:1246-1249, 1989.

25. Cohen IS, Anderson DW, Virmani R, et al: Congestive cardiomyopathy in association with the acquired immunodeficiency syndrome. N Engl J Med 315:628-630, 1986.

26. Himelman R, Chung W, Chernoff D, et al: Cardiac manifestations of human immunodeficiency virus infection: A two-dimensional echocardiographic study. J Am Coll Cardiol 13:1030-1036, 1989.

27. Levy WS, Simon GL, Rios JC: Prevalence of cardiac abnormalities in human immunodeficiency virus infection. Am J Cardiol 63:86-89, 1989.

28. Raffanti S, Chiaramida A, Sen P, et al: Assessment of cardiac function in patients with acquired immunodeficiency syndrome. Chest 93:592-594, 1988.

29. LaFont A, Darwiche H, Sayegh F, et al: At which stage of human immunodeficiency virus infection is echocardiography useful in diagnosing cardiac injury? Circulation 1988;78(suppl II):II-458.

30. Stewart JM, Kaul A, Gromisch DS, et al: Symptomatic cardiac dysfunction in children with human immunodeficiency virus infection. Am Heart J 117:140-144, 1989.

31. Lipshultz SE, Chanock S, Sanders SP, et al: Cardiovascular manifestations of human immunodeficiency virus infection in infants and children. Am J Cardiol 63:1489-1497, 1989.

32. Lopez JA, Ross RS, Fishbein MC, Siegel RJ: Nonbacterial thrombotic endocarditis: A review. Am Heart J 113:773-784, 1987.

33. Lopez JA, Fishbein MC, Siegel RJ: Echocardiographic features of nonbacterial thrombotic endocarditis. Am J Cardiol 59:478-480, 1987.

34. Henochowicz S, Mustafa M, Laivrinson WE, et al: Cardiac aspergillosis in acquired immune deficiency syndrome. Am J Cardiol 55:1239-1240, 1985.

35. Joshi VV, Pawel B, Connor E, et al: Arteriopathy in children with acquired immune deficiency syndrome. Pediatr Pathol 7:261-275, 1987.

36. Calabrese LH, Estes M, Yen-Lieberman B, et al: Systemic vasculitis in association with human immunodeficiency virus infection. Arthritis Rheum 32:569-576, 1989.

37. Bharati S, Joshi VV, Connor EM, et al: Conduction system in children with acquired immunodeficiency syndrome. Chest 96:406-413, 1989.

38. DiCarlo FJ, Anderson DW, Virmani R, et al: Rheumatic heart disease in a patient with acquired immunodeficiency syndrome. Hum Pathol 20:917-920, 1989.

39. Krumholz H, Cheitlin M: Cardiac disease in persons with acquired immunodeficiency syndrome. Clin Cardiol 3:249-252, 1990.

40. Andress JD, Polish LB, Clark DM, Hossack KF: Transvenous biopsy diagnosis of cardiac lymphoma in an AIDS patient. Am Heart J 118:421-423, 1989.

11

PATHOLOGY OF THE KIDNEYS

Arthur H. Cohen and Cynthia C. Nast

Lesions of the kidneys in HIV-infected patients are extremely varied in pathogenesis, pathology, and clinical significance.[8,10,11,22,27,29,38,45,50,52,56,60,69,70] The abnormalities may result from such widely diverse mechanisms as disseminated opportunistic infections and neoplasms, effects of therapeutic agents and hemodynamic alterations, immunologic abnormalities, and perhaps direct HIV infection of renal cells. In this chapter we consider the various diseases and address pathogenesis or morphogenesis when known. Some of the lesions are discovered at autopsy and have little direct clinical significance, some are the effects of nephrotoxic therapeutic agents and are also encountered in postmortem examinations, and some have profound clinical manifestations and are often diagnosed by renal biopsy during life. The renal lesion known as HIV-associated nephropathy may be the initial manifestation of HIV infection.

HIV-ASSOCIATED NEPHROPATHY

In 1984 three independent reports described a glomerulopathy in patients with AIDS. Rao et al.[55] from Downstate Medical Center in Brooklyn, Pardo et al.[51] from the University of Miami, and Gardenswartz et al.[27] from Lenox Hill Hospital in New York all found that some AIDS patients have heavy proteinuria associated with a glo-

merular lesion, focal and segmental glomerulosclerosis. Although this was initially termed AIDS-associated focal and segmental glomerulosclerosis or AIDS-associated nephropathy, it is now known that the tubules and interstitium may also be abnormal in this disorder and that it can occur in HIV-infected individuals without manifestations of AIDS or AIDS-related complex (ARC).[11,17,18,24] Hence most workers in this field now prefer the term "HIV-associated nephropathy."[11,15,17,18,24,29,37,65] The clinical characteristics include heavy proteinuria, often with features of the nephrotic syndrome, and rapid evolution to end-stage renal failure.[11,15,29] Hypertension is uncommon.

Many other glomerular lesions with heavy proteinuria have been reported in HIV-infected patients (see later discussion), including immune complex–mediated glomerulonephritides such as membranous glomerulonephritis or membranoproliferative glomerulonephritis.[29,30] Unfortunately, some investigators have termed all proteinuria-producing glomerulopathies "HIV-associated nephropathy."[58] This has led to confusion concerning classification and pathogenesis of the diverse group of glomerular lesions. For the sake of clarity we use the term "HIV-associated nephropathy" to refer only to the renal lesion characterized by focal and segmental glomerulosclerosis with accompanying tubular and interstitial damage and ultrastructural peculiarities.[29] We refer to the other glomerular disorders by their usual designation, such as membranous glomerulonephritis.

HIV-associated nephropathy has been observed in many cities in the United States and throughout the world. As of late 1990, this lesion had been reported in New York,[15,16,24,27,42,55] Miami,[11,15] Detroit,[54] Boston,[1] Los Angeles,[18] Newark,[22] San Francisco,[45] Washington, D.C.,[14] and Cincinnati,[29]; in addition, we are aware of unreported cases in Pittsburgh, San Diego, Kansas City, Rochester, N.Y., and Philadelphia.[29] Other countries where HIV-associated nephropathy has been observed include Canada,[50] Brazil, Trinidad,[29] Mexico,[34] Spain,[11] Italy,[28] France,[25] and Senegal.[35] The majority of cases are from the New York metropolitan area. Over 200 cases have been formally reported and probably considerably more exist. More than 95% of reported cases are in blacks, although blacks constitute a much smaller percentage of HIV-infected patients in the United States.[9,11] Presumably this racial predilection explains the rarity of the lesion in San Francisco, where the majority of HIV-infected patients are white.[37] Although perhaps as much as 50% of the U.S. patients are intravenous drug abusers, the remainder of the patients acquired HIV infection by other means, including maternal-fetal transmission, receipt of infected transfused blood, and heterosexual or male homosexual transmission. All age groups are affected, and most patients are male.[11,29]

At the time renal dysfunction becomes apparent, patients may have any manifestation of infection with HIV: AIDS, ARC, or the carrier state.[11,18,29] However, because clinicians now have greater knowledge of HIV-associated nephropathy and its typical presentation with heavy proteinuria, progressive renal insufficiency, and enlarged kidneys, patients with AIDS or ARC rarely undergo renal biopsy for diagnostic purposes.[24,29] Most biopsies for the diagnosis of this disorder are performed in patients not previously known to be infected with HIV. Because of the characteristic morphologic features in the kidney tissue, the pathologist can recommend a determination of the patient's HIV status.[18,24,52] Although there is no effective therapy for the kidney disorder, early reports have indicated that azidothymidine (AZT) may slow progression to end-stage renal failure.[25]

Gross examination at autopsy indicates the kidneys to be normal or bilaterally enlarged,

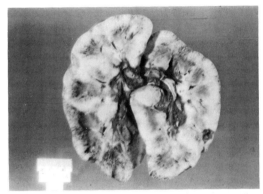

Figure 11–1. Gross appearance of HIV-associated nephropathy. Kidney is enlarged; cortex is pale.

even in patients with end-stage renal disease.[10,11,24,52,53] In the series of Pardo et al.[52,53] the mean two-kidney weight in 18 patients was 487 g. The capsular surfaces are smooth, and the parenchyma is pale (Fig. 11–1). Small cysts may be observed at the corticomedullary junction.[52] Although concomitant infections and neoplasms have been observed at postmortem examination in some series,[24] this has not been a regular finding in HIV-associated nephropathy.

Microscopic examination shows prominent abnormalities in glomeruli, tubules, and to a lesser degree the interstitium.[16,18,24] The glomerular lesion, focal and segmental sclerosis, is often in an *early stage* of evolution at the time of tissue examination.[16,18,24,29,30] Visceral epithelial cells are segmentally or globally hyperplastic and enlarged and contain large cytoplasmic vacuoles and numerous protein reabsorption droplets (Fig. 11–2 to

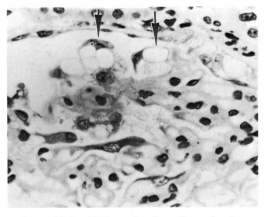

Figure 11–2. HIV-associated nephropathy in very early stage of evolution. A few greatly enlarged and coarsely vacuolated visceral epithelial cells can be seen (*arrows*) in one segment of this glomerulus. (Hematoxylin and eosin, ×400.)

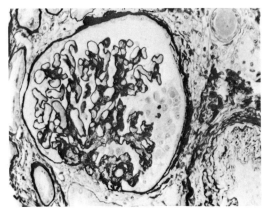

Figure 11–3. Glomerulus with segmental increase in visceral epithelial cells associated with partial capillary wall collapse; remainder of tuft is unremarkable. (Periodic acid–methenamine silver, ×180.)

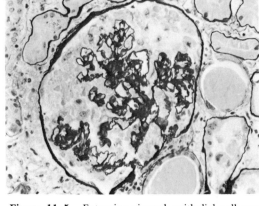

Figure 11–5. Extensive visceral epithelial cell proliferation simulating crescent. Relatively minor degree of capillary wall collapse is present. (Periodic acid–methenamine silver, ×200.)

11–5). Some cells are the sites of mitotic figures. (Fig. 11–6). Underlying capillary walls are usually collapsed. In some glomeruli few capillaries are affected, whereas in others all or nearly all are collapsed (Fig. 11–5). As the lesion progresses *(middle stage)*, in addition to collapse (Fig. 11–7), lipid-containing macrophages (foam cells) accumulate in capillaries (Fig. 11–8 to 11–10). Ultimately a combination of mesangial matrix–basement membrane material and plasma protein precipitates (insudative lesions) obliterates capillaries *(late stage)* (Fig. 11–11). As we[17,18,29,30] and others[21] have stressed, the abnormalities most commonly are in the early stage, and visceral epithelial cell lesions are most prominent. Even in later stages the epithelial cells still have many abnormal features.

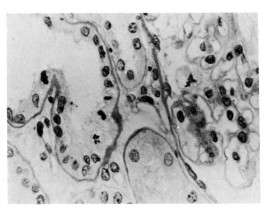

Figure 11–6. Early-stage glomerular lesion with simultaneous epithelial cell mitotic figures in glomerulus and adjacent tubules. Proximal tubular cells lack distinct brush border staining. (Periodic acid–Schiff, ×400.)

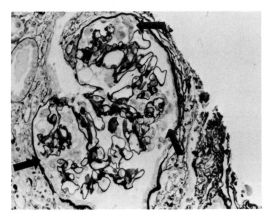

Figure 11–4. Glomerulus in which multiple segments have visceral epithelial cell hyperplasia *(arrows)*. (Periodic acid–methenamine silver, ×180.)

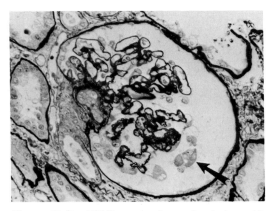

Figure 11–7. Middle-stage glomerular lesion with early obliteration of capillaries by mesangial matrix–basement membrane. Overlying visceral epithelial cells are hyperplastic and vacuolated *(arrow)*. (Periodic acid–methenamine silver, ×160.)

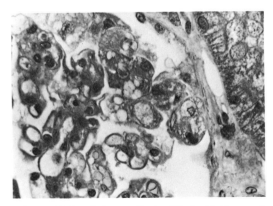

Figure 11–8. A few capillaries filled with foam cells and adherent to Bowman's capsule. Visceral epithelium shows persistent abnormalities. (Masson's trichrome, ×400.)

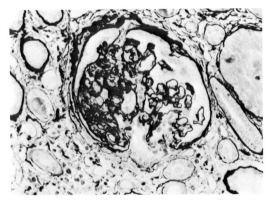

Figure 11–11. Late stage of glomerular abnormality. Segmental sclerosis is well-formed; abnormal segment is adherent to Bowman's capsule. (Periodic acid–methenamine silver, ×200.)

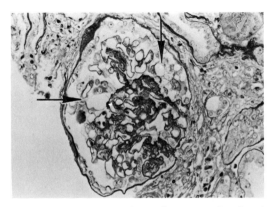

Figure 11–9. More advanced segmental sclerosis with combined collapse and increased mesangial matrix. Visceral epithelial cells are persistently enlarged and coarsely vacuolated *(arrows).* (Periodic acid–methenamine silver, ×200.)

Tubular epithelium is also distinctly abnormal.[11,17,18,24,52] At the onset of the disease, tubular cells undergo degeneration and necrosis; proximal tubular cells lack brush border staining (Fig. 11–6). Cells of all tubular segments are flattened, and lumina are slightly dilated. Overt necrosis of single cells is unusual. Mitotic figures are common. A prominent feature is microcystic dilatation of clusters of tubules (usually representing the same nephron sectioned at different levels) filled with pale-staining cast material (Fig. 11–12). While the "cysts" are most prominent at the corticomedullary junction, they may be found throughout the kidneys and may achieve considerable size (Fig. 11–13). Dilated proximal tubules are usually in direct continuity with dilated Bowman's spaces of glomeruli (Fig. 11–14). Many tubules of all sizes are

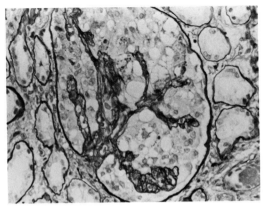

Figure 11–10. Extensive visceral epithelial cell proliferation and vacuolization with widespread capillary collapse and multiple segments of sclerosis. Compare with Figure 11–5, which is slightly earlier view. (Periodic acid–methenamine silver, ×215.)

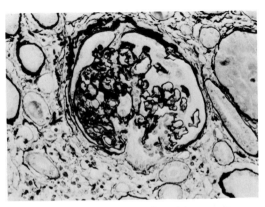

Figure 11–12. Numerous pale-staining casts in many dilated tubules and Bowman's spaces. (Periodic acid–Schiff, ×36.)

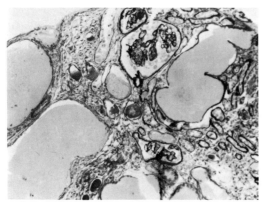

Figure 11–13. Several cystically dilated tubules filled with plasma protein–containing casts and dwarfing adjacent glomeruli. (Periodic acid–methenamine silver, ×100.)

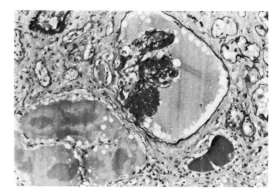

Figure 11–15. Dark-staining cast *(lower right)* is typical hyaline cast, which is strongly periodic acid–Schiff positive. Compare with other tubular "casts" and contents of Bowman's space. (Periodic acid–Schiff, ×90.)

filled with pale-staining casts, which may also be found in Bowman's spaces.[18,24,52] Proximal cells contain numerous protein reabsorption droplets.[18] The interstitium is diffusely edematous and infiltrated by small numbers of lymphocytes.[18] Arteries and arterioles are not abnormal.

The composition of the cast material has been determined.[18] Unlike typical hyaline casts, which are strongly periodic acid–Schiff (PAS) positive, these luminal masses are PAS negative and fuchsin positive with Masson's trichrome stain. Hyaline casts are composed of Tamm-Horsfall protein, IgA and both light chains. The casts in the dilated tubules and enlarged Bowman's spaces consist of all plasma proteins sought and not Tamm-Horsfall protein (Figs. 11–15 and 11–16).

This suggests that they are precipitates of filtered plasma protein and, by inference, that the glomerular lesion results in nonselective proteinuria.

Immunofluorescence staining of the glomeruli usually discloses segmental granular to amorphous deposits of IgM and C3 corresponding to the insudative lesions of segmental sclerosis (Fig. 11–17). In some instances mesangial deposits of IgM and C3 are also present (Fig. 11–18).[7,11,16,18,24,29,51-53,55,58] Segmental localization of immunoglobulin and complement does not indicate an immune-mediated process. Most investigators agree that these proteins are possibly trapped at sites of injury. This segmental pattern of fluorescence should be contrasted with a more typical one in an immune com-

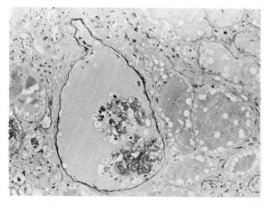

Figure 11–14. Dilated Bowman's space filled with "cast," which is also in adjoining proximal tubule. Segmental sclerosis and collapse of glomerular tuft can be seen. (Periodic acid–Schiff, ×100.)

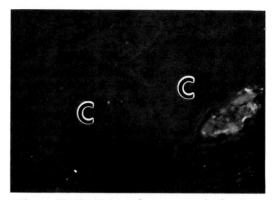

Figure 11–16. Immunofluorescent stain for Tamm-Horsfall protein. Single cast is positive for the protein, whereas two plasma protein "casts" *(C)* are negative. (×200.)

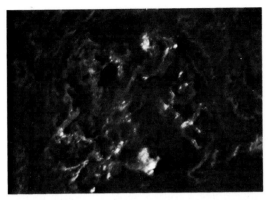

Figure 11–17. Segmental coarsely granular staining for immunoglobulin M in glomerular capillary walls. (×100.)

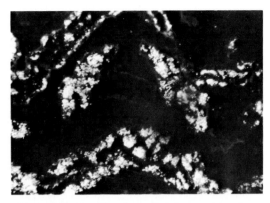

Figure 11–19. Abundant albumin protein reabsorption droplets in many tubular cells. (×250.)

plex–mediated glomerulonephritis (see later discussion). Tubular epithelial cells contain abundant albumin in the form of protein reabsorption droplets (Fig. 11–19).[18]

Ultrastructural abnormalities are commonly observed.[16,18,24,53,60,65] The foot processes of glomerular visceral epithelial cells are completely effaced, as might be expected in focal and segmental glomerulosclerosis of any cause (Figs. 11–20 and 11–21). Some of the epithelial cells are considerably enlarged, with large, round, single membrane–bound vacuoles, and contain numerous rounded dense and medium-dense secondary lysosomes (protein reabsorption droplets) (Figs. 11–21 to 11–23). The cells may be partially detached from underlying basement membranes, which are often partly collapsed. In later stages, thin layers of new basement membrane material separate the podocytes from the original basement membrane (Figs. 11–22 and 11–24).

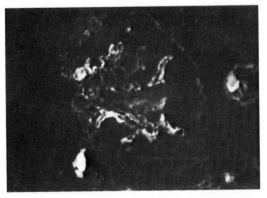

Figure 11–18. Diffuse granular staining for immunoglobulin M in glomerular mesangium. (×120.)

Endothelial cells of glomeruli, peritubular capillaries, arteries, and veins contain numerous, large, complex tubuloreticular structures (Figs. 11–24 and 11–25).[1,16,18,24,52,65] These structures, consisting of interanastomosing tubules 25 nm in diameter found within cisternae of endoplasmic reticulum and composed of lipid and acidic glycoprotein, appear to result from interferon alfa's effect on the cells.[41,63] They are also in the cytoplasm of circulating and tissue-infiltrating lymphocytes and monocytes, and less commonly in the cytoplasm of vascular smooth muscle and interstitial cells. Tubuloreticular structures occur in many other forms of renal disease, but only in systemic lupus erythematosus are they as common and widespread as in HIV-infected patients. In both HIV infection and systemic lupus erythematosus, many cells throughout the body contain tubuloreticular structures; they are not solely features of renal disease.[29,41,53] In addition, they are usually present in renal endothelium of HIV-infected patients with some other forms of renal disease, including immune complex glomerulonephritis and interstitial nephritis.[18] In yet other renal diseases they are exceedingly rare and, when present, are limited to very few glomerular endothelial cells.[1]

Other abnormal cytoplasmic inclusions, emphasized primarily by Chander et al.,[16,65] consist of parallel stacks of closely apposed membranes with intervening electron-dense material in some tubular epithelial cells, and cylindrical confronting cisternae, also known as test-tube and ring-shaped forms, in tubular epithelium and interstitial cells. These also are noted in cells of other organs and tissues from HIV-infected patients.[41,63]

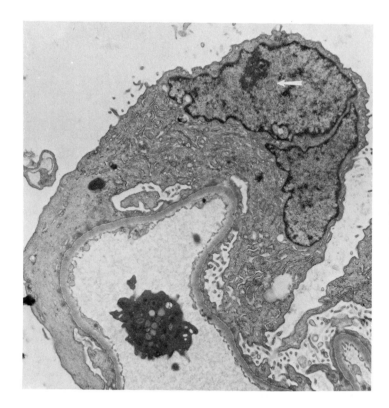

Figure 11–20. Capillary wall with complete effacement of foot processes of visceral epithelial cells. Nuclear body is present *(arrow)*. (×6000.)

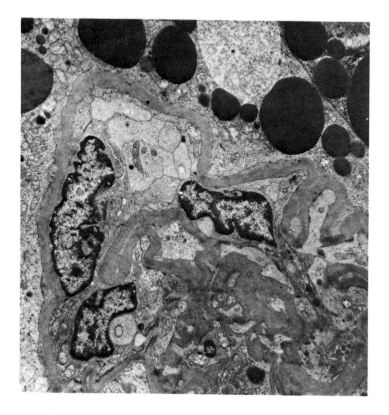

Figure 11–21. Collapsing glomerular capillary wall; foot processes are completely effaced. Epithelial cell contains numerous dense secondary lysosomes (protein reabsorption droplets). (×6000.)

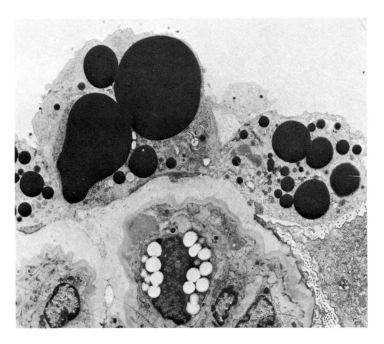

Figure 11–22. Later stage of segmental glomerular sclerosis than that shown in Figure 11–21. Protein reabsorption droplets are in epithelial cells, which are separated from original basement membrane by thin layers of pale basement membrane material. Cell with numerous clear lipid vacuoles can be seen in remnant of lumen. (×3500.)

The nuclei have a variety of abnormalities defined by electron microscopy.[16] Nuclear bodies, classified into at least five different types based on structural characteristics,[12] are found frequently in tubular, interstitial, and glomerular cells (Fig. 11–26).[16,24] Transformation of nuclei to peculiar granular (Fig. 11–27) and granulofibrillar (Fig. 11–28) structures, with loss of peripheral heterochromatin, is common in tubular and interstitial

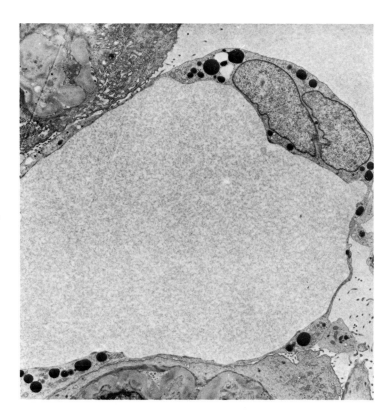

Figure 11–23. Greatly enlarged visceral epithelial cell with very large "vacuole" and numerous small protein reabsorption droplets. Basement membrane, at bottom of photograph, is partially collapsed. (×3750.)

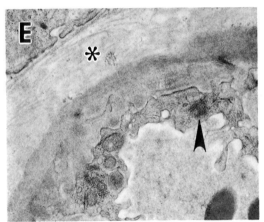

Figure 11–24. Portion of capillary wall in which visceral epithelial cell *(E)* is separated from original basement membrane by new layers of basement membrane *(asterisk)*. Tubuloreticular structure is in endothelial cell *(arrowhead)*. (×11,500.)

cells.[16] These alterations may affect the entire nucleus or a portion thereof; the nuclear membranes are sometimes ruptured, spilling nuclear contents into the cytoplasm. This may be associated with swelling of mitochondria and other organelles. In our experience fibrillar transformation is most commonly noted in postmortem tissue. The nuclear changes are not limited to renal cells but are evident in cells from other tissues in HIV-infected patients, especially those with full-blown AIDS.[63] However, nuclear abnormalities are rare in glomerular epithelium. We and other investigators have been unable to identify virions in any renal cell despite careful search.[16,18,24,52]

Electron-dense (immune complex–type) deposits in the mesangium are found in a few biopsy specimens, mainly from patients shown to have concomitant granular mesangial deposits by immunofluorescence.[51-53]

The combination of the light microscopic abnormalities—focal and segmental glomerulosclerosis in an early stage, tubular cell degeneration, microcystically dilated tubules, and Bowman's spaces filled with plasma protein casts—with ultrastructural features, especially numerous large tubuloreticular structures, is considered virtually pathognomonic of HIV-associated nephropathy.[18] Indeed, as pointed out previously, this unique constellation of findings allows the pathologist to diagnose HIV infection in an otherwise asymptomatic patient.[18,24] Furthermore, as Alpers et al.,[1] noted, the presence of tubuloreticular structures in a patient with focal and segmental glomerulosclerosis is sufficient evidence to suggest HIV infection, since tubuloreticular structures in this glomerular lesion are otherwise virtually unknown.

Some investigators have implicated the tubular lesions of necrosis and obstructing casts to be responsible for progressive renal insufficiency[18,29]; focal and segmental glomerulosclerosis alone would be unlikely to cause such rapid loss of function.[42]

Few studies of the pathogenesis of HIV-associated nephropathy have been published.[10] We were struck by the profound simultaneous changes in glomerular visceral and tubular epithelial cells.[19] Some of the cellular changes noted on light or electron microscopy may be considered morphologic

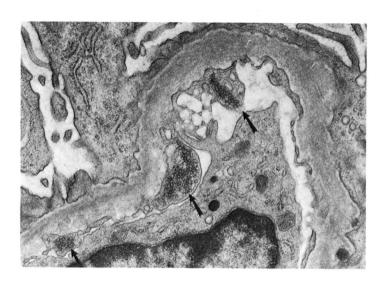

Figure 11–25. Numerous tubuloreticular structures *(arrows)* in glomerular endothelial cell. (×20,300.)

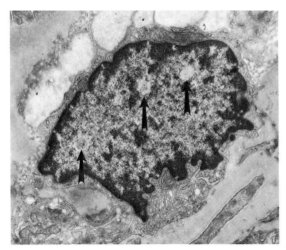

Figure 11–26. Glomerular endothelial cell with three nuclear bodies *(arrows).* (×8100.)

markers of viral infection, although they do not necessarily indicate the presence of viral protein.[16] Consequently, we wondered whether direct infection of renal epithelium by HIV might play a role in the genesis of the disorder. In an initial study using in situ hybridization and complementary DNA, we found HIV genome in both tubular and glomerular epithelium in biopsy and autopsy tissues from patients with HIV-associated nephropathy (Fig. 11–29). This contrasted sharply both in extent of distribution and in frequency of positive cells in kidneys from HIV-infected patients who had immune complex–mediated glomerulonephritis

or who had no functional or structural evidence of renal disease. This difference suggested to us that HIV is involved in the genesis or progression of HIV-associated nephropathy; whether only HIV is responsible or cofactors, such as simultaneous infection with other viruses, (e.g., CMV, herpes, and hepatitis B) hereditary factors, concomitant drugs, or toxins, are involved is not known.[19,29]

We also used immunohistochemistry to search for p24 antigen in cells in paraffin-embedded sections.[19] We observed considerably fewer cells positive for the antigen with this method than with in situ hybridization. The positivity was limited to tubular epithelium (Fig. 11–30). Our group had similar findings in other tissues.[62,67] A preliminary study from Italy failed to demonstrate HIV antigens p18, p25, gp45, and gp110 in renal cells stained with immunoperoxidase; other methods were not used.[28]

Although renal epithelial cells do not express CD4 antigen, the presence of virus in these cells is not surprising.[44] In the study perhaps most relevant to ours,[19] Nelson et al.[48] found HIV genome in duodenal and large intestinal epithelium and enterochromaffin cells in biopsy specimens from AIDS patients with diarrhea of no obvious cause. This observation indicated that HIV can infect epithelium not expressing CD4 and can cause clinical manifestations that presumably result from cell dysfunction. Renal cellular lesions possibly have a similar pathogenesis and

Figure 11–27. Interstitial cells with large nuclear bodies *(arrowheads)* and granular transformation of nucleus *(arrow).* (×12,000.)

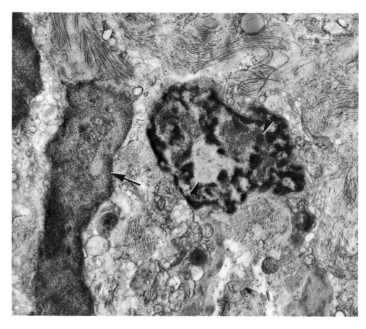

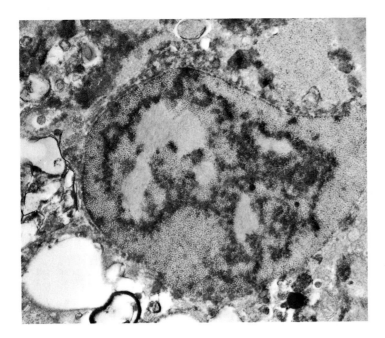

Figure 11–28. Interstitial cell with granulofibrillar transformation of nucleus. This is from postmortem material. (×20,000.)

effect: proteinuria and segmental sclerosis developing from infection of glomerular epithelium, and progressive renal failure from infection of tubular epithelium.[17] Langs et al.[42] have suggested an alternative mechanism for the tubular cell changes and glomerular capillary wall collapse. They postulate, without functional data, that renal ischemia is responsible for both sets of structural and clinical abnormalities.

A preliminary report recently described immunohistochemical and electron microscopic localization of *Mycoplasma incognitus* in many intracellular and extracellular sites throughout the kidneys in HIV-associated nephropathy. The investigators suggested that renal parenchymal infection with *M. incognitus* is necessary for the development of this disorder.[5] This observation needs confirmation.

A renal abnormality known as heroin-associated nephropathy may develop in heroin users. This disorder is characterized clinically by heavy proteinuria and renal failure and pathologically by focal and segmental glomerulosclerosis.[23] Because of these fea-

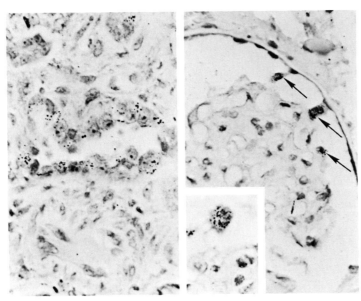

A   B

Figure 11–29. In situ hybridization using cDNA probe in HIV-associated nephropathy. *A,* Numerous positive cells in single tubule. *B,* Hybridization product *(dark grains)* are in several glomerular visceral epithelial cells *(arrows). Inset,* Enlargement showing positive visceral epithelial cell overlying few patent capillaries. (*A,* ×400; *B,* ×350; *inset,* ×480.) (From Cohen AH, Sun NCJ, Shapshak P, Imagawa DT: Demonstration of human immunodeficiency virus in renal epithelium in HIV associated nephropathy. Mod Pathol 2:125-128, 1989. © by U.S. and Canadian Academy of Pathology, Inc.)

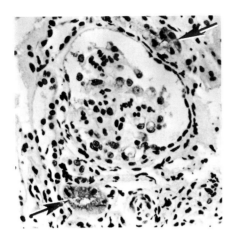

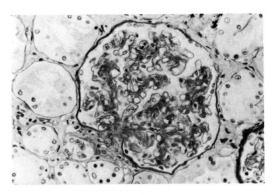

Figure 11–31. Glomerulus with mild diffuse mesangial hypercellularity. (Periodic acid–Schiff, × 180.)

Figure 11–30. Localization of p24 antigen in tubular cells *(arrows)* in HIV-associated nephropathy; glomerular epithelia are negative for p24 antigen. (Avidin-biotin immunoperoxidase, × 215.) (From Cohen AH, Sun NCJ, Shapshak P, Imagawa DT: Demonstration of human immunodeficiency virus in renal epithelium in HIV associated nephropathy. Mod Pathol 2:125-128, 1989. © by U.S. and Canadian Academy of Pathology, Inc.)

tures and because many of the patients initially described with HIV-associated nephropathy were heroin addicts, some concern was expressed that the lesions of HIV-associated nephropathy were in fact heroin-associated nephropathy in HIV-infected patients.[3] Several studies addressed this problem; all concluded that qualitative and quantitative pathologic differences separate these two forms of renal disease.[16,18,24] With the passage of time and with increased reports, it has become clear that HIV-associated nephropathy is not limited to heroin abusers.[11] The condition has been reported in all risk groups, including children with perinatally acquired HIV infection.[11,18,22,52,53,66]

OTHER GLOMERULAR LESIONS

Perhaps the second most common form of glomerular disease in HIV-infected patients is characterized morphologically by diffuse mesangial hypercellularity (Fig. 11–31).[51-53] This disorder has been noted especially in children, although Pardo et al.[51] and Gardenswartz et al.[27] described it in their early reports, which included adults. Patients generally manifest low-grade proteinuria and normal or slightly impaired renal function.[11] Mesangial immunoglobulin and complement granular deposits are observed by immunofluorescence, and in many biopsy specimens small mesangial electron-dense deposits are also noted.[51-53,66]

The significance and frequency of these changes are debated; whether they are precursors to or early lesions of focal and segmental sclerosis is uncertain. One explanation for this lesion is that it represents a mild form of immune complex–mediated glomerulonephritis unrelated to HIV-associated nephropathy (see later discussion). Several isolated cases of minimal change disease have been reported in HIV-infected patients.[11,29,64]

A large variety of morphologically better defined and characterized immune complex–mediated glomerulonephritides have been documented in HIV-infected patients, not all of whom have had full-blown AIDS.[11,18,20,21,27,29,30,40,45,56,57,60,66] Some patients were also infected with hepatitis B virus.[33] The lesions include membranous glomerulonephritis, membranoproliferative glomerulonephritis type I, acute proliferative (postinfectious) glomerulonephritis (Fig. 11–32), and IgA nephropathy.[4,39] The clinical

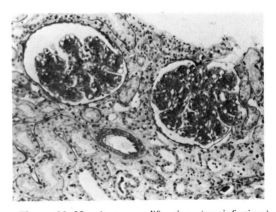

Figure 11–32. Acute proliferative (postinfectious) glomerulonephritis. Both glomeruli are hypercellular. Note lack of tubular and interstitial changes. (Periodic acid–Schiff, × 80.)

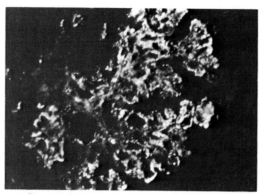

Figure 11–33. Immunofluorescence in immune complex–mediated glomerulonephritis. Granular capillary wall and mesangial staining. (Anti-C3, ×200.)

presentations are similar to those in non-HIV-infected individuals: proteinuria often with hematuria and variable renal insufficiency.[29,30] The light microscopic changes in the glomeruli are virtually the same as those occurring in the absence of HIV infection and are easily diagnosed. Immunofluorescence microscopy shows granular capillary wall or mesangial deposits of immunoglobulins and complement (Fig. 11–33). However, the ultrastructural abnormalities are different from those in non-HIV-infected patients; cytoplasmic tubuloreticular structures are regularly observed in endothelial cells (Fig. 11–34), and the other ultrastructural cellular and nuclear abnormalities described previously are also evident in HIV-infected patients.[18]

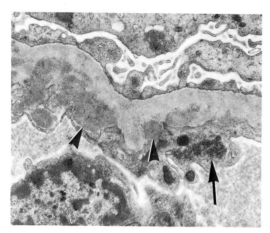

Figure 11–34. Immune complex glomerulonephritis in HIV-infected patient. This portion of glomerular capillary wall contains several subendothelial electron-dense deposits *(arrowheads);* tubuloreticular structures *(arrow)* are in endothelial cell. (×12,000.)

The antigen(s) in the immune complexes are being investigated. In one well-studied case of membranous glomerulonephritis, the nature of the antigens in the immune complexes was determined; Collins et al.[21] found hepatitis B surface and e antigens in glomeruli from a patient with AIDS and hepatitis. We searched for HIV core (p17, p24) and envelope (gp41, gp120) antigens in glomerular deposits from three patients with immune complex glomerulonephritis but were unable to find them.[20] Whether most of the immune complex glomerular disorders are induced by HIV immune complexes or are caused by other antigens in HIV-infected patients remains to be elucidated; perhaps more sensitive techniques for identifying antigens are required.

Several HIV-infected patients have been reported to have coexisting IgA-mediated glomerular disease, including IgA nephropathy and Henoch-Schönlein purpura.[9,39] An attempt to identify HIV antigen(s) in three patients was unsuccessful.[4] Again, this may represent an immune complex–mediated glomerulonephritis not directly related to HIV infection. Lupus glomerulonephritis has occurred in several children with perinatally acquired AIDS; the glomerulopathies have included mesangial proliferative, diffuse proliferative,[66] and membranous glomerulonephritis.[24] The affected patients all had usual serologic markers of systemic lupus erythematosus. No glomerulopathies other than HIV-associated nephropathy are associated with tubulointerstitial abnormalities. This difference was addressed specifically in our study[18]; furthermore, other reports of immune complex–mediated glomerulonephritis neither describe nor illustrate these lesions.

The coexistence of HIV infection and either hemolytic-uremic syndrome or thrombotic thrombocytopenic purpura has been reported with increasing frequency, although this still is a relatively uncommon association.[43,47] Clinical signs of renal involvement vary; the microscopic abnormalities in the kidneys are similar to those in non-HIV-infected patients with thrombotic microangiopathies. Small arterial and arteriolar thrombi with concomitant endothelial cell swelling, as well as glomerular capillary wall and luminal fibrin, also with endothelial cell swelling, are the usual pathologic findings. When the condition is severe, as in hemolytic-uremic syndrome, cortical necrosis may ensue.

TUBULOINTERSTITIAL LESIONS

A variety of abnormalities involving the renal tubules and interstitium are observed in HIV-infected patients, most commonly in postmortem material and less frequently in renal biopsy specimens. Interstitial nephritis with varying degrees of interstitial edema and less commonly fibrosis has been noted in 3%[56,57] to 38%[60] of AIDS patients at autopsy, occurring in about one third of those who died with clinically evident renal disease.[27,46,56,69] Acute tubular necrosis (ATN) is identified in one fourth to one third of patients dying of AIDS with renal complications[27,46] and is often associated with interstitial nephritis. Acute interstitial nephritis (AIN) is also a common finding in patients without clinically significant renal disease.[52] Both ATN and AIN are frequently related to renal infections or the administration of nephrotoxic drugs (Fig. 11–35), which also induce renal injury in patients without AIDS.[8,11,46,50] Acute renal failure resulting from tubular and interstitial injury is more prevalent in white homosexual or bisexual patients.[45]

Direct renal infection is encountered in approximately 20% to 25% of AIDS patients at autopsy.[24,49,59,60,71] CMV is observed frequently, since it is the most common infection at the time of death.[32,39,60,71] Intracellular inclusions are within tubular epithelium (Fig. 11–36) and glomerular endothelial cells,[24,50,71] with some patients having only glomerular inclusions.[45,49] As with all infections in immunocompromised patients, there

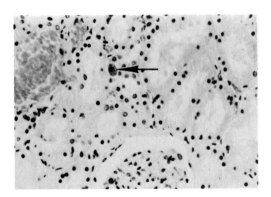

Figure 11–36. Renal cytomegalovirus infection. Tubular epithelial cell has large nucleus containing dense intranuclear inclusion *(arrow)*. (Hematoxylin and eosin, ×160.)

may be associated interstitial inflammation or virtually no host response.[71] Glomerular infection is not associated with hypercellularity unless a corresponding immune complex–mediated disease process is present. Renal involvement in disseminated cryptococcosis[24,27,46,60,71] and candidiasis[11,24,49] occurs in 5% to 10% of patients, with organisms identified in the tubulointerstitium as well as in glomeruli (Fig. 11–37). Infection with *M. tuberculosis* or *M. avium-intracellulare* may be accompanied by well or poorly formed granulomas[49,60] or no specific inflammatory response (Fig. 11–38).[27,71] The organisms may be observed in any part of the renal parenchyma. Renal invasion has also occurred with *Pneumocystis, Nocardia, Histoplasma, Toxoplasma,* and *Aspergillus* organisms, herpes virus,[11,60] and bacteria.[36] When significant epithelial injury is present, tubular necrosis with or without

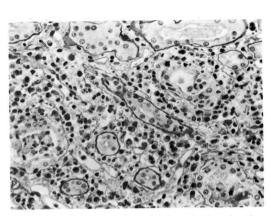

Figure 11–35. Acute interstitial nephritis related to drug hypersensitivity. Interstitium is edematous and infiltrated by numerous mononuclear leukocytes; many mononuclear leukocytes are also in tubule walls. (Periodic acid–Schiff, ×200.)

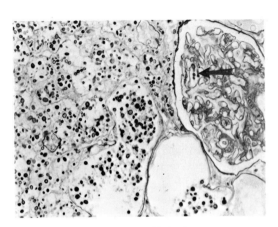

Figure 11–37. Cryptococcal infection. Numerous organisms are present in dilated tubules, interstitium, and few glomerular capillaries *(arrow)*. (Periodic acid–Schiff, ×200.)

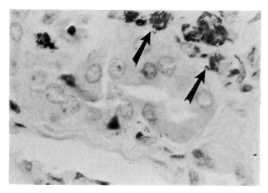

Figure 11–38. *Mycobacterium avium-intracellulare* infection. Many organisms are in cells within interstitium. (Ziehl-Neelsen, ×350.)

interstitial inflammation may accompany the infection. Renal invasion by microorganisms may impair renal function; however, CMV infection is often clinically unsuspected[36] and in the absence of interstitial nephritis there may be few clinical indications of renal disease.

Drug-induced lesions including tubular necrosis and AIN are identified in both biopsy- and autopsy-derived material. These findings may be associated with acute renal failure. Pentamidine, an agent used to treat *Pneumocystis* infection, is implicated in 5% to 10% of patients with drug-induced renal failure,[2,11,27,56] particularly those with concomitant hypoglycemia.[50] Chronic interstitial nephritis is also observed with pentamidine therapy[24]; the mechanism of this injury is unknown. Sensakovic et al.[61] reported myoglobinuria associated with pentamidine administration in one patient. Rhabdomyolysis, also noted with AZT administration, has not been associated with renal failure.[10] Aminoglycoside, trimethoprim-sulfamethoxazole, and amphotericin B therapies used to treat infections commonly observed in AIDS induce acute tubulointerstitial nephritides (Fig. 11–35).[11,24,27,31,50] Other agents implicated in acute renal failure with tubulointerstitial lesions include nonsteroidal antiinflammatory drugs, radiocontrast media, rifampin, foscarnet, and sulfadiazine.[11,13,60] Using less nephrotoxic agents such as ketoconazole and gancyclovir whenever possible may prevent acute tubulointerstitial nephritis in already compromised patients.[11]

AIDS patients may have episodes of renal ischemia for a variety of reasons; up to one third of those with renal failure have an associated ischemic episode.[45] Fever and dehydration are frequent events and result in hypo-volemia with tubular necrosis. Terminal hypoperfusion may explain why many kidneys display an ischemic pattern of tubular injury at autopsy.[56,71] Sepsis followed by hypotension and shock also causes tubular necrosis with renal failure.[45,56] In addition, patients with sepsis may have renal infarcts, probably as a result of infected emboli.[71] Infarcts also may be related to necrotic foci of lymphomatous infiltrates following chemotherapy. The presence of ischemia for more prolonged periods may induce chronic changes, including tubular atrophy and interstitial fibrosis with mononuclear leukocytic infiltrates.[69]

Tissue deposition of calcium in multiple organs is a common finding in necropsy specimens,[46] with nephrocalcinosis occurring in 5%[45] to 40%[24] of autopsy series. Niedt et al.[49] reported the association of nephrocalcinois with amphotericin B. However, others have noted renal calcium deposition with myocobacterial infection[26] or without any specific drug or infectious association.[24,27,46,60] There is no concomitant stone formation,[24] and the calcifications occur in the tubules and interstitium of the cortex and medulla (Fig. 11–39).[60] D'Agati et al.[24] observed an association with pulmonary granulomatous inflammation. The finding of nephrocalcinosis is often of morphologic interest only; it is associated with hypocalcemia, possibly resulting from excess tissue calcium deposition.[60]

NEOPLASMS

The kidneys are the site of neoplastic processes in a relatively small percentage of AIDS patients. Kaposi's sarcoma has been noted in 1% to 6% of patients, generally as a part of

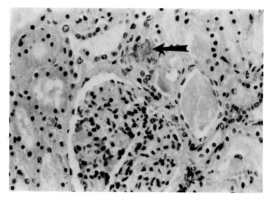

Figure 11–39. Small focus of interstitial calcification (*arrow*). (Hematoxylin and eosin, ×220.)

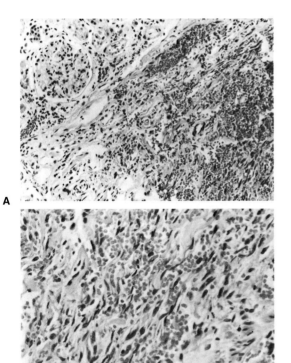

A

B

Figure 11–40. Renal Kaposi's sarcoma. *A*, Portion of cortical parenchyma is replaced by this malignancy. *B*, Higher magnification shows proliferating spindle cells with many extravasated erythrocytes. (Hematoxylin and eosin, *A*, ×120; *B*, ×240.)

disseminated disease.[24,69,71] The malignancy may be multifocal or in a single renal location (Fig. 11–40).[24,17] Like Kaposi's sarcoma in other sites, renal Kaposi's sarcoma is almost exclusively observed in homosexual or bisexual men.[45] Intravenous drug abuse, when the only source of HIV infection, is not associated with this neoplasm. Non-Hodgkin's lymphoma involving the kidney is part of widespread disease[45,60,69] and is found in approximately 2% of autopsy specimens. A single case of myeloma in the kidney with IgA kappa production has been reported.[68] Renal cell carcinoma in AIDS is found at an earlier age than the usual sixth decade of presentation.[6,45,46]

REFERENCES

1. Alpers CE, Harawi S, Rennke HG: Focal glomerulosclerosis with tubuloreticular inclusions: Possible predictive value for acquired immunodeficiency syndrome (AIDS). Am J Kidney Dis 12:240-242, 1988.
2. Anderson R, Boedicker M, Ma M, et al: Adverse reactions associated with pentamidine isethionate in AIDS patients. Drug Intell Clin Pharm 20:862-868, 1986.
3. Balow JE, Macher AM, Rook AH: Paucity of glomerular disease in acquired immunodeficiency syndrome (AIDS) [abstract]. Kidney Int 29:178, 1986.
4. Bargman JM, Katz A: IgA-associated nephropathy in HIV positive patients [abstract]. Kidney Int 37:254, 1990.
5. Bauer FA, Wear DJ, Angritt P, et al: *Mycoplasma incognitus* infection in kidneys of AIDS patients with AIDS-associated nephropathy [abstract]. Abstracts of the Sixth International Conference on AIDS 1:255, 1990.
6. Bleiweiss IJ, Pervez NK, Hammer GS, et al: Cytomegalovirus-induced adrenal insufficiency and associated renal cell carcinoma in AIDS. Mt Sinai J Med 53:676-679, 1986.
7. Bourgoignie JJ, Meneses R, Pardo V: The nephropathy related to the acquired immune deficiency syndrome. Adv Nephrol 17:113-126, 1988.
8. Bourgoignie JJ, Meneses R, Ortiz C, et al: The clinical spectrum of renal disease associated with human immunodeficiency virus. Am J Kidney Dis 12:131-137, 1988.
9. Bourgoignie JJ, Ortiz-Interiam C, Green DF, et al: Race, a cofactor in HIV-I-associated nephropathy. Transplant Proc 21:3899-3901, 1989.
10. Bourgoignie JJ, Ortiz-Interiam C, Green DF, et al: Renal complications of human immunodeficiency virus-type I. In Andreucci VE (ed): International Yearbook of Nephrology 1990. Kluwer Academic Publishers, Boston, 1990, pp 73-88.
11. Bourgoignie JJ: Renal complications of human immunodeficiency virus type I. Kidney Int 37:1571-1584, 1990.
12. Bouteille M, Kalifar SR, Delarue J: Ultrastructural variations of nuclear bodies in human disease. J Ultrastruct Res 19:474-486, 1967.
13. Cacoub O, Deray G, Baumelow A, et al: Acute renal failure induced by foscarnet: 4 cases. Clin Nephrol 29:315-318, 1988.
14. Cantor ES, Kimmel PK, Bosch JP: Impact of race on renal disease in patients with AIDS [abstract]. Kidney Int 35:222, 1989.
15. Carbone L, D'Agati V, Cheng J-T, et al: Course and prognosis of human immunodeficiency virus–associated nephropathy. Am J Med 87:389-395, 1989.
16. Chander P, Soni A, Suri A, et al: Renal ultrastructural markers in AIDS-associated nephropathy. Am J Pathol 126:513-526, 1987.
17. Cohen AH: Considerations of pathogenesis of HIV-associated nephropathy. In Proceedings of the XIth International Congress of Nephrology. Springer-Verlag Tokyo, Inc., in press.
18. Cohen AH, Nast CC: HIV-associated nephropathy: A unique combined glomerular, tubular, and interstitial lesion. Mod Pathol 1:87-97, 1988.
19. Cohen AH, Sun NCJ, Shapshak P, et al: Demonstration of human immunodeficiency virus in renal epithelium in HIV associated nephropathy. Mod Pathol 2:125-128, 1989.
20. Cohen AH, Sun NJS, Shapshak P, et al: Immune complex (IC) glomerulonephritis (GN) in HIV-infected patients: Lack of HIV antigens in immune complexes [abstract]. Lab Invest 60:18A, 1989.
21. Collins AB, Bhan AK, Dienstag JL, et al: Hepatitis B

immune complex glomerulonephritis: Simultaneous glomerular deposition of hepatitis B surface and e antigens. Clin Immunol Immunopathol 24:137-153, 1983.

22. Connor E, Gupta S, Joshi V, et al: Acquired immunodeficiency-associated renal disease in children. J Pediatr 113:39-44, 1988.

23. Cunningham EE, Brentjens JR, Zielezny MA, et al: Heroin nephropathy: A clinico-pathologic and epidemiologic study. Am J Med 68:47-53, 1989.

24. D'Agati V, Suh J-I, Carbone L, et al: Pathology of HIV-associated nephropathy: A detailed morphologic and comparative study. Kidney Int 35: 1358-1370, 1989.

25. Dosquet P, Michel C, Elyaszewica M, et al: Focal and segmental glomerulosclerosis (FSG) among HIV infected (HIV+) patients: Possible favourable effect of treatment with azidothymidine (AZT). Abstracts of the Eleventh International Congress on Nephrology, Tokyo, 1990, p 14A.

26. Falkoff GE, Rigsby CM, Rosenfield AT, et al: Partial, combined cortical and medullary nephrocalcinosis, US and CT patterns in AIDS-associated MAI infection. Radiology 162:343-344, 1987.

27. Gardenswartz MH, Lerner CW, Seligson GR, et al: Renal disease in patients with AIDS: A clinicopathologic study. Clin Nephrol 21:197-204, 1984.

28. Genderini A, Vago L, Bertoli S, et al: HIV-associated-nephropathy: Absence of HIV-antigens [abstract]. Abstracts of the Sixth International Conference on AIDS 2:208, 1990.

29. Glassock RJ, Cohen AH, Danovitch G, et al: Human immunodeficiency virus (HIV) infection and the kidney. Ann Intern Med 112:35-49, 1990.

30. Glassock RJ, Nast CC, Cohen AH: The renal response to infection. Adv Exp Med Biol 252: 163-172, 1988.

31. Gordin FM, Simon GL, Wofsky CB, et al: Adverse reactions to trimethoprim-sulfamethoxazole in patients with the acquired immunodeficiency syndrome. Ann Intern Med 100:495-499, 1985.

32. Guarda LA, Luna MA, Smith JL, et al: Acquired immune deficiency syndrome: Postmortem findings. Am J Clin Pathol 81:549-557, 1984.

33. Guerra IL, Abraham AA, Kimmel PL, et al: Nephrotic syndrome associated with chronic persistent hepatitis B in an HIV antibody positive patient. Am J Kidney Dis 10:385-388, 1987.

34. Heredia JB, Angeles AA, Gutierrez ER, et al: Nephropatia associada al sindrome di immunodeficiencia acquirida. Rev Invest Clin 39:105-115, 1987.

35. Hory B, Bresson C, Lorge JF, et al: Associated focal and segmental glomerulosclerosis in the acquired immunodeficiency syndrome. Am J Kidney Dis 12:169, 1988.

36. Hui AN, Koss MN, Meyer PR: Necropsy findings in acquired immunodeficiency syndrome: A comparison of premortem diagnoses with postmortem findings. Hum Pathol 15:670-676, 1984.

37. Humphreys MH: Human immunodeficiency virus-associated nephropathy: East is east and west is west? Arch Intern Med 150:253-255, 1990.

38. Humphreys MH, Schoenfeld PY: Renal complications in patients with the acquired immune deficiency syndrome. Am J Nephrol 7:1-7, 1987.

39. Kenouch S, Delhousse M, Meny J-P, et al: Mesangial IgA deposits in two patients with AIDS-related complex. Nephron 54:338-340, 1990.

40. Kim KK, Factor SM: Membranoproliferative glom-erulonephritis and plexogenic pulmonary arteriopathy in a homosexual man with acquired immunodeficiency syndrome. Hum Pathol 18: 1293-1296, 1987.

41. Kostianovsky M, Orenstein JM, Schaff Z, et al: Cytomembranous inclusions observed in acquired immunodeficiency syndrome. Arch Pathol Lab Med 111:218-223, 1987.

42. Langs C, Gallo GR, Schacht RG, et al: Rapid renal failure in AIDS-associated focal glomerulscoerosis. Arch Intern Med 150:287-292, 1990.

43. Leaf AN, Lamberstein J, Raphael B, et al: Thrombotic thrombocytopenic purpura associated with human immunodeficiency virus type I (HIV-I) infection. Ann Intern Med 109:194-197, 1989.

44. Levy JA: The human immunodeficiency viruses: Detection and pathogenesis. In AIDS: Pathogenesis and Treatment. Marcel Dekker, New York, 1989, pp 159-229.

45. Mazbar SA, Schoenfeld PY, Humphreys MH: Renal involvement in patients infected with HIV: Experience at San Francisco General Hospital. Kidney Int 37:1325-1332, 1990.

46. Mobley K, Rotterdam HZ, Lerner CW, et al: Autopsy findings in the acquired immune deficiency syndrome. In Sommers SC, Rosen PP, Fechner RE (eds): Pathology Annual (part 1). Appleton-Century-Crofts, Norwalk, Conn, 1985, pp 45-65.

47. Nair JMG, Bellevue R, Bertoni M, et al: Thrombotic thrombocytopenic purpura in patients with the acquired immunodeficiency syndrome (AIDS)-related complex: A report of two cases. Ann Intern Med 109:209-212, 1989.

48. Nelson JA, Wiley CA, Reynolds-Kohler C, et al: Human immunodeficiency virus detected in bowel epithelium from patients with gastrointestinal symptoms. Lancet 1:259-262, 1988.

49. Niedt GW, Schinella RA: Acquired immunodeficiency syndrome. Arch Pathol Lab Med 109:727-734, 1985.

50. O'Regan S, Russo P, LaPointe N, et al: AIDS and the urinary tract. J AIDS 3:244-251, 1990.

51. Pardo V, Aldana M, Colton M, et al: Glomerular lesions in the acquired immunodeficiency syndrome. Ann Intern Med 101:429-434, 1984.

52. Pardo V, Bell M, Malaga S, et al: Renal manifestations of human immunodeficiency virus infection. In Damjanov I, Cohen AH, Mills SE, Young RD (eds): Progress in Reproductive and Urinary Tract Pathology, vol II. Field & Wood, New York, 1990, pp 137-155.

53. Pardo V, Meneses R, Ossa L, et al: AIDS-related glomerulopathy: Occurrence in specific risk groups. Kidney Int 31:1167-1173, 1987.

54. Provenzano R, Kupin W, Santiago GC: Renal involvement in the acquired immunodeficiency syndrome: Presentation, clinical course, and therapy. Henry Ford Hosp Med J 35:38-41, 1989.

55. Rao TKS, Filippone EJ, Micastri AD, et al: Associated focal and segmental glomerulosclerosis in the acquired immunodeficiency syndrome. N Engl J Med 310:669-673, 1984.

56. Rao TKS, Friedman EA, Nicastri AD: The types of renal disease in the acquired immunodeficiency syndrome. N Engl J Med 316:1062-1068, 1987.

57. Rao TKS, Friedman EA: Renal syndromes in the acquired immunodeficiency syndrome (AIDS): Lessons learned from analysis over 5 years. Artif Organs 12:206-209, 1988.

58. Rao TKS, Friedman EA: AIDS (HIV)-associated nephropathy: Does it exist? An in-depth review. Am J Nephrol 9:441-453, 1989.

59. Reichert CM, O'Leary TJ, Levens DI, et al: Autopsy pathology in the acquired immune deficiency syndrome. Am J Pathol 112:357-382, 1983.

60. Seney FD Jr, Burns DK, Silva FG: Acquired immunodeficiency syndrome and the kidney. Am J Kidney Dis 16:1-13, 1990.

61. Sensakovic JW, Suarez M, Perez G, et al: Pentamidine treatment of *Pneumocystis carinii* pneumonia in the acquired immunodeficiency syndrome: Association with acute renal failure and myoglobinuria. Arch Intern Med 145:2247, 1985.

62. Shapshak R, Sun NCJ, Resnick L, et al: The detection of HIV by in situ hybridization. Mod Pathol 3:146-153, 1990.

63. Sidhu GS, Stahl RE, El-Sadr W, et al: The acquired immunodeficiency syndrome: An ultrastructural study. Hum Pathol 16:377-386, 1985.

64. Singer DR, Jenkins AP, Gupta S, et al: Minimal change nephropathy in the acquired immune deficiency syndrome. Br Med J 291:868, 1985.

65. Soni A, Agarwal A, Chander P, et al: Evidence for an HIV-related nephropathy: A clinico-pathological study. Clin Nephrol 31:12-17, 1989.

66. Straus J, Abitbol C, Zilleruelo G, et al: Renal disease in children with the acquired immunodeficiency syndrome. N Engl J Med 321:625-630, 1989.

67. Sun NCJ, Shapshak P, Lachant NA, et al: Bone marrow examination in patients with AIDS and AIDS-related complex (ARC): Morphologic and *in situ* hybridization studies. Am J Clin Pathol 92:589-594, 1989.

68. Thomas MA, Ibels LS, Wells JV, et al: IgA kappa multiple myeloma and lymphadenopathy syndrome associated with AIDS virus infection. Aust N Z J Med 16:401-404, 1986.

69. van der Reijden HJ, Schipper MEI, Danner SA, et al: Glomerular lesions and opportunistic infections of the kidney in AIDS: An autopsy study of 47 cases. Adv Exp Med Biol 252:181-188, 1988.

70. Vaziri ND, Barbari A, Licorish K, et al: Spectrum of renal abnormalities in acquired immune-deficiency syndrome. J Natl Med Assn 77:369-375, 1985.

71. Welch K, Finkbeiner W, Alpers CE, et al: Autopsy findings in the acquired immune deficiency syndrome. JAMA 252:1152-1159, 1984.

12

ASSOCIATED CUTANEOUS DISEASES

Theodore H. Kwan and Antoinette F. Hood

A number of diseases affecting the skin and mucous membranes have been described in patients with AIDS, AIDS-related complex (ARC), or HIV seropositivity. Indeed, HIV-positive patients have a high prevalence of skin disease. Coldiron and Bergstresser[1] found that 92% of 100 serial HIV-seropositive patients had skin diseases. Interestingly, prevalence and severity were similar among AIDS, ARC, and asymptomatic patients. The major categories of skin diseases preceding or occurring with HIV infection are malignancies and atypical hyperplasias, infections, and dermatoses (Table 12–1). The list of diseases is growing and can be considered only provisional at this time. For the most part the themes of neoplasia, infection, and dermatoses associated with other immunodeficiency states are recapitulated in HIV patients, but often as unusual and sometimes extravagant variations. For example, Kaposi's sarcoma (KS) in an AIDS patient may have a pityriasis rosea–like distribution, or disseminated histoplasmosis may have the features of a transepidermal elimination disorder. Of course, some diseases described as occurring in HIV-infected hosts may be only coincidentally related. Time and additional knowledge will help to exclude such diseases.

AIDS and HIV infection are commonly manifest in the skin and mucocutaneous areas. KS, chronic candidiasis, severe herpes simplex and varicella-zoster infections, xerosis, asteatotic eczema, and severe forms of seborrheic dermatitis lead the list of cutaneous signs of AIDS and ARC.

NEOPLASIAS AND ATYPICAL HYPERPLASIAS

Kaposi's Sarcoma

Before the AIDS epidemic, KS was classified as either a rare, European, usually indolent variety or a common, African, usually aggressive variety. In addition, a number of cases occurred in patients with iatrogenically induced or other immune deficiency, for example, in renal transplant patients,[2] patients treated with high-dose corticosteroids for such diseases as asthma[3] and temporal arteritis,[4] and patients with other deficiencies or malignancies of the hematopoietic and lymphoreticular systems.[5] Correction of the iatrogenically induced immunodeficiency resulted in regression of KS in many cases. Before the AIDS era, the reported incidence of KS in the United States was no more than 0.061 per 100,000 population.[6] Figures for the African form are not readily available, but in Uganda KS accounted for 9% of tumors diagnosed.[6] This disease is more common in men in a ratio of up to 15:1. Associations with cytomegalovirus (CMV) and possibly Epstein-Barr virus have been proposed.[7] A role for immune response genes, as defined by human lymphocyte antigen phenotypes, has also been proposed.[8] The most convincing evidence pertaining to the cell of origin of this tumor has only recently been forthcoming. Beckstead et al.,[9] based on a profile of antigens defined by immunoperoxidase studies, have proposed a lymphatic derivation.

Table 12–1. Cutaneous and Mucocutaneous Disorders Described in Association with HIV Infection

Neoplasms and Atypical Hyperplasias
Kaposi's sarcoma
Bacillary epithelioid angiomatosis
Non-Hodgkin's lymphoma
Hodgkin's lymphoma
Squamous cell carcinoma in situ
Basal cell carcinoma
Malignant melanoma
Infectious diseases
Viruses: herpes simplex, varicella-zoster,
    cytomegalovirus, molluscum contagiosum,
    papillomavirus, HIV (see HIV exanthem and
    enanthem), adenovirus (see granuloma annulare),
    Epstein-Barr virus (see oral hairy leukoplakia)
Fungi: *Candida* species, *Cryptococcus neoformans,*
    Histoplasma capsulatum, Cladosporium, Sporothrix,
    Coccidioides immitis, Aspergillus, dermatophytes
Mycobacterial infection
Pyogenic bacterial infection
Syphilis
Amebiasis
? Toxoplasmosis
Scabies
Pneumocystis carinii
Protothecosis
Other Dermatoses and Mucocutaneous Disorders
HIV exanthem and enanthem
Dermatitis medicamentosa (including neutrophilic
    eccrine hidradenitis, pigmentation, oral ulcers,
    keratoderma)
Seborrheic dermatitis–like eruption
Chronic pruritus
Eosinophilic pustular folliculitis
Bacterial and fungal folliculitis
Vasculitis
Papular granulomatous eruption and granuloma
    annulare
Yellow nail syndrome
Oral hairy leukoplakia
Hyperalgesic pseudothrombophlebitis
Thrombocytopenic purpura
Others: xerosis, nutritional deficiencies, miliaria,
    psoriasis, keratosis pilaris, hyperpigmentation,
    Reiter's syndrome, reactive perforating collagenosis,
    erythema dyschromium perstans, vitiligo, dermatitis
    herpetiformis, porphyria cutanea tarda, anorectal
    inflammation and proctitis, exfoliative erythroderma
    and flagellate plaques associated with
    hypereosinophlic syndrome, neutrophilic eccrine
    hidradenitis with sweat gland necrosis, ichthyosis,
    asteatotic eczema, focal acantholytic dyskeratosis,
    aphthous stomatitis, telangiectasias

In 1981 reports of KS in young, previously healthy homosexual men began to accumulate.[10,11] In contrast to the type of KS usually seen in the United States, this form was widely disseminated on the skin, mucocutaneous areas, and viscera. Not surprisingly, this KS was sometimes fulminant. The incidence of KS in AIDS patients varies among series.[12-16] Prob-ably the most comprehensive figures are those compiled by the Centers for Disease Control (CDC) in Atlanta.[10] From June 1981 to August 1983, 2008 AIDS cases were recorded. KS was present in 533 (27%) of these. Autopsy studies of AIDS and ARC patients indicate that the incidence of KS at death is probably higher, with figures up to 94% in one series.[17] In the same series KS involving the skin was seen in only 26%, a figure similar to that of the CDC given previously. Preliminary data indicate that the incidence of KS is highest in the AIDS subgroup of homosexual or bisexual men and lowest in the subgroup of hemophiliacs.[16,18,19] Differences in life-style, including the use of amyl nitrates, have been invoked to explain these epidemiologic differences.[20] Since these data were collected, incidence of KS in homosexual men has dropped.[21,22]

The clinical manifestations of KS include cutaneous and mucocutaneous lesions, which may occur anytime during the course of AIDS or may be the initial sign of the disease. The lesions may be single, grouped, or widely dispersed. Because they are usually asymptomatic, they may go unnoticed for a long time. The lesions may occur anywhere on the body but have a predilection for the head (Figs. 12–1 and 12–2) and trunk. Mucosal involve-

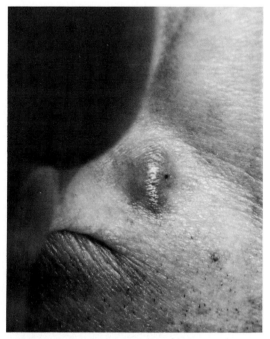

Figure 12–1. Posterior auricular lesion of Kaposi's sarcoma in AIDS patient. Such a lesion could be mistaken for folliculitis or acne.

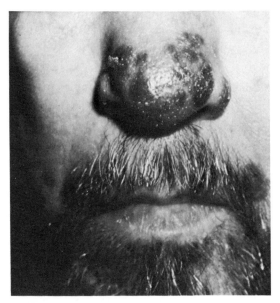

Figure 12–2. Kaposi's sarcoma in AIDS patient: facial papules and plaques. (Courtesy R. Shapiro, MD.)

ment, especially of the hard palate, is relatively common in this form of KS.

Individual lesions begin as small, red-purple macules resembling ecchymoses. Unlike ecchymoses, however, they do not fade but gradually enlarge and become palpable. Round, oval, or irregularly shaped plaques and nodules vary in color from pink to violaceous to red-brown. Individual lesions range from 2 mm to several centimeters in diameter. The tumors rarely become ulcerated and, as

mentioned previously, are usually asymptomatic. Very large lesions may be tender, especially if over a bony prominence.

A linear configuration of lesions has been proposed as a useful morphologic clue to KS associated with HIV infection.[23] A peculiar distribution of lesions on the trunk has also been described in AIDS-associated KS. Individual round or oval lesions tend to arise bilaterally along skin cleavage lines and give the eruption a pityriasis rosea–like appearance (Figs. 12–3 and 12–4).[24]

Lesions may regress, sometimes apparently in response to treatment, leaving red-brown rusty areas with varying degrees of scarring.

The histopathologic features of fully evolved lesions are indistinguishable from those of non-AIDS-associated KS.[6] A dermal proliferation of atypical spindle cells with erythrocytes in slitlike spaces unlined by endothelial cells is characteristic (Fig. 12–5). This proliferation may form a dermal nodule or patchy, small aggregates within the dermis and subcutis. Occasionally these atypical spindle cells form an irregular trabecular pattern as they infiltrate between collagen bundles. Also notable are hyaline eosinophilic globules that are smaller than erythrocytes and are present both extracellularly and within macrophages and tumor cells. Associated with these are lymphectasia and varying degrees of vascular proliferation without cytologic atypia. Lymphocytic and plasma cellular infiltrates are sometimes seen but are seldom prominent. In lesions of longer duration, hemo-

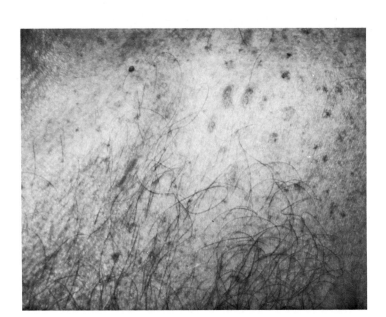

Figure 12–3. Pityriasis rosea-like lesions of Kaposi's sarcoma on chest of AIDS patient.

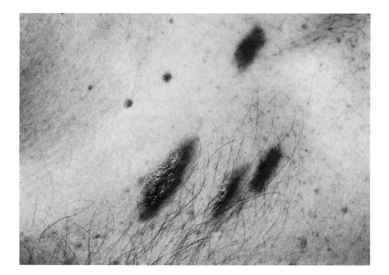

Figure 12–4. Pityriasis rosea-like lesions of Kaposi's sarcoma adjacent to clavicle of AIDS patient.

siderin deposition may be noted. In our opinion, cytologic atypia of the spindle cells is the feature necessary for the definitive diagnosis of KS. We have had the opportunity to review biopsies of lesions that were considered to be KS and resolved following interferon therapy. Findings include a disordered pattern of vessels (Fig. 12–6) or fibrosis with extensive hemosiderin deposition (Fig. 12–7). Atypical cells are absent in these regressed lesions. Poulsen et al.,[25] Real and Krown,[26] and Niedt and Schinella[27] have reported similar histologic findings. The phenomenon of spontane-

ously healing KS in AIDS patients has also been discussed by Maurice et al.,[28] Levy et al.,[29] and Janier et al.[30]

An inflammatory variant of KS usually occurs in lymph nodes and viscera and is only infrequently observed in skin.[17] These lesions have the usual histopathologic characteristics of KS, with well-formed nodular aggregates of atypical spindle cells and erythrocytes in slit-shaped spaces. Admixed with these tumor cells are prominent lymphocytes, plasma cells, eosinophils, and macrophages. The inflammation may be so dense that it apparently

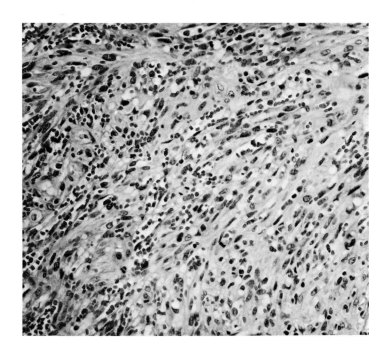

Figure 12–5. Biopsy specimen of Kaposi's sarcoma showing proliferation of atypical spindle cells and erythrocytes within slitlike spaces and poorly formed vascular spaces. Lymphocytic infiltrates are also present throughout tumor. This histopathologic pattern is typical and easy to recognize.

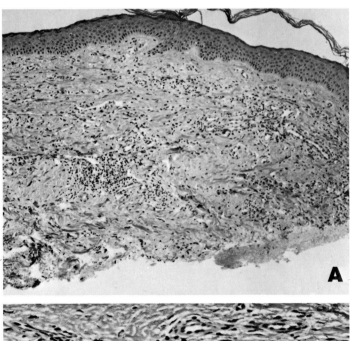

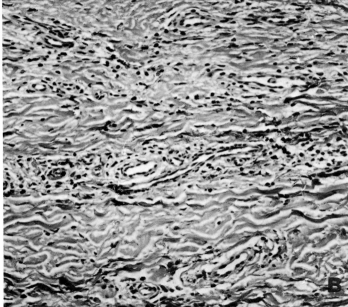

Figure 12–6. Low power, *A*, and high power, *B*, photomicrographs of biopsy specimen from suspected regressed lesions of Kaposi's sarcoma following alpha interferon therapy. Dermal vessels are disordered and increased in number with patchy lymphocytic infiltrates.

obscures the proliferation of tumor cells and vessels. Scattered tumor cells with marked nuclear anaplasia are also present. Vascular proliferation may be prominent, with arborizing, thickened, hyalinized vessels reminiscent of angioimmunoblastic lymphadenopathy.

Biopsy specimens are sometimes inconclusive from individuals at risk for AIDS in whom KS is suspected. These have consisted of vascular proliferations, some clearly benign hemangiomas, and other unusual congeries of poorly formed vessels in a patchy distribution

but without cytologic atypia (Fig. 12–8). Because the latter is absent, we are cautious about the diagnosis of KS. We respond to such biopsy specimens with a description and a comment about the lesion's unusual nature and possible relationship to KS. We believe strongly that patients with inconclusive diagnoses should be followed up carefully for the possible development of more diagnostic lesions. The entity of pseudo-KS was described in the pre-AIDS era[31-33] and should not be overlooked. Also relevant to this discussion is the report of Schwartz et al.,[34] who described, in a

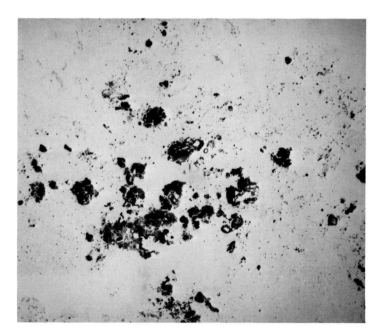

Figure 12–7. Biopsy specimen of regressed Kaposi's sarcoma showing dense fibrosis with hemosiderin deposits.

biopsy specimen of clinically normal skin from an AIDS patient with KS, an unusual proliferation of plump endothelial cells and scant spindle cells around irregularly branching vessels, which they called pre-Kaposi's sarcoma. Fukunaga and Silverberg[35] presented DNA flow cytometry data showing that AIDS-associated KS from 21 patients were all diploid with a low S-phase fraction. On the basis of these data

they suggested that KS may be a proliferative process rather than a malignant neoplasm.

A possible animal model of KS in pig-tailed macaques with an AIDS-like syndrome has been described.[36,37] Another possible animal model is avian hemangiomatosis induced by a retrovirus; indeed, Dictor and Järplid[38] suggest that a parallel etiopathologic retrovirus be sought in human KS.

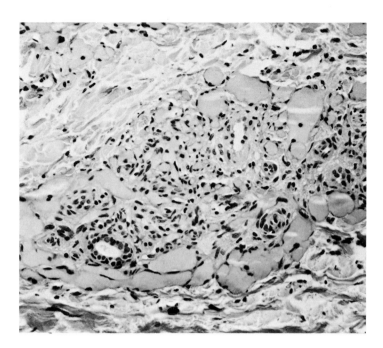

Figure 12–8. Proliferation of dilated thin-walled vessels and spindle cells from AIDS patient. These histopathologic findings strongly suggest Kaposi's sarcoma.

Bacillary Epithelioid Angiomatosis

In 1983 Stoler et al.[39] described an AIDS patient with multiple subcutaneous vascular nodules inhabited by small bacillary forms seen on Warthin-Starry stain. From subsequent reports by Cockerell et al.,[40] LeBoit et al.,[41] Knobler et al.,[42] and Koehler et al.,[43] an entity has emerged that clinically and histologically resembles pyogenic granuloma and histiocytoid hemangioma and is probably associated with the cat-scratch bacillus. The lesions are usually asymptomatic papules, plaques, or nodules. Filiform and skin tag–like lesions have also been described. The lesions are more often multiple but may be solitary. They may be exophytic or nodular, ulcerated or not. They may occur anywhere on the skin. Mucosal surfaces, viscera, and bone may also be involved. About half the cases described are associated with a history of a cat scratch. Cockerell[44] reported bird scratches associated with this entity in an otherwise healthy, HIV-seronegative patient without risk factors for AIDS. The lesions are reported to resolve with erythromycin therapy.[45]

The histologic features of bacillary epithelioid angiomatosis (BEA) consist of a proliferation of vessels, often with the architecture of a pyogenic granuloma, that is, an exophytic papulonodule with an epidermal collarette. Alternatively, BEA may form a deep, dermal or subcutaneous vascular nodule or, more rarely, filiform or skin tag–like lesions. The cells of the frequently ectatic vessels are cytologically benign and are frequently epithelioid. The stroma between the vessels may contain a mixture of neutrophils, lymphocytes, and histiocytes. Clumps of basophilic bacillary forms 1 to 2 µm long may be seen on hematoxylin and eosin–stained sections. Warthin-Starry stain has been the stain of choice for identifying these organisms in tissue sections. Although the organisms are described as gram negative, they have not been seen with tissue Gram's stains such as the Brown and Brenn stain. Electron microscopy has confirmed that the organisms are bacteria.[39] An immunoperoxidase reagent raised against the cat-scratch bacillus reacted with organisms in tissue sections.[41,43] To date, cat-scratch organisms have not been grown on cultures from these lesions. When the polymerase chain reaction and oligonucleotide primers complementary to the 16S ribosomal RNA genes of eubacteria were used to amplify gene fragments directly from tissue samples, the results suggested that bacillary angiomatosis is caused by a previously uncharacterized rickettsia-like organism closely related to *Rochalimaea quintana*.[46] The histologic resemblance of BEA to pyogenic granulomas and histiocytoid hemangioma (Kimura's disease) is evident. There is no resemblance to KS; no spindle cell component and no slitlike spaces are present.

The similarity of BEA to verruga peruana, a disease endemic to certain regions of Peru and caused by *Bartonella bacilliformis*, was noted by Omura and Omura.[47] This disorder is associated with high fevers (Oroya fever) and is sometimes fatal. Vascular papules, plaques, and nodules, known as Peruvian warts, develop in this disorder. It is transmitted by an insect vector.[48] BEA differs from verruga peruana in that fevers are usually absent or ascribed to other causes in BEA; as far as we know, BEA is not transmitted by an insect vector (the Peruvian vector does not exist in North America); and *B. bacilliformis* has never been grown on cultures from BEA lesions.

BEA also does not resemble typical cat-scratch disease affecting the skin and lymph nodes.[49,50] Cat-scratch disease is usually associated with a cutaneous nodule followed weeks to months later by regional adenopathy. Sometimes the nodule becomes ulcerated. Other cutaneous lesions reported to occur with cat-scratch disease include erythema multiforme, erythema nodosum, and vague macular and papular eruptions. Vascular lesions were not reported before the advent of AIDS. The histopathologic characteristics of the cutaneous lesions of typical cat-scratch disease are not well described. The lymphadenopathy shows stellate granulomas with central neutrophilic microabscesses. The bacillus can be seen by Warthin-Starry stain in some cases and can also be grown on cultures.

Interestingly, cat-scratch disease affecting the conjunctiva can be associated with the development of vascular tissue reactions similar to BEA.

In some ways BEA resembles the clinical and histologic reaction pattern seen in response to a variety of infectious agents. Chancroid, for example, shows an ulcerated nodule and lymphadenopathy. A histologic feature of chancroid is a trilevel pattern including a prominent vascular or granulation tissue layer. Admittedly the vascular proliferation usually does not closely resemble the histiocytoid hemangioma–like pattern of BEA.

Non-Hodgkin's Lymphoma

The incidence of non-Hodgkin's lymphoma in patients with AIDS or ARC is higher than in the general population. Parallels may be drawn to lymphomas occurring in patients with congenital or acquired immunodeficiency, iatrogenic immunodeficiency (as in renal transplant patients), or certain viral infections.[51] Loss of normal T-cell function, polyclonal expansion of B-cells, and infection by Epstein-Barr virus and CMV[52] is well described in patients with AIDS and ARC. The emergence of a monoclonal lymphoma from the polyclonal B-cell expansion in the face of viral infections known to be associated with lymphomas is not surprising. That the non-Hodgkin's lymphomas in AIDS and ARC have all been undifferentiated or B-cell in type is noteworthy.[53-55]

Non-Hodgkin's lymphomas in the HIV-infected population follow a more aggressive course than lymphomas of similar types in patients without AIDS or ARC. Ziegler et al.[53] report that the mortality rate in AIDS and ARC patients is more than twice that of homosexual men without prodromal symptoms. In this same series, extranodal disease was remarkably common. Cutaneous involvement, however, reported in 14 of 88 patients (16%), was not appreciably different in incidence from skin involvement in lymphomas during the pre-AIDS era.[56]

Individual lesions in the skin are erythematous nodules and plaques, either single or multiple, and localized or diffuse. In the study cited previously the most common sites of lesions were (in descending order) intraoral, anorectal, thigh, popliteal fossa, earlobes, multiple cutaneous nodules, and scalp.[53] This contrasts with lymphoma cutis in patients without AIDS or ARC, in which the head and neck are the most common sites of involvement.[57] Also worth noting is the initial site of lymphoma in the series of Ziegler et al.[53] In seven men intraoral and anorectal areas were the initial sites. As an example of another unusual presentation, Ragni et al.[58] report lymphoma occurring as a traumatic hematoma in a hemophiliac who had antibody to human T-cell lymphotropic virus type III (HTLV-III).

Lymphoma cutis is characterized histopathologically by dermal infiltrates of lymphoma cells. The differential diagnosis of lymphocytic infiltrates in the skin includes many diseases; features that favor lymphoma are extensive involvement of the dermis, cytologic atypia (nuclear hyperchromasia, high nuclear/cytoplasmic ratio), and a monomorphous population of lymphoid cells, which reflects the monoclonality of the lymphoma. Unfortunately, not all biopsy specimens reflect these features. In some cases the infiltrate is patchy with a primarily perivenular distribution. Cytologic atypia may be absent in well-differentiated lymphomas. The monomorphous nature of the lymphoma may be obscured by inflammatory cells reacting to the lymphoma. Lymphocyte marker studies sometimes help to distinguish monoclonal from polyclonal lymphocyte populations in the skin. Knowledge of the differential diagnosis of lymphocytic infiltrates in the skin is a complex matter but is helpful in evaluating these biopsies. In all cases consideration of extracutaneous disease, especially in lymph nodes, spleen, bone marrow, and the central nervous system, is important.

Atypical Lymphoid Hyperplasias

Atypical lymphoid hyperplasias—angioimmunoblastic lymphadenopathy,[59,60] angiofollicular lymph node hyperplasia (Castleman's disease),[61,62] and lymphadenopathy—have been described in association with AIDS and ARC. Cutaneous involvement has been described in non-HIV-infected patients with angioimmunoblastic lymphadenopathy, but we are unaware of any reports of skin involvement in patients with AIDS or ARC. We have reviewed biopsy findings from a male homosexual who had had lymphomatoid papulosis for 4 years before the onset of AIDS. Although these two diseases may have occurred coincidentally in this patient, it is interesting that both are diseases of T-lymphocytes.

Hodgkin's Disease

Schoeppel et al.[63] described Hodgkin's disease in four homosexual men, one of whom had cutaneous involvement in contiguity with underlying lymph nodes involved by tumor. The clinical and histologic features of the cutaneous lesions were not detailed in this report. Descriptions of Hodgkin's disease in the skin without reference to AIDS or ARC are available elsewhere.[64,65]

Squamous Cell Carcinoma in Situ and Basal Cell Carcinoma

Single cases of squamous cell carcinoma (SCC) in situ of the penis, basal cell carcinoma (Fig. 12–9), and SCC of the tongue have been

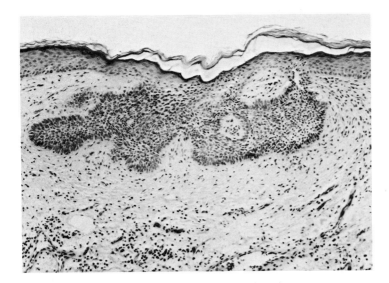

Figure 12–9. Basal cell carcinoma from asymptomatic 48-year-old male homosexual infected with HIV.

described in AIDS patients.[66,67] As noted by Slazinski et al.,[66] the association is not so much between AIDS and these tumors as the known and more plausible association between immunodeficiency states in general and these tumors. The clinical and histologic features of these cases did not appear to differ appreciably from those in non-AIDS patients. However, human papillomavirus (HPV) subtypes not ordinarily associated with malignancy may be seen.[68] As AIDS patients' lives are prolonged, more of these and other tumors may be reported.

Malignant Melanoma

Malignant melanoma has been reported in HIV-seropositive patients.[69,70] Whether an association between melanoma and HIV infection exists or the reports represent two common diseases occurring in these patients remains to be seen.

INFECTIOUS DISEASES OF PATIENTS WITH AIDS AND ARC

Alterations of many aspects of immunity,[71] including Langerhans' cells,[72] macrophages,[73] and B- and T-lymphocytes, occur in HIV-infected individuals. The prospective study of Murray et al.[74] suggests that the risk of opportunistic infections may correlate with the inability to generate antigen-induced gamma interferon. In the face of this severely compromised immune system, it is perhaps surprising that more infectious agents have not been described in the skin. Additional in-

fectious agents with unusual clinical presentations in the skin will probably be added to the literature as time goes by.

As noted by Hatcher,[75] the infectious diseases that follow are not specific for AIDS and ARC. They have been observed in both immunocompetent and immunosuppressed populations. These diseases tend to appear in unusual or unusually severe forms in the latter population. Such a presentation in a person at risk for AIDS indicates the need for close monitoring for the development of serious opportunistic infections.

In addition to routine histologic studies and special stains, a number of other studies may be useful in the diagnosis of cutaneous infections. These include immunofluorescence and immunoperoxidase techniques, DNA hybridization studies, electron microscopy, and appropriate cultures. As a minimal workup of biopsy specimens from patients with AIDS or ARC, we recommend special stains for bacteria, fungi, and acid-fast organisms. Special stain for spirochetes also merits consideration.

Viral Infections

Evidence by histology or culture or both has been described for the following viruses in the skin: herpes simplex and varicella-zoster, CMV, molluscum contagiosum, papillomavirus, HIV, and adenovirus.[14,17,75-91] Evidence suggests that Epstein-Barr virus also replicates in oropharyngeal epithelial cells.[90] Many of these reports emphasize clinical features of unusual extent or chronicity. These unusual presentations are sometimes seen in other immunosuppressed states[92] and are not unique to AIDS and ARC. One feature more common in patients with AIDS or ARC than in other immunosuppressed patients is simultaneous infection of the skin by multiple agents.[83,84]

Herpesvirus Infection

Herpes Simplex. The characteristic lesion of herpes simplex is a cluster of vesicles on a slightly erythematous, elevated base. After 2 to 3 days the vesicles become cloudy and subsequently eroded and crusted. Primary infection may involve a large area of skin and typically resolves in 2 weeks. Recurrent (reactivation) lesions usually involve a smaller area of skin and last only 7 to 10 days. The face, lips, and genitals are commonly affected areas; however, infection may occur anywhere on the mucocutaneous surface of the body. The causative organisms are herpes simplex virus types 1 and 2. Infection with herpes simplex virus type 2 appears to be a risk factor for subsequent or concurrent HIV infection.[86]

Herpes simplex infection in the HIV-infected host may be much more extensive and heal much more slowly than in an immunocompetent individual.[83,88] Atypical clinical presentations, such as absence of vesicles and mucocutaneous dissemination, have also been described.[89,91] Although the use of acyclovir in HIV-positive hosts with severe herpes virus infection has reduced the considerable morbidity of this disease, the emergence of acyclovir-resistant strains[91,93] has been described and presents a new challenge to the treatment of herpes simplex infections.

Herpes Varicella-Zoster. Severely immunosuppressed individuals are susceptible to primary HVZ infection and reactivation of latent infection. Varicella is classically manifested by scattered clear vesicles on a slightly erythematous base (Figure 12–10). The vesicles soon collapse, become umbilicated, and form an erosion with overlying crust. Reactivation of HVZ virus produces similar vesicles arranged in a unilateral dermatomal distribution. Often zoster vesicles become hemorrhagic and necrotic. These lesions resolve, leaving scars with hypopigmentation or hyperpigmentation. Disseminated HVZ infection (Fig. 12–11) is also well known. Postherpetic neuralgia, a debilitating complication of herpes zoster, lasts months to years after the initial eruption clears. HIV-infected hosts, especially those previously taking acyclovir, may have disseminated, nodular, necrotic, hyper-

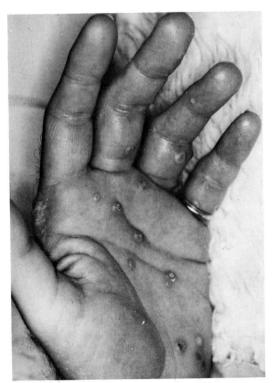

Figure 12–10. Disseminated varicella-zoster on palm of AIDS patient. (Courtesy R. Shapiro, MD.)

keratotic, or poxlike lesions instead of the more usual lesions.[94-97] A prolonged course, multiple relapses, and death have occurred.

Tzanck's Smear. In herpes simplex, varicella, and zoster, smears from the vesicle floors or from erosions reveal balloon and multinucleated giant epithelial cells. Nuclear viral inclusion bodies are usually not visualized with the Tzanck technique.

Biopsy. Mature lesions show an intraepidermal vesicle containing serum, neutrophils, mononuclear cells, and acantholytic epidermal cells. The base or floor of the blister cavity is lined with infected epidermal cells that may be large, irregular, ballooned, or multinucleated. These cells show nuclear margination of chromatin with a violet, "ground-glass" appearance. Viral inclusion bodies surrounded by a faint, clear halo may occasionally be seen within nuclei. The necrosis and cytopathic keratinocyte changes often extend down appendages (Fig. 12–12), particularly hair follicles. In the dermis there is a moderately intense to severe, predominantly mononuclear perivascular infiltrate. This inflammatory cell response may be absent or appreciably diminished in leukopenic individuals. Severe infection may be accompanied by a

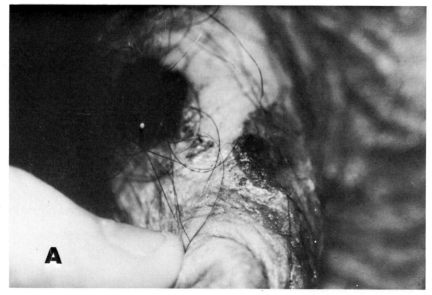

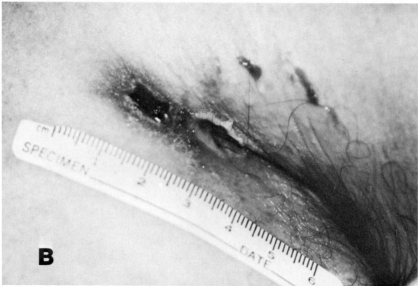

Figure 12–11. Herpetic ulcers, *A,* on penis and *B,* in axilla of AIDS patient.

leukocytoclastic vasculitis involving the deep vessels in the reticular dermis. Herpesvirus infections caused by varicella-zoster and simplex viruses cannot be distinguished from each other microscopically.[98]

Human Papillomavirus Infection. Warts caused by HPV are common in both immunocompetent and immunodeficient or immunocompromised individuals.[99,100] In the latter groups the lesions may be quite extensive, do not regress spontaneously, and are often recalcitrant to traditional modes of therapy. Common warts, or verruca vulgaris, are round, well-demarcated papules with hyperkeratotic,

irregular surfaces that favor the extensor surfaces of the hands and fingers. Flat warts are small, round papules occurring most commonly on the face and extremities. Condyloma acuminatum begins as a small, verrucous papule that gradually enlarges to form exophytic, verrucous nodules and plaques. These lesions are seen most commonly in the anogenital area, including the mucosa of the vagina, rectum, and urethra.

Over the past decade the ability to classify warts has been enhanced by serologic typing and nucleic acid hybridization techniques. To date, over 30 different types of HPV have

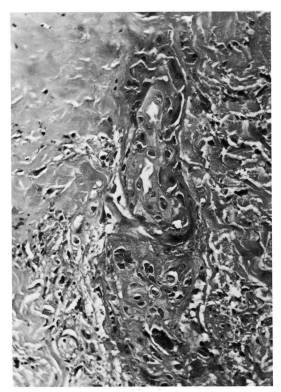

Figure 12–12. Herpetic lesion from patient in Figure 12–11. Collagen necrobiosis and viral cytopathic changes within eccrine duct can be seen.

been identified. Common warts, including plantar lesions, are associated with HPV types 1, 2, and 4, flat warts are associated with HPV-3, and condylomata acuminata are associated with HPV-6 and HPV-16. Oncogenic HPV-5 has been identified in squamous cell carcinomas of renal transplant patients who have been immunosuppressed with azathioprine and corticosteroids.[101] Disseminated warts and apparent evolution to squamous cell carcinoma have been described in an AIDS patient.[68] In this patient DNA sequences related to HPV-6/11 were seen in a verrucous penile lesion interpreted as evolving squamous cell carcinoma. These sequences are rarely associated with squamous cell carcinoma. HPV-16 and HPV-13 sequences, most commonly associated with malignancy, were not seen.

The histologic appearance of warts varies with the morphology and serologic type of the infecting virus.[102] Common warts are characterized by orthokeratosis and parakeratosis, acanthosis with papillomatosis, prominent hypergranulosis with condensation of keratohyalin granules, and moderate koilocytosis of granular cells at the top of the papillae. Flat

warts exhibit orthohyperkeratosis, acanthosis, and prominent koilocytosis of cells in the upper malphigian layer. This so-called bird's eye vacuolization is characterized by perinuclear vacuoles and a centrally located pyknotic, basophilic nucleus. Features of condyloma acuminatum include parakeratosis, pronounced acanthosis with rounded papillomatosis, and perinuclear vacuolization (koilocytosis) with marginated, crescent-shaped nuclei in the upper malphigian layers. Spherical, deep, eosinophilic nucleolus-like inclusion bodies are occasionally seen in young common and plantar warts.

Cytomegalovirus Infection. Although CMV infection is common in immunocompromised individuals, skin lesions are uncommon or unrecognized. In patients with disseminated CMV infection, ulcers occasionally develop, most frequently in the genital or perineal region. The lesions in many ways resemble the indolent ulcerations caused by HSV in immunosuppressed patients.[103] In other immunosuppressed patients with disseminated CMV infection, a widespread papular, exanthematous eruption develops.[104,105] None of the patients with this particular cutaneous manifestation of CMV infection have survived the acute infection; this type of cutaneous involvement has been associated with multiorgan involvement at autopsy. AIDS patients may show the previously described clinical lesions with CMV infection, but proliferative, keratotic, verrucous lesions have also been seen.[106] Segal et al.[107] describe a case of thrombotic thrombocytopenic purpura in a patient with AIDS and CMV infection.

The characteristic histologic finding in both ulcerative and exanthematous eruptions, as well as keratotic lesions, is the presence of CMV inclusions within the nuclei of enlarged endothelial cells or macrophages in the dermis. The inclusion bodies are finely granular and surrounded by halos. In AIDS patients, CMV cytopathic changes may affect keratinocytes as well.[106] There is a prominent perivascular and interstitial infiltrate composed of lymphocytes, histiocytes, and in some cases neutrophils. Cytoplasmic inclusions are less commonly seen. Notably, no epidermal changes occur similar to those in herpes simplex or herpes varicella-zoster infection such as balloon cells, nuclear moulding, and multinucleated giant cells. Horn and Hood[108] point out that CMV inclusions are commonly present in ulcers from immunosuppressed patients, but that this does not establish CMV as the cause of the ulcer. Appropriate cultures, serologic studies, or both should be obtained in all cases of suspected infection, since they will identify the organism and can provide information about the appropriate agent for treatment.

Fungal Infections

Cutaneous infection with *Candida* species, *Cryptococcus neoformans, Histoplasma capsulatum, Cladosporium, Sporothrix, Coccidioides immitis, Aspergillus,* and dermatophytes have been described in AIDS and ARC patients.[13,14,67,75,77,78,109-120] Unusually extensive and persistent candidal infection is considered to be one of the cardinal signs of immunodeficiency.[111] The theme of unusual cutaneous presentations is again emphasized in many of these reports. Examples include histoplasmosis occurring as a transepidermal elimination disorder,[120] *Cryptococcus* infection resembling molluscum contagiosum,[110] and herpetiform cryptococcosis.[109] These three cases were notable in that they all represented cutaneous involvement in patients with disseminated fungemia. Histopathologic examination of the skin in these cases showed the characteristic morphology of the organism and usually sparse inflammation.

Mycobacterial Infections

Most reports of mycobacterial infection focus on noncutaneous sites of infection.[121,122] In reports of mycobacterial cutaneous infection, the organism was not always diagnosed clinically. Pennys and Hicks[77] described a patient whose clinical findings suggested KS and whose pathologic findings included innumerable acid-fast organisms in histiocytes, with adjacent granulomas and KS. Kwan and Kaufman[84] described biopsy findings of acid-fast bacilli with granulomas, a mixed inflammatory infiltrate, and CMV inclusions (Fig. 12–13) in a patient who also had clinical signs of KS. This latter patient had previously had *M. avium-intracellulare* grown on cultures of the lung. He subsequently died of intestinal obstruction, and innumerable cytomegalic inclusions with vasculitis were present in the bowel at autopsy. We have observed an AIDS patient with clinically unremarkable papules on the chest (Fig. 12–14), which showed rare acid-fast bacilli on a background of poorly formed granulomas and a mixed inflammatory infiltrate. Mehlmauer[123] described a patient with ARC who had keratotic papules and nodules and hyperkeratosis of palms and soles; tuberculosis was unrecognized in this patient because of the unusual clinical presentation. We advocate the use of special stains in

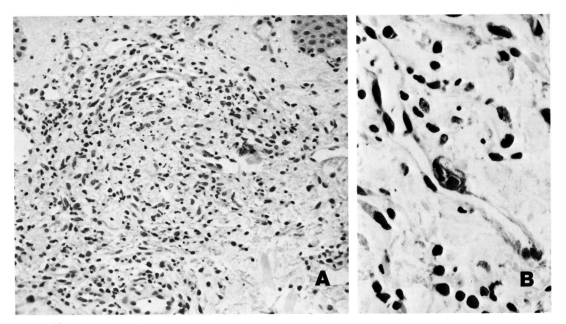

Figure 12–13. Biopsy specimen from lesion suspected of being Kaposi's sarcoma shows, *A,* poorly formed granulomas and, *B,* large nuclear inclusions of cytomegalovirus. Acid-fast bacilli were observed on special stains (not illustrated here).

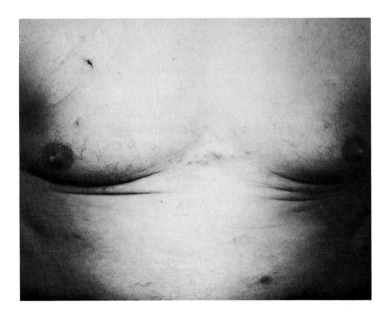

Figure 12–14. Ill-defined papules on central chest, probably caused by atypical mycobacterial infection. Biopsy specimens taken from left pectoral area showed acid-fast bacilli. (Courtesy Suzanne Olbricht, MD.)

histologic examinations of skin of all AIDS patients to detect occult infections with atypical *Mycobacterium*.

Pyogenic Bacterial Infections

The incidence of pyogenic bacterial infection is difficult to assess. Most reports do not describe pyogenic infections in patients with AIDS or ARC. Hatcher[75] however, described impetigo and other pyodermas as common in HIV-infected patients, particularly on the head and neck and in intertriginous areas. The histologic features of these lesions are not given, presumably because the clinical appearance and microbiology cultures were typical. Dermal abscesses with *Staphylococcus aureus*, CMV, and acid-fast bacilli were described by Boudreau et al.[124] Bacterial sepsis secondary to severe scabetic infestation has also been described.[125] Botryomycosis has been found in AIDS patients as well.[126,127]

Syphilis

Already known for its diverse clinical manifestations before the AIDS era, syphilis has become even more difficult to diagnose with the AIDS epidemic. Gregory et al.[128] summarized salient features of syphilis in HIV-infected patients: misleading antibody titers, increased severity of the disease, including rapid progression to the tertiary phase, and unexpected relapse after standard treatment with penicillin. Antibody titers to *Treponema pallidum* may be unusually high, low, or absent

in the phase of active infection; biopsy specimens stained with appropriate silver stains (Warthin-Starry, Dieterle's, modified Steiner's) or immunoperoxidase reagents can demonstrate the spirochetes when the serologic response is absent.[129] Increased severity of syphilis in HIV-infected patients may be manifest as ulceronodular lesions,[130] rapid progression from secondary to tertiary phases of the infection, as evidenced histopathologically by granulomas,[130,131] and rapid development of neurosyphilis.[132] Relapse after treatment with standard doses of penicillin is thought to occur because of reservoirs of infection in the CNS and other sites and because of the markedly altered immune system. Thus syphilis in HIV-infected individuals has important clinical features, but the histopathologic patterns are the same as those described before AIDS. In this time of AIDS the biopsy has assumed greater importance in the diagnosis of syphilis because of the variability of the serologic response.

Protozoal Infections

Pennys and Hicks[77] described an AIDS patient from whom an incisional biopsy of a thigh papule (noted at autopsy) disclosed numerous amebic trophozoites within suppurative inflammation. In this AIDS patient disseminated *Acanthamoeba castellani* infection had been diagnosed during life. Hirschmann and Chu[133] described a widespread papulovesicular rash in a patient with disseminated toxoplasmosis. Biopsy examination of this rash showed a perivascular lymphocytic and histiocytic infiltrate without organisms.

Scabetic *(Sarcoptes Scabiei)* Infestation

Scabetic infestation can occur in patients with HIV infection. The severe, extensively crusted form, also known as Norwegian scabies, is especially notable, since it can be confused clinically with seborrheic dermatitis or drug reactions and can serve as the portal of entry for secondary bacterial infection, resulting in sepsis and even death.[125,134-136] The clinical and histologic findings are similar to those in patients without HIV infection.

OTHER DERMATOSES AND MUCOCUTANEOUS DISORDERS OF HIV-POSITIVE PATIENTS

HIV Exanthem and Enanthem

Primary infection with HIV may be associated with a mononucleosis-like illness. This illness may be present in over 90% of patients who become seropositive for HIV. Fever, sweats, lethargy, malaise, anorexia, nausea, myalgia, arthralgia, headache, photophobia, sore throat, diarrhea, lymphadenopathy, and a rash have been described. In two prospective studies the exanthem occurred in 50% of 12 seroconverters[137] and in 23% of 39 seroconverters.[138] The cutaneous eruption has been described as erythematous, maculopapular, and usually truncal or generalized. The cutaneous lesions may be papulosquamous with scaling, may show hemorrhage, and may involve palms and soles. Desquamation of palms and soles has also been described. The rash has been likened to that of roseola[139] and syphilis.[140] The enanthem may include superficial erosions and glossitis. Skin biopsies have shown a superficial perivascular lymphocytic infiltrate with exocytosis; hemorrhage, parakeratosis, spongiosis, basal layer vacuolar changes, necrosis, and vascular ectasia have also been noted.[140] These histologic changes are not specific, but they resemble those in other viral exanthems with the possible exception of the described necrosis.

Dermatitis Medicamentosa

Cutaneous drug reactions to trimethoprim-sulfamethoxazole have occurred with a surprisingly high incidence in AIDS patients be-ing treated for *Pneumocystis carinii* pneumonia, up to 69%[141,142] as compared with 5.9%[143] in earlier series of non-AIDS patients. De-Hovitz et al.,[144] however, recorded a 4.8% rate of cutaneous reactions to a comparable high-dose regimen in their series of 21 Haitian AIDS patients being treated for *Isospora belli* or intestinal *Cryptosporidium* infection. Dermatitis medicamentosa is characterized by an erythematous maculopapular eruption affecting the entire body. The rash appears in 1 to 9 days and remains as long as 14 to 21 days following initiation of therapy.[144] These eruptions may be associated with constitutional symptoms such as fever. Leukopenia, thrombocytopenia, and hepatitis are also among the toxic reactions associated with trimethoprim-sulfamethoxazole. The cutaneous reaction may subside spontaneously or, more commonly, following withdrawal of the drug. The histologic features of the cutaneous reaction have not been described.

Pentamidine is associated with a high incidence of systemic toxic reaction but a low incidence of cutaneous eruptions.[142]

Neutrophilic eccrine hidradenitis of unknown pathogenesis has been reported in two HIV patients taking zidovudine.[145] Grau-Massanes et al.[146] described mucocutaneous pigmentation and longitudinal, bandlike pigmentation of the nails in HIV-positive patients taking zidovudine. These changes began after 6 weeks of drug administration. These pigmentary changes subsided after treatment was discontinued in one of the three patients described.

McNeely et al.[147] described a mucocutaneous eruption with oral ulcers in reaction to 2'-3'-dideoxycytidine.

Keratoderma in 6 of 20 AIDS patients receiving glucan has been reported by Duvic et al.[148] Palmoplantar keratosis has been seen in a wide variety of systemic and cutaneous conditions in both HIV- and non-HIV-infected individuals.

Cutaneous drug reactions are common in other immunocompromised populations. At first glance it seems paradoxical that a patient who cannot fend off an opportunistic infectious agent is able to react against a drug. However, as Wintroub and Stern[149] pointed out, drug reactions are mediated by many mechanisms, both immunologic and nonimmunologic.

Interface dermatitis, whether drug related or not, is a common but seldom reported finding in AIDS patients.[150] This histologic pattern in AIDS patients probably represents a variety of disorders as it does in non-HIV-infected patients.

Seborrheic Dermatitis–Like Eruption

Seborrheic dermatitis in AIDS patients and other HIV-positive individuals has been noted in numerous reports.[77,78,151-153] In a small series of AIDS patients examined by a dermatologist, seborrheic dermatitis was noted in up to 46%, compared with 5% for a large number of non-AIDS patients examined during the same period.[151] Mathes and Douglass[152] observed seborrheic dermatitis in 86% of their series of 18 AIDS patients. The clinical features include a scaling, erythematous, oily rash affecting any or all of the following areas: scalp, eyebrows, ears, periauricular areas, central face, central upper chest and back, axilla, groin, and genitalia. Seborrheic dermatitis in the HIV-positive population is sometimes "explosive" in onset and is often more inflammatory and less responsive to therapy than in most other patients. For example, dandruff usually consists of mild scaling, but in this population, heavy, greasy scales and marked erythema are common. In the report of Eisenstadt and Wormser,[151] the facial eruption was described as a butterfly rash, leading some of the nondermatologists to consider lupus erythematosus. Because of its distinctive clinical appearance, seborrheic dermatitis rarely requires biopsy for diagnosis, and only one of the preceding reports includes histopathologic findings.[153] These were psoriasiform hyperplasia, parakeratosis with neutrophils and exudate, exocytosis of lymphocytes, dyskeratotic cells in some cases, superficial perivenular lymphocytic, plasma-cellular and neutrophilic infiltrates, vascular ectasia, and follicular plugging. In contrast, the histologic features of seborrheic dermatitis in non-AIDS patients include a mixed psoriasis–eczematous dermatitis picture: psoriasiform epidermal hyperplasia with hyperkeratosis and parakeratosis, Munro's microabscesses, spongiosis, and a superficial perivascular lymphocytic infiltrate. Dyskeratotic cells and plasma cells are not often seen in the non-AIDS type. Soeprono et al.[153] concluded that the seborrheic dermatitis–like eruption observed in AIDS patients is an entity distinct from the seborrheic dermatitis of non-AIDS patients. Groisser et al.[115] suggested a possible association between *Pity-*

rosporum orbiculare and seborrheic dermatitis in AIDS patients.

As noted previously, seborrheic dermatitis occurs in some other immunodeficiency states, as well as Parkinson's disease, other neurologic disorders, chronic alcoholism, cardiac failure, and zinc deficiency. The pathogenesis is unclear.

Seborrheic dermatitis, especially the severe forms, is common in HIV-positive patients, and severe seborrheic dermatitis correlated with a poor prognosis in one series.[152]

Chronic Pruritus

Pruritus in HIV-infected patients has many causes, such as drug reactions, ectoparasite infestation, and eosinophilic pustular folliculitis. A persistent, nonspecific, macular, papular, and nodular erythematous rash of unknown cause has also been described.[154,155] This rash is most often on the extremities but sometimes appears on the trunk and face. Biopsy of these lesions has shown a lymphocytic and eosinophilic perivascular and perifollicular infiltrate. This histologic pattern often represents a hypersensitivity reaction in non-HIV-infected patients. The eruption is unusually persistent and unresponsive to treatment. Gorin et al.[156] reported successful treatment with psoralens plus ultraviolet A phototherapy. In 134 Haitian patients studied by Liataud et al.,[155] these lesions were seen in 79% of patients with AIDS, and often appeared before the diagnosis of KS or opportunistic infection was established.

Pennys et al.[157] hypothesized that this chronic pruritic eruption associated with AIDS may represent a chronic "recall" reaction to an antigen, a further expression of altered immunity.

Eosinophilic Pustular Folliculitis

In 1986 Soeprono et al.[158] reported eosinophilic pustular folliculitis in three patients with AIDS. Before the advent of AIDS this disorder was reported mostly in Japanese patients[159,160] and a few patients from Europe[161,162] but not in the United States. In non-AIDS patients it affects mostly males from infancy to the mid-seventies.[163,164] The clinical and histologic features of this disease are similar in non-AIDS and AIDS patients. Clinical examination shows a pruritic folliculocentric dermatosis with sterile follicular pustules on an expanding erythematous plaque. The lesions are usually 3 to 5 cm in diameter, with a tendency to central healing and peripheral pustules. Some patients also have fever, leukocytosis, and eosinophilia. Resolution may occur spontaneously over months or years. Response to dapsone,[165] corticosteroids,[158,164] and ultraviolet B phototherapy[166] has been reported.

Biopsy of the pustules at the advancing edge of the plaque shows an eosinophilic abscess within the hair follicle or sebaceous gland. Neutrophils and lymphocytes may be mingled with the eosinophils. Bacteria and fungi are not found in these abscesses. *Demodex* mites are sometimes found within or adjacent to the infiltrate,[158,167] but whether they are directly involved in causing this dermatosis is not clear. The follicular epithelium may show a distinctive histologic pattern of spongiosis and necrosis. Multiple sections are frequently necessary to demonstrate the distinctive follicular or sebaceous gland eosinophilic pustule. Biopsy specimens from the plaque away from the advancing edge may simply show a nonspecific perivascular and interstitial mixed infiltrate with eosinophils.

Bacterial and Fungal Folliculitis

Erythematous follicular papules and nodules, sometimes with production of pus, are considered the typical clinical appearance of folliculitis. Cultures grow pyogenic and, less commonly, gram-negative organisms. In one series of AIDS and HIV-positive patients, folliculitis was noted in 10 of 53.[78] In some patients the severity has been notable, with acnelike eruptions. Axillary and perianal involvement has also been noted. Biopsy of these lesions is not often performed, but perhaps it should be, because the clinical appearance is relatively nonspecific. Farthing et al.[78] described one patient with a pustular eruption typical of folliculitis but negative for organisms when cultured and showing KS on biopsy. In addition, eosinophilic pustular folliculitis must be distinguished from folliculitis of infectious etiology. The usual histologic picture of folliculitis is superficial or deep neutrophilic or lymphohistiocytic infiltrates in and around pilar follicles with or without abscess formation and foreign body reaction. Organisms are sometimes difficult to demonstrate in histologic sections, and cultures identify the organism and provide information for specific therapy.

Vasculitis

Leukocytoclastic vasculitis in the skin has been noted in several AIDS patients. Farthing et al.[78] described two cases, both with immunofluorescence studies. When initially examined both patients had purpura, widespread in one and localized to the feet in the other. Both had CMV pneumonia, but no CMV antigens could be demonstrated in cutaneous vessels. In one case, bright fluorescence was seen in vessels when a reaction of tissue to high-titer anti-HIV serum was produced. Niedt and Schinella[27] described arteritis in the bowel wall associated with CMV inclusions but no vasculitis in the skin. A purpuric lesion on the thigh of another AIDS patient with CMV infection showed evidence of septic embolic infarction.[168] We have observed leukocytoclastic vasculitis adjacent to a herpetic blister and herpetic folliculitis in a patient with CMV inclusions and acid-fast bacilli in the skin.[84] Vasculitis subjacent to a herpetic blister is a fairly common occurrence in severe herpetic infection.

Vasculitis has many causes, and its presence is not surprising in any population of hospitalized patients, especially those prone to infection. To date, we are unaware of any increased incidence of vasculitis in HIV-positive patients. Possibly pertinent to the subject of vasculitis are reports of circulating immune complexes in patients with AIDS or ARC.[169,170] Chren et al.[171] described asymptomatic HIV infection, elevated immunoglobulin E levels, and leukocytoclastic vasculitis in a 9-year-old girl.

Papular Granulomatous Eruption and Granuloma Annulare

A clinically distinctive papular eruption has been reported in 7 of 35 patients with AIDS or ARC.[172] Numerous, occasionally pruritic, 2 to 5 mm, skin-colored papules were present, usually on the head, neck, and upper trunk, waxing and waning over periods up to or exceeding 1 year. This dermatosis did not correlate with severity of disease or presence of infection. Four of the seven patients underwent biopsy. Most had only a superficial perivascular mononuclear cell infiltrate with occasional swollen endothelial cells. Three biopsy specimens from one patient showed epithelioid cell granulomas distributed around hair follicles and vessels and interstitially. In addition, there were scattered mononuclear and plasma cells, as well as eosinophils adjacent to the granulomas. Cultures and Giemsa, Fite-Farco, and periodic acid–Schiff stains were negative for organisms. James et al.[172] concluded that this eruption is clinically distinctive for human retrovirus infection. A lichenoid granulomatous papular dermatitis has also been described.[173] Heymann[174] pointed out that secondary syphilis can mimic these clinical and microscopic findings. The importance of excluding a treatable infection from the diagnosis cannot be overemphasized.

We have seen two patients whose histologic findings included granulomas and scattered lymphocytic, plasma cellular, and eosinophilic infiltrates that contained acid-fast bacilli, but the clinical appearance of the lesions did not conform to that described previously.[84]

Pennys and Hicks[77] described a disseminated papular eruption in two homosexual men. Biopsy findings were extensive palisading granulomas, which these authors considered to be similar to granuloma annulare. No organisms were identified in these two lesions. Photodistributed, localized, generalized, and perforating variants have been described.[175-177] Adenovirus has been isolated from a granuloma annulare–like lesion.[178] These lesions have been described as remarkably transient.[177] Remission with zidovudine therapy has been seen.[179]

Yellow Nail Syndrome

Yellow nails have been previously associated with lymphedema and other diseases.[180,181] Chernosky and Finley[182] reported that four of eight patients with AIDS showed discoloration of the distal portions of one or more nails. In addition, some patients had ridges, absent or small lunulae, violaceous or erythematous darkening of subungual areas distally, and occasional opacity. These patients did not have conditions previously associated with yellow nails. However, some patients had, when examined or subsequently, *Pneumocystis carinii* pneumonia, chronic sinusitis, pleural effusion, tuberculosis, and KS.

In one patient examination of the nail plate by use of a high-speed dental burr showed that the pigmentation involved the entire nail thickness. Wood's lamp examination for fluorescence, potassium hydroxide preparations, and cultures were all negative for organisms. In all cases the yellow pigment had been present for less than a year. The pathogenesis of yellow nail syndrome is unclear. Chernosky and Finley[182] suggest that yellow nails are an important sign of early disease in persons at risk for AIDS.

Oral Hairy Leukoplakia

In 1984 Greenspan et al.[183] reported a series of 37 homosexual men with a distinctive leukoplakia of the tongue and, less commonly, the buccal mucosa. The lesions, designated oral hairy leukoplakia (OHL), were poorly demarcated, slightly elevated white areas with a corrugated or hairy surface (Fig. 12–15). The lesions were single or multiple and ranged in size from a few millimeters to a few centimeters. Only rarely was soreness a

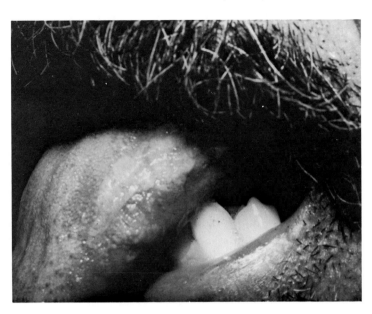

Figure 12–15. Oral hairy leukoplakia of tongue.

complaint. All patients were well at the time the lesions appeared. AIDS subsequently developed in eight patients within the 33-month period of the study. Thirty-five biopsy specimens were obtained from 30 of the patients. These showed hyperkeratosis, parakeratosis, papillomatosis, koilocytosis, and ballooning cytoplasmic changes. Mild cytologic atypia was seen in six patients. Candidiasis was found in 26 of the 37 patients. Immunoperoxidase staining showed papillomavirus in 23 of 30 patients. Six patients were examined by electron microscopy. None was found to have papillomavirus, but five had viruses interpreted as probably of the herpesvirus group. In a 1985 follow-up study,[184] papillomavirus-like particles (25 of 25 specimens) and herpesvirus-like particles (23 of 25 specimens) were seen on electron microscopy. Most notably, evidence for Epstein-Barr virus infection was established for the first time in this study by immunofluorescence staining and DNA hybridization techniques. The authors speculated that the pathogenesis of OHL may involve multiple infectious agents, including papillomavirus and Epstein-Barr virus, as well as possible interactions among these agents. Langerhans' cells are absent or greatly decreased in lesions of OHL.[185]

Evidence of Epstein-Barr virus infection has been found in ulcers of the oropharynx and esophagus.[186] Infection of the oral tissues by this virus may be more common than is generally perceived.[187]

Treatment with various antifungal agents does not cause involution of the OHL, although the fungi disappear.[183] Resolution of OHL has been reported in a few patients treated with azidothymidine.[188-191] Spontaneous resolution has also been reported,[183,192] but lesions tend to recur.

OHL is regarded as a sensitive and possibly specific indicator of HIV infection.[193-195] Survival analysis and other studies[192,194,196] indicate that OHL is highly predictive for the development of AIDS.

Hyperalgesic Pseudothrombophlebitis

A unique syndrome of unilateral calf swelling associated with incapacitating pain, exquisite tenderness, and fever has been described in five men, four with AIDS and one with chronic giardiasis and lymphopenia.[197] Physical examination of four of these patients disclosed the presence of a superficial cord. Venography was performed in all five pa-

tients because of suspected thrombophlebitis, but no evidence of venous obstruction could be found. Three patients were treated with ibuprofen; the other two were not treated for this disorder. All gradually improved, with resolution of the fever in several days in most cases; however, the edema, erythema, and discomfort persisted for many weeks. Biopsy of these lesions was not performed. The pathogenesis of hyperalgesic pseudo-thrombophlebitis is unclear. It may be an unusual manifestation of AIDS and should be added to the list of diseases mimicking thrombophlebitis so that unnecessary anticoagulation can be avoided.

Thrombocytopenic Purpura

Walsh et al.[170] and Strickler et al.[198] reported on thrombocytopenic purpura in homosexual men with and without AIDS. The incidence of this disorder in homosexual men is unknown. These reports described laboratory studies and the mechanism of the disease but did not include clinical or histologic findings. The patients may have had signs or symptoms of thrombocytopenia, since the platelet count (mean ± SD) was $16,000 \pm 3,000/mm^3$.[199] Since purpura can represent a variety of diseases, biopsy and cultures are strongly recommended in patients with this finding. Segal et al.[107] reported thrombotic thrombocytopenic purpura in an AIDS patient with widespread CMV infection.

Miscellaneous Cutaneous Disorders Reported in HIV-Infected Patients

Langerhans' cells are markedly decreased in the skin of HIV patients.[200] The consequences of this alteration are not entirely understood.

Xerosis[78] and cutaneous changes suggestive of nutritional deficiencies, probably pellagra and scurvy,[77] are not surprising given the multitude of gastrointestinal problems, wasting, and cachexia associated with AIDS. Other common dermatologic conditions may be unrelated to HIV infection but have been noted in various reports: severe tinea pedis, miliaria, psoriasis, keratosis pilaris, postinflammation hyperpigmentation,[151] Reiter's syndrome,[201] reactive perforating collagenosis,[202] erythema dyschromium perstans,[203] vitiligo,[204] dermatitis herpetiformis,[205,206] porphyria cutanea tarda,[207-210] anorectal inflammation and

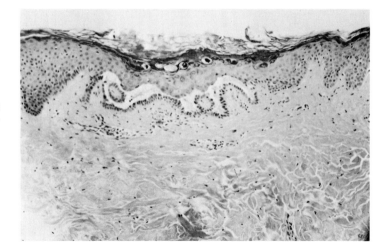

Figure 12–16. Focal acantholytic change consistent with transient acantholytic dermatosis.

proctitis,[211] exfoliative erythroderma and flagellate plaques associated with hypereosinophilic syndrome,[212] neutrophilic eccrine hidradenitis with sweat gland necrosis,[145] and acquired ichthyosis and asteatotic eczema.[77] Psoriasis and exacerbation of preexisting psoriasis have also been reported.[201,213,214] McNutt et al.[215] found dyskeratotic cells, lymphocytoclasis, and a lack of suprapapillary thinning in biopsy specimens of psoriasis in HIV-infected patients. Horn et al.[216] noted that plasma cells are more commonly observed in biopsy specimens from HIV-positive psoriatic patients. We have observed focal acantholytic dyskeratosis in an HIV-seropositive male homosexual (Fig. 12–16). Aphthous stomatitis has been reported.[217,218] Telangiectasia of the anterior chest has been noted in HIV-positive and HIV-negative homosexual men.[219] Jimenez-Acosta et al.[220] reported similar findings in an HIV-positive hemophiliac man (without a history of drug abuse or homosexuality) who was successfully treated with tetracyline.

REFERENCES

1. Coldiron BM, Bergstresser PR: Prevalence and clinical spectrum of skin disease in patients infected with human immunodeficiency virus. Arch Dermatol 125:357-361, 1989.
2. Hardy MA, Goldfarb P, Levine S, et al: *De novo* Kaposi's sarcoma in renal transplantation. Cancer 38:144-148, 1976.
3. Howshaw RA, Schwartz RA: Kaposi's sarcoma after immunosuppressive therapy with prednisone. Arch Dermatol 116:1280-1282, 1980.
4. Leung F, Fam AG, Osoba D: Kaposi's sarcoma complicating corticosteroid therapy for temporal arteritis. Am J Med 71:320-322, 1981.
5. Ulbright TM, Santa Cruz DJ: Kaposi's sarcoma: Relationship with hematologic, lymphoid and thymic neoplasia. Cancer 47:963-973, 1981.
6. Modlin RL, Hofman FM, Kempf RA, et al: Kaposi's sarcoma in homosexual men: An immunohistochemical study. J Am Acad Dermatol 8:620-627, 1983.
7. Giraldo G, Beth E, Huang ES, et al: Kaposi's sarcoma and its relationship to cytomegalovirus. II. CMV-DNA and CMV early antigens in Kaposi's sarcoma. Int J Cancer 26:23, 1980.
8. Prince HE, Schroff RW, Ayoub G, et al: HLA studies in acquired immune deficiency syndrome patients with Kaposi's sarcoma. J Clin Immunol 4:242-245, 1984.
9. Beckstead JH, Wood GS, Fletcher V: Evidence for the origin of Kaposi's sarcoma from lymphatic endothelium. Am J Pathol 119:294-300, 1985.
10. Curran JW: AIDS—two years later [editorial]. N Engl J Med 309:609-610, 1983.
11. Urmacher C, Myskowski P, Ochoa M, et al: Outbreak of Kaposi's sarcoma with cytomegalovirus infection in young homosexual men. Am J Med 72:569-575, 1982.
12. Haverkos HW, Drotman DP: Prevalence of Kaposi's sarcoma among patients with AIDS [letter]. N Engl J Med 312:1518, 1985.
13. Hui AN, Koss MN, Meyer PR: Necropsy findings in acquired immunodeficiency syndrome: A comparison of premortem diagnosis with postmortem findings. Hum Pathol 15:670-676, 1984.
14. Reichert CM, O'Leary TJ, Levens DL, et al: Autopsy pathology in the acquired immunodeficiency syndrome. Am J Pathol 112:357, 1983.
15. Welch K, Finkbeiner W, Alpers CE, et al: Autopsy findings in the acquired immune deficiency syndrome. JAMA 252:1152-1159, 1984.
16. DeJarlais DC, Marmor M, Thomas P, et al: Kaposi's sarcoma among four different AIDS risk groups [letter]. N Engl J Med 310:1119, 1984.
17. Moskowitz L, Hensley GT, Chan JC, et al: Immediate causes of death in acquired immunodeficiency syndrome. Arch Pathol Lab Med 109:735-738, 1985.
18. Cohn DL, Judson FN: Absence of Kaposi's sarcoma in hemophiliacs with the acquired immunodefi-

ciency syndrome [letter]. Ann Intern Med 101: 401, 1984.

19. Evatt BL, Ramsey RB, Lawrence DN, et al: The acquired immunodeficiency syndrome in patients with hemophilia. Ann Intern Med 100: 499-504, 1984.

20. Safai B, Sarngadharan MG, Koziner B, et al: Spectrum of Kaposi's sarcoma in the epidemic of AIDS. Cancer Res 45(suppl):4646S-4648S, 1985.

21. Haverkos HW, Friedman-Kien AE, Drotman DP, et al: The changing incidence of Kaposi's sarcoma among patients with AIDS. J Am Acad Dermatol 22:1250-1253, 1990.

22. Friedman-Kien AE, Saltzman BR: Clinical manifestations of classical, endemic African and epidemic AIDS-associated Kaposi's sarcoma. J Am Acad Dermatol 22:1237-1250, 1990.

23. Rendon MJ: Linear cutaneous lesions of Kaposi's sarcoma: A clinical clue to the diagnosis of acquired immunodeficiency syndrome. Arch Dermatol 124:327-329, 1988.

24. Friedman-Kien AE, Ostreicher R: Overview of classical and epidemic Kaposi's sarcoma. In Friedman-Kien AE, Laubenstein LF (eds): AIDS, the epidemic of Kaposi's sarcoma and opportunistic infections, New York, Masson, 1984.

25. Poulsen A, Hultberg B, Thomsen K, et al: Regression of Kaposi's sarcoma in AIDS after treatment with dapsone [letter]. Lancet 1[8376]:560, 1984.

26. Real FX, Krown SE: Spontaneous regression of Kaposi's sarcoma in patients with AIDS [letter]. N Engl J Med 313:1659, 1985.

27. Niedt GW, Schinella RA: Acquired immunodeficiency syndrome. Arch Pathol Lab Med 109: 727-734, 1985.

28. Maurice PD, Smith NP, Pinching AJ: Kaposi's sarcoma with benign course in a homosexual [letter]. Lancet 1[8271]:571, 1982.

29. Levy EM, Beldekas JC, Black PH, et al: Patients with Kaposi's sarcoma who opt for no treatment [letter]. Lancet 2:223, 1985.

30. Janier M, Vignon MD, Cottenot F: Spontaneously healing Kaposi's sarcoma in AIDS [letter]. N Engl J Med 312:1638-1639, 1985.

31. Bluefarb SM, Adams LA: Arteriovenous malformation with angiodermatitis. Arch Dermatol 96:176-181, 1967.

32. Earhart RM, Aeling JA, Nuss DD, et al: Pseudo-Kaposi's sarcoma. Arch Dermatol 110:907, 1974.

33. Brenner S, Ophir J, Krakowski A, et al: Kaposi-like arteriovenous malformation and angiodermatitis (pseudo-Kaposi). Cutis 30:240-256, 1982.

34. Schwartz JL, Muhlbauer JE, Steigbigel RT: Pre-Kaposi's sarcoma. J Am Acad Dermatol 11: 377-380, 1984.

35. Fukunaga M, Silverberg SG: Kaposi's sarcoma in patients with acquired immune deficiency syndrome: A flow cytometric DNA analysis of 26 lesions in 21 patients. Cancer 66:758-764, 1990.

36. Giddens WE, Tsai C-C, Morton WR, et al: Retroperitoneal fibromatosis and acquired immunodeficiency syndrome in macaques: Pathologic observations and transmission studies. Am J Pathol 119:253-263, 1985.

37. Tsai CC, Warner TFCS, Uno H, et al: Subcutaneous fibromatosis associated with an acquired immune deficiency syndrome in pig-tailed macaques. Am J Pathol 120:30-37, 1985.

38. Dictor M, Järplid B: The cause of Kaposi's sar-

coma: An avian retroviral analogue. J Am Acad Dermatol 18:398-402, 1988.

39. Stoler MH, Bonfiglio TA, Steigbigel RT, et al: An atypical subcutaneous infection associated with acquired immune deficiency syndrome. Am J Clin Pathol 80:714-718, 1983.

40. Cockerell CJ, Webster GF, Whitlow MA, et al: Epithelioid angiomatosis: A distinct vascular disorder in patient with the acquired immunodeficiency syndrome or AIDS-related complex. Lancet 2:634, 1987.

41. LeBoit PE, Egbert BA, Stoler MH, et al: Epithelioid hemangioma-like vascular proliferation in AIDS: Manifestation of cat-scratch disease bacillus infection? Lancet 1:961, 1988.

42. Knobler EH, Silvers DN, Fine KC, et al: Unique vascular skin lesions associated with human immunodeficiency virus. JAMA 260:524-527, 1988.

43. Koehler JE, LeBoit PE, Egbert BM, et al: Cutaneous vascular lesions and disseminated cat-scratch disease in patients with the acquired immunodeficiency syndrome (AIDS) and AIDS-related complex. Ann Intern Med 109:449-455, 1988.

44. Cockerell CJ: Bacillary epithelioid angiomatosis occurring in an immunocompetent individual. Arch Dermatol 126:787-790, 1990.

45. Rudikoff D, Phelps RG, Gordon RE, et al: Acquired immunodeficiency syndrome–related bacillary vascular proliferation (epithelioid angiomatosis): Rapid response to erythromycin therapy. Arch Dermatol 125:706-707, 1989.

46. Relman DA, Loutit JS, Schmidt TM, et al: The agent of bacillary angiomatosis: An approach to the identification of uncultured pathogens. N Engl J Med 323:1573-1580, 1990.

47. Omura EF, Omura GA: Human immunodeficiency virus–associated skin lesions. JAMA 261:991, 1989.

48. Dooley JR: Bartonellosis. In Binford CH, Connor DH (eds): Pathology of Tropical and Extraordinary Diseases, vol 2. Washington, DC, Armed Forces Institute of Pathology, 1976, pp 190-193.

49. Wear DJ, Margileth AM, Hadfield TL, et al: Cat-scratch disease: A bacterial infection. Science 221:1403-1404, 1983.

50. Margileth AM, Wear DJ, English CK: Systemic cat scratch disease: Report of 23 patients with prolonged or recurrent severe bacterial infection. J Infect Dis 155:390-401, 1987.

51. Louie S, Daoust PR, Schwartz RS: Immunodeficiency and the pathogenesis of non-Hodgkin's lymphoma. Semin Oncol 7:267-284, 1980.

52. Binkes RL, Gal AA, Stewart ML, et al: Simultaneous occurrence of *Pneumocystis carinii* pneumonia, cytomegalovirus infection, Kaposi's sarcoma and B-immunoblastic sarcoma in a homosexual man. JAMA 253:3425-3428, 1985.

53. Ziegler JL, Beckstead JA, Volberding PA, et al: Non-Hodgkin's lymphoma in 90 homosexual men, relation to generalized lymphadenopathy and the acquired immunodeficiency syndrome. N Engl J Med 311:565-570, 1984.

54. Ioachim JL, Cooper MC, Hellman GC: Lymphomas in men at high risk for acquired immune deficiency syndrome (AIDS), a study of 21 cases. Cancer 56:2831-2842, 1985.

55. Levine AM, Meyer PR, Begandy MK, et al: Development of B-cell lymphoma in homosexual men: Clinical and immunologic findings. Ann Intern Med 100:7-13, 1984.

56. Rosenberg SA, Diamond HD, Jaslowitz B, et al: Lymphosarcoma: A review of 1269 cases. Medicine (Baltimore) 40:31-84, 1961.

57. Long JC, Mihm MC, Qazi R: Malignant lymphoma of the skin. Cancer 38:1282-1296, 1976.

58. Ragni MV, Lewis JH, Bontempo FA, et al: Lymphoma presenting as a traumatic hematoma in an HTLV-III antibody–positive hemophiliac [letter]. N Engl J Med 312:640, 1985.

59. Blumenfeld W, Beckstead JH: Angioimmunoblastic lymphadenopathy with dysproteinemia in homosexual men with acquired immune deficiency syndrome. Arch Pathol Lab Med 107:567, 1983.

60. Kluin-Nelemans H, Elbers HRJ, Ramselaar CG: Angioimmunoblastic lymphadenopathy followed by Kaposi's sarcoma. Arch Dermatol 120:958-960, 1984.

61. Lachant NA, Sun NC, Leong LA, et al: Multicentric angiofollicular lymph node hyperplasia (Castleman's disease) followed by Kaposi's sarcoma in two homosexual males with the acquired immunodeficiency syndrome (AIDS). Am J Clin Pathol 83:27-33, 1985.

62. Perlow LS, Taff ML, Orsini JM, et al: Kaposi's sarcoma in a young homosexual man: Association with angiofollicular lymphoid hyperplasia and a malignant lymphoproliferative disorder. Arch Pathol Lab Med 107:510-513, 1983.

63. Schoeppel SL, Hoppe RT, Dorfman RF, et al: Hodgkin's disease in homosexual men at risk for the acquired immune deficiency syndrome. Ann Intern Med 102:68-70, 1985.

64. Reddy S, Pellettiere E, Saxena V, et al: Extranodal non-Hodgkin's lymphoma. Cancer 46:1925-1931, 1980.

65. Smith JL Jr, Butler JJ: Skin involvement in Hodgkin's disease. Cancer 45:354-361, 1980.

66. Slazinski L, Stall JF, Matthews CR: Basal cell carcinoma in a man with acquired immunodeficiency syndrome [letter]. J Am Acad Dermatol 11:140-141, 1984.

67. Gottlieb MS, Groopman JE, Weinstein WM, et al: The acquired immunodeficiency syndrome: UCLA conference. Ann Intern Med 99:208, 1983.

68. Milburn PB, Brandsma JL, Goldsmann CI, et al: Disseminated warts and evolving squamous cell carcinoma in a patient with acquired immunodeficiency syndrome. J Am Acad Dermatol 19:401-405, 1988.

69. Krause W, Mittag H, Gieler U, et al: A case of malignant melanoma in AIDS-related complex. Arch Dermatol 123:867-868, 1987.

70. Tindall B, Findlayson R, Mutimer K, et al: Malignant melanoma associated with human immunodeficiency virus infection in three homosexual men. J Am Acad Dermatol 20:587-591, 1989.

71. Lane HC, Depper JM, Greene WC, et al: Quantitative analysis of immune function in patients with the acquired immunodeficiency syndrome. N Engl J Med 313:79-84, 1985.

72. Belsito DV, Sanchez MR, Baer RL: Reduced Langerhans' cell Ia antigen and ATPase activity in patients with the acquired immunodeficiency syndrome. N Engl J Med 310:1279-1282, 1984.

73. Smith PD, Ohura K, Masur H, et al: Monocyte function in the acquired immune deficiency syndrome: Defective chemotaxis. J Clin Invest 74:2121-2128, 1984.

74. Murray HW, Hillman JK, Rubin BY, et al: Patients at risk for AIDS-related opportunistic infections. N Engl J Med 313:1504-1510, 1985.

75. Hatcher VA: Mucocutaneous infections in acquired immune deficiency syndrome. In Friedman-Kien AE, Laubenstein AJ (eds): AIDS, the epidemic of Kaposi's sarcoma and opportunistic infections, New York, Masson, 1984.

76. Siegal FP, Lopez C, Hammer GS, et al: Severe acquired immunodeficiency in male homosexuals, manifested by chronic perianal ulcerative herpes simplex lesions. N Engl J Med 305:1439-1444, 1981.

77. Pennys NS, Hicks B: Unusual cutaneous lesions associated with acquired immunodeficiency syndrome. J Am Acad Dermatol 13:845-852, 1985.

78. Farthing CF, Staughton RCD, Rowland Payne CME: Skin disease in homosexual patients with acquired immune deficiency syndrome (AIDS) and lesser forms of human T cell leukaemia virus (HTLV III) disease. Clin Exp Dermatol 10:3-12, 1985.

79. Sarma DP, Weilbaecher TG: Molluscum contagiosum in the acquired immunodeficiency syndrome [letter]. J Am Acad Dermatol 13:682-683, 1985.

80. Douglass MC, Mathes B, Thomas L: Molluscum contagiosum in the acquired immunodeficiency syndrome. J Am Acad Dermatol 13:683, 1985.

81. Lombardo PC: Molluscum contagiosum and acquired immunodeficiency syndrome. Arch Dermatol 121:834-835, 1985.

82. Redfield RR, James WD, Wright DC, et al: Severe molluscum contagiosum infection in a patient with human T cell lymphotrophic (HTLV III) disease. J Am Acad Dermatol 13:821-823, 1985.

83. Quinnan GV, Masur H, Rook AH, et al: Herpesvirus infections in the acquired immunodeficiency syndrome. JAMA 252:72-77, 1984.

84. Kwan TH, Kaufman HW: Acid-fast bacilli with cytomegalovirus and herpesvirus inclusions in the skin of an AIDS patient. Am J Clin Pathol 85:236-238, 1986.

85. Forman AB: Association of human immunodeficiency virus seropositivity and extensive perineal condylomata acuminata in a child. Arch Dermatol 124:1010-1011, 1988.

86. Holmberg SD, Stewart JA, Gerber AR, et al: Prior herpes simplex virus type 2 infection as a risk factor for HIV infection. JAMA 259:1048-1050, 1988.

87. Gilson IH, Barnett JH, Conant MA, et al: Disseminated ecthymatous herpes varicella-zoster virus infection in patients with acquired immunodeficiency syndrome. J Am Acad Dermatol 20:637-642, 1989.

88. Norris SA, Kessler HA, Fife KH: Severe, progressive herpetic whitlow caused by an acyclovir-resistant virus in a patient with AIDS [letter]. J Infect Dis 157:209-210, 1988.

89. Schneiderman H, Robert NJ, Walker S, et al: Herpes without vesicles: Limited, recurrent genital lesions in an immunodebilitated host. South Med J 79:368-370, 1986.

90. Sixbey JW, Nedrud JG, Raab-Traub N, et al: Epstein-Barr virus replication in oropharyngeal epithelial cells. N Engl J Med 310:1225-1230, 1984.

91. Marks GL, Nolan PE, Erlich KS, et al: Mucocutaneous dissemination of acyclovir-resistant herpes simplex virus in a patient with AIDS. Rev Infect Dis 11:474-476, 1989.

92. Wong DT, Ogra PL: Viral infections in immuno-compromised patients. Med Clin North Am 67:1075-1092, 1983.

93. Erlich KS, Mills J, Chatis P, et al: Acyclovir-resistant herpes simplex virus infections in patients with the acquired immunodeficiency syndrome. N Engl J Med 320:293-296, 1989.

94. Disler RS, Dover JS: Chronic localized herpes zoster in the acquired immunodeficiency syndrome. Arch Dermatol 126:1105-1106, 1990.

95. Gulick RM, Heath-Chiozzi M, Crumpacker CS: Varicella-zoster disease in patients with human immunodeficiency virus infection. Arch Dermatol 126:1086-1088, 1990.

96. Hoppenjans WB, Bibler MR, Orme RL, et al: Prolonged cutaneous herpes zoster in acquired immunodeficiency syndrome. Arch Dermatol 126:1048-1050, 1990.

97. Perronne C, Lazanas M, Leport C, et al: Varicella in patients infected with the human immunodeficiency virus. Arch Dermatol 126:1033-1036, 1990.

98. McSorley J, Shapiro L, Brownstein MH, et al: Herpes simplex and varicella-zoster: Comparative histopathology of 77 cases. Int J Dermatol 13:69-75, 1974.

99. Koranda FC, Dehmel EM, Kahn G, et al: Cutaneous complications in immunosuppressed renal homograft recipients. JAMA 229:419-424, 1974.

100. Morison WL: Survey of warts, herpes zoster and herpes simplex in patients with secondary immune deficiencies and neoplasms. Br J Dermatol 10:18-19, 1974.

101. Lutzner R, Croissant O, Ducasse MF, et al: A potentially oncogenic human papillomavirus (HPV-5) found in two renal allograft recipients. J Invest Dermatol 75:353-356, 1980.

102. Gross G, Pfister H, Hagedorn M, Gissman L: Correlation between human papillomavirus (HPV) type and histology of warts. J Invest Dermatol 78:160-164, 1982.

103. Pariser RJ: Histologically specific skin lesions in disseminated cytomegalovirus infection. J Am Acad Dermatol 9:937-946, 1983.

104. Walker JD, Chesney TM: Cytomegalovirus infection of the skin. Am J Dermatopathol 4:263-265, 1982.

105. Lin CS, Penha PD, Krishnan MN, et al: Cytomegalic inclusion disease of the skin. Arch Dermatol 117:282-284, 1981.

106. Bournerias I, Boisnic S, Patey O, et al: Unusual cutaneous cytomegalovirus involvement in patients with acquired immunodeficiency syndrome. Arch Dermatol 125:1243-1246, 1989.

107. Segal GH, Tubbs RR, Ratliff NB, et al: Thrombotic thrombocytopenic purpura in a patient with AIDS. Cleve Clin J Med 57:360-366, 1990.

108. Horn TD, Hood AF: Cytomegalovirus is predictably present in perineal ulcers from immunosuppressed patients. Arch Dermatol 126:642-644, 1990.

109. Borton LK, Wintroub BU: Disseminated cryptococcosis presenting as herpetiform lesions in a homosexual man with acquired immunodeficiency syndrome. J Am Acad Dermatol 10:387-390, 1984.

110. Rico MJ, Pennys NS: Cutaneous cryptococcosis resembling molluscum contagiosum in a patient with AIDS. Arch Dermatol 121:901-902, 1985.

111. Klein RS, Harris CA, Small CB, et al: Oral candidiasis in high-risk patients as the initial manifestation of the acquired immunodeficiency syndrome. N Engl J Med 311:354-358, 1984.

112. Kaplan MH, Sadick N, McNutt NS, et al: Dermatologic findings and manifestation of acquired immunodeficiency syndrome (AIDS). J Am Acad Dermatol 16:485-506, 1987.

113. Bibler MR, Luber HJ, Glueck HI, et al: Disseminated sporotrichosis in a patient with HIV infection after treatment for acquired factor VIII inhibitor. JAMA 256:3125-3126, 1986.

114. Lipstein-Kresch E, Isenberg HD, Singer C, et al: Disseminated *Sporothrix schenkii* infection with arthritis in a patient with acquired immunodeficiency syndrome. J Rheumatol 12:805-808, 1985.

115. Groisser D, Bottone EJ, Lebwohl M, et al: Association of *Pityrosporum orbiculare (Malassezia furfur)* with seborrheic dermatitis in patients with acquired immunodeficiency syndrome (AIDS). J Am Acad Dermatol 20:770-773, 1989.

116. Shaw JC, Levinson W, Montanaro A, et al: Sporotrichosis in the acquired immunodeficiency syndrome. J Am Acad Dermatol 21:1145-1147, 1989.

117. Cohen PR, Bank DE, Silvers DN, et al: Cutaneous lesions of disseminated histoplasmosis in human immunodeficiency virus–infected patients. J Am Acad Dermatol 23:422-428, 1990.

118. Wheat LJ, Small CB: Disseminated histoplasmosis in the acquired immune deficiency syndrome. Arch Intern Med 144:2147-2149, 1984.

119. Drabick JJ, Gomatos PJ, Solis JB: Cutaneous cladosporiosis as a complication of skin testing in a man positive for human immunodeficiency virus. J Am Acad Dermatol 22:135-136, 1990.

120. Mayoral F, Pennys NS: Disseminated histoplasmosis presenting as a transepidermal elimination disorder in an AIDS victim [letter]. J Am Acad Dermatol 13:842-844, 1985.

121. Pitchenik AE, Cole C, Russel BW, et al: Tuberculosis, atypical mycobacteriosis and the acquired immunodeficiency syndrome among Haitian and non-Haitian patients in south Florida. Ann Intern Med 101:641-645, 1984.

122. Sohn CC, Schroff RW, Kliewer KE, et al: Disseminated *Mycobacterium avium intracellulare* infection in homosexual men with acquired cell-mediated immunodeficiency: A histologic and immunologic study of two cases. Am J Clin Pathol 79:247-252, 1983.

123. Mehlmauer MA: Keratotic papules and nodules and hyperkeratosis of palms and soles in a patient with tuberculosis and AIDS-related complex. J Am Acad Dermatol 23:381-385, 1990.

124. Boudreau S, Hines HC, Hood AF: Dermal abscesses with *Staphylococcus aureus*, cytomegalovirus and acid-fast bacilli in a patient with acquired immunodeficiency syndrome (AIDS). J Cutan Pathol 15:53-57, 1988.

125. Glover A, Young L, Goltz AW: Norwegian scabies in acquired immunodeficiency syndrome: Report of a case resulting in death from associated sepsis. J Am Acad Dermatol 16:396-399, 1987.

126. Paterson JW, Kitces EN, Neafie RC: Cutaneous botryomycosis in a patient with acquired immunodeficiency syndrome. J Am Acad Dermatol 16:238-242, 1987.

127. Weitzner JM, Dhawan SS, Rosen LB, et al: Successful treatment of botryomycosis in a patient with acquired immunodeficiency syndrome. J Am Acad Dermatol 21:1312-1314, 1989.

128. Gregory N, Sanchez M, Buchness MR: The spectrum of syphilis in patients with human immunodeficiency virus infection. J Am Acad Dermatol 22:1061-1067, 1990.

129. Hicks CB, Benson PM, Lupton GP, et al: Seronegative secondary syphilis in a patient infected with the human immunodeficiency virus with Kaposi's sarcoma. Ann Intern Med 107:492-494, 1987.

130. Bari MM, Shulkin DJ, Abell E: Ulcerative syphilis in acquired immunodeficiency syndrome: A case of precocious tertiary syphilis in a patient infected with human immunodeficiency virus. J Am Acad Dermatol 21:1310-1312, 1989.

131. Breneman DL, Amornsiripanitch S, Barron DR, et al: Granulomatous secondary syphilis in a patient with human immunodeficiency virus infection. Cutis 44:377-381, 1989.

132. Johns DR, Tierney M, Felsenstein D: Alteration in the natural history of neurosyphilis by concurrent infection with the human immunodeficiency virus. N Engl J Med 316:1569-1572, 1987.

133. Hirschmann JV, Chu AC: Skin lesions with disseminated toxoplasmosis in a patient with the acquired immunodeficiency syndrome. Arch Dermatol 124:1446-1447, 1988.

134. Rau RC, Baird IM: Crusted scabies in a patient with acquired immunodeficiency syndrome. J Am Acad Dermatol 15:1058-1059, 1986.

135. Hall JC, Brewer JH, Appl BA: Norwegian scabies in a patient with acquired immune deficiency syndrome. Cutis 43:325-329, 1989.

136. Jucowicz P, Ramon ME, Don PC, et al: Norwegian scabies in an infant with acquired immunodeficiency syndrome. Arch Dermatol 125:1670-1671, 1989.

137. Cooper DA, MacLean P, Finlayson R, et al: Acute AIDS retrovirus infection: Definition of a clinical illness with seroconversion. Lancet 1:537-540, 1985.

138. Tindall B, Barker S, Donovan B, et al: Characterization of the acute clinical illness associated with human immunodeficiency virus infection. Arch Intern Med 148:945-949, 1988.

139. Lindskov R, Orskov Lindhardt B, Weismann K, et al: Acute HTLV-III infection with roseola-like rash [letter]. Lancet 1:447, 1986.

140. Hulsebosch HJ, Claessen FAP, van Ginkel CJW, et al: Human immunodeficiency virus exanthem. J Am Acad Dermatol 23:483-486, 1990.

141. Mitsuyasu R, Groopman J, Volberding P: Cutaneous reaction to trimethoprim-sulfamethoxazole in patients with AIDS and Kaposi's sarcoma [letter]. N Engl J Med 308:1535-1536, 1983.

142. Gordin FM, Simon GL, Wopsy CB, et al: Adverse reactions to trimethoprim-sulfamethoxasole in patients with the acquired immunodeficiency syndrome. Ann Intern Med 100:495-499, 1984.

143. Arndt KA, Jick H: Rates of cutaneous reactions to drugs. JAMA 235:915-923, 1976.

144. DeHovitz JA, Johnson WD, Pape JW: Cutaneous reactions to trimethoprim-sulfamethoxzole in Haitians [letter]. Ann Intern Med 103:479-480, 1985.

145. Smith KJ, Skelton HG, James WD, et al: Neutrophilic eccrine hidradenitis in HIV-infected patients. J Am Acad Dermatol 23:945-947, 1990.

146. Grau-Massanes M, Millan F, Febrer MI, et al: Pigmented nail bands and mucocutaneous pigmentation in HIV-positive patients treated with zidovudine. J Am Acad Dermatol 22:687-688, 1990.

147. McNeely MC, Yarchoan R, Broder S, et al: Dermatologic complications associated with administration of 2′,3′-dideoxycytidine in patients with human immunodeficiency virus infection. J Am Acad Dermatol 21:1213-1217, 1989.

148. Duvic M, Reisman M, Finley V, et al: Glucan-induced keratoderma in acquired immunodeficiency syndrome. Arch Dermatol 123:751-756, 1987.

149. Wintroub B, Stern R: Cutaneous drug reactions: Pathogenesis and clinical classification. J Am Acad Dermatol 13:167-179, 1985.

150. Rico MJ, Kory WP, Gould EW, et al: Interface dermatitis in patients with the acquired immunodeficiency syndrome. J Am Acad Dermatol 16:1209-1218, 1989.

151. Eisenstadt BA, Wormser GP: Seborrheic dermatitis and butterfly rash in AIDS [letter]. N Engl J Med 311:189, 1984.

152. Mathes BM, Douglass MC: Seborrheic dermatitis in patients with acquired immunodeficiency syndrome. J Am Acad Dermatol 13:947-951, 1985.

153. Soeprono FF, Schinella RA, Cockerell CJ, et al: Seborrheic-like dermatitis of acquired immunodeficiency syndrome. J Am Acad Dermatol 14:242-248, 1986.

154. Shapiro RS, Samorodin C, Hood AF: Pruritus as a presenting sign of acquired immunodeficiency syndrome. J Am Acad Dermatol 16:1115-1117, 1987.

155. Liataud B, Pape JW, DeHovitz JA, et al: Pruritic skin lesions, a common initial presentation of acquired immunodeficiency syndrome. Arch Dermatol 125:629-633, 1989.

156. Gorin I, Lessana-Leibowitch M, Fortier P, et al: Successful treatment of the pruritus of human immunodeficiency virus infection and acquired immunodeficiency syndrome with psoralens plus ultraviolet A therapy. J Am Acad Dermatol 20:511-513, 1989.

157. Pennys NS, Nayar JK, Bernstein H, et al: Chronic pruritic eruption in patients with acquired immunodeficiency syndrome associated with increased antibody titers to mosquito salivary gland antigens. J Am Acad Dermatol 21:421-425, 1989.

158. Soeprono FF, Shinella RA: Eosinophilic pustular folliculitis in patients with acquired immunodeficiency syndrome: Report of three cases. J Am Acad Dermatol 14:1020-1022, 1986.

159. Ise S, Ofuji S: Subcorneal pustular dermatosis: A follicular variant? Arch Dermatol 92:169-171, 1965.

160. Ofuji S, Ogino A, Horio T, et al: Eosinophilic pustular folliculitis. Acta Derm Venereol (Stockh) 50:195-203, 1970.

161. Holst R: Eosinophilic pustular folliculitis: Report of a European case. Br J Dermatol 95:661-664, 1976.

162. Orfanos CE, Sterry W: Sterile eosinophile pustulose. Dermatologica 157:193-205, 1978.

163. Lucky AW, Esterly NB, Heskel W, et al: Eosinophilic pustular folliculitis in infancy. Pediatr Dermatol 1:202-206, 1984.

164. Takematsu H, Nakamura K, Igarashi M, et al: Eosinophilic pustular folliculitis. Arch Dermatol 121:917-920, 1985.

165. Steffen C: Eosinophilic pustular folliculitis (Ofuji's disease) with response to dapsone therapy. Arch Dermatol 121:921-923, 1985.

166. Buchness MR, Lim HW, Hatcher VA, et al: Eosinophilic pustular folliculitis in the acquired immunodeficiency syndrome. N Engl J Med 318:1183-1186, 1988.

167. Ashack RJ, Frost ML, Norins AL: Papular pruritic eruption of Demodex folliculitis in patients with acquired immunodeficiency syndrome. J Am Acad Dermatol 21:306-307, 1989.

168. Case records of the MGH. N Engl J Med 309:359-364, 1983.

169. Gupta S, Licorish K: Circulating immune complexes in AIDS [letter]. N Engl J Med 310:1530-1531, 1984.

170. Walsh CM, Nardi MA, Karpatkin S: On the mechanism of thrombocytopenic purpura in sexually active homosexual men. N Engl J Med 311:635-639, 1984.

171. Chren M-M, Silverman RA, Sorensen RU, et al: Leukocytoclastic vasculitis in a patient infected with human immunodeficiency virus. J Am Acad Dermatol 21:1161-1164, 1989.

172. James WD, Redfield RR, Lupton GP, et al: A papular eruption associated with human T cell lymphotropic virus type III disease. J Am Acad Dermatol 13:563-566, 1985.

173. Viraben R, Dupré A: Lichenoid granulomatous papular dermatosis associated with human immunodeficiency virus infection: An immunohistochemical study. J Am Acad Dermatol 18:1140-1141, 1988.

174. Heymann WR: Lichenoid granulomatous papular dermatosis associated with human immunodeficiency virus infection [letter]. J Am Acad Dermatol 21:584, 1989.

175. Cohen PR, Grossman ME, Silvers DN, et al: Generalized granuloma annulare on sun-exposed areas in a human immunodeficiency virus–seropositive man with ultraviolet B photosensitivity. Arch Dermatol 126:830-831, 1990.

176. Huerter CJ, Bass J, Bergfeld W, et al: Perforating granuloma annulare in a patient with acquired immunodeficiency syndrome. Arch Dermatol 123:1217-1220, 1987.

177. Ghadially R, Sibbald RG, Walter JB, et al: Granuloma annulare in patients with human immunodeficiency virus infections. J Am Acad Dermatol 20:232-235, 1989.

178. Coldiron B, Freeman RG, Beaudoing DL: Isolation of adenovirus from a granuloma annulare–like lesion in the acquired immunodeficiency syndrome–related complex. Arch Dermatol 124:654-655, 1988.

179. Leenutaphong V, Hölzle E, Erckenbrecht J, et al: Remission of human immunodeficiency virus–associated generalized granuloma annulare under zidovudine therapy. J Am Acad Dermatol 19:1126-1127, 1988.

180. Pavlidakey GP, Hashimoto K, Blum D: Yellow nail syndrome. J Am Acad Dermatol 11:509-512, 1984.

181. Venencie PY, Dicken CH: Yellow nail syndrome: Report of five cases. J Am Acad Dermatol 10:187-192, 1984.

182. Chernosky ME, Finley VK: Yellow nail syndrome in patients with acquired immunodeficiency disease. J Am Acad Dermatol 13:731-736, 1985.

183. Greenspan D, Conant M, Silverman S, et al: Oral "hairy" leukoplakia in male homosexuals: Evidence of association with both papillomavirus and herpes-group virus. Lancet 2:831-834, 1984.

184. Greenspan JS, Greenspan D, Lenette ET, et al: Replication of Epstein-Barr virus within the epithelial cells of oral "hairy" leukoplakia, an AIDS-associated lesion. N Engl J. Med 313:1564-1571, 1985.

185. Daniels TE, Greenspan D, Greenspan JS, et al: Absence of Langerhans' cells in oral hairy leukoplakia, an AIDS associated lesion. J Invest Dermatol 89:178-182, 1987.

186. Logan RPH, Polson RJ, Kitchen VS, et al: Oral leucoplakia and HIV. Lancet 335:170, 1990.

187. Loning T, Henke RP, Reichart P, et al: In situ hybridization to detect Epstein-Barr virus DNA in oral tissues of HIV-infected patients. Virchows Arch [A] 412:127-133, 1987.

188. Friedman-Kien AE: Viral origin of hairy leukoplakia [letter]. Lancet 2(8508):694-695, 1986.

189. Phelan JA, Klein RS: Resolution of oral hairy leukoplakia during treatment with azidothymidine. Oral Surg Oral Med Oral Pathol 65:717-720, 1988.

190. Kessler HA: Regression of oral hairy leukoplakia during zidovudine therapy. Arch Intern Med 148:2496-2497, 1988.

191. Greenspan JS, Greenspan D: Oral hairy leukoplakia: Diagnosis and management. Oral Surg Oral Med Oral Pathol 67:396-403, 1989.

192. Alessi E, Berti E, Cusini M, et al: Oral hairy leukoplakia. J Am Acad Dermatol 22:79-86, 1990.

193. Greenspan D, Greenspan JS, Hearst NG, et al: Oral hairy leukoplakia: Human immunodeficiency virus status and the risk for developing AIDS. J Infect Dis 155:475-481, 1987.

194. Lupton GP, James WD, Redfield RR, et al: Oral hairy leukoplakia: A distinctive marker of human T-cell lymphotropic virus type III (HTLV-III) infection. Arch Dermatol 123:624-628, 1987.

195. Schiodt M, Greenspan D, Daniels TE, et al: Clinical and histologic spectrum of oral hairy leukoplakia. Oral Surg Oral Med Oral Pathol 64:716-720, 1987.

196. Morfeldt-Manson L, Julander I, Nilsson B: Dermatitis of the face, yellow toe nail changes, hairy leukoplakia and oral candidiasis are clinical indicators of progression to AIDS/opportunistic infection in patients with HIV infection. Scand J Infect Dis 21:497-505, 1989.

197. Abramson SB, Odajnyk CM, Grieco AJ, et al: Hyperalgesic pseudothrombophlebitis: New syndrome in male homosexuals. Am J Med 78:317-320, 1985.

198. Strickler RB, Abrams DI, Corash L, et al: Target platelet antigen in homosexual men with immune thrombocytopenia. N Engl J Med 313:1375-1380, 1985.

199. Morris L, Distenfeld A, Amorosi E, et al: Autoimmune thrombocytopenic purpura in homosexual men. Ann Intern Med 96:714-717, 1982.

200. Stingl G, Rappersberger K, Tschachler E, et al: Langerhans' cells in HIV-I infection. J Am Acad Dermatol 22:1210-1217, 1990.

201. Duvic M, Johnson TM, Rapini RP, et al: Acquired

immunodeficiency syndrome: Associated psoriasis and Reiter's syndrome. Arch Dermatol 123: 1622-1632, 1987.

202. Bank DE, Cohen PR, Kohn SR: Reactive perforating collagenosis in a setting of double disaster: Acquired immunodeficiency syndrome and end-stage renal disease. J Am Acad Dermatol 21: 371-374, 1989.

203. Venencie PY, Laurian Y, Lamarchand-Venencie F, et al: Erythema dyschromium perstans following human immunodeficiency virus seroconversion in a child with hemophilia B. Arch Dermatol 124:1013, 1988.

204. Duvic M,. Rapini R, Hoots WK, et al: Human immunodeficiency virus–associated vitiligo: Expression of autoimmunity with immunodeficiency. J Am Acad Dermatol 17:656-662, 1987.

205. Mitsuhashi Y, Hohl D: Dermatitis herpetiformis in a patient with acquired immunodeficiency syndrome–related complex. J Am Acad Dermatol 18:583, 1988.

206. Hasson A, Gutierrez MC, Martin L, et al: Dermatitis herpetiformis and AIDS-related complex. J Am Acad Dermatol 22:1117-1119, 1990.

207. Hogan D, Card RT, Ghadially MB, et al: Human immunodeficiency virus infection and porphyria cutanea tarda. J Am Acad Dermatol 126:642-644, 1990.

208. Wissel PS, Sordillo P, Anderson KL, et al: Porphyria cutanea tarda associated with the acquired immune deficiency syndrome. Am J Hematol 25: 107-113, 1987.

209. Lobato MN: Porphyria cutanea tarda associated with the acquired immunodeficiency syndrome. Arch Dermatol 124:1009-1010, 1988.

210. Nip-Sakamoto CJ, Wong RHW, Izumi AK: Porphyria cutanea tarda and AIDS. Cutis 44:470-471, 1989.

211. Lenhard B, Naher H, Petzoldt D: Anorectal inflammation and periproctitis in HIV infections. Hautarzt 38:361-363, 1987.

212. May LP, Kelly J, Sanchez M: Hypereosinophilic syndrome with unusual cutaneous manifestations in two men with HIV infection. J Am Acad Dermatol 23:202-204, 1990.

213. Johnson TM, Duvic M, Rapini RP, et al: AIDS exacerbates psoriasis [letter]. N Engl J Med 313: 1415, 1985.

214. Lazar AP, Roenigk HH: Acquired immunodeficiency syndrome (AIDS) can exacerbate psoriasis. J Am Acad Dermatol 18:144, 1988.

215. McNutt NS, Hsu A, Sadick NS, et al: Psoriasiform dermatitis of AIDS. J Cutan Pathol 16:317, 1989.

216. Horn TD, Herzberg GZ, Hood AF: Characterization of the dermal infiltrate in human immunodeficiency virus-–infected patients with psoriasis. Arch Dermatol 126:1462-1465, 1990.

217. Bach MC, Valenti AJ, Howell DA, et al: Odynophagia from aphthous ulcers of the pharynx and esophagus in the acquired immunodeficiency syndrome (AIDS). Ann Intern Med 109:338-339, 1988.

218. Radeff B, Kuffer R, Samson J: Recurrent aphthous ulcer in patient infected with human immunodeficiency virus: Successful treatment with thalidomide. J Am Acad Dermatol 23:523-525, 1990.

219. Fallon T, Abell E, Kingsley L, et al: Telangiectasias of the anterior chest in homosexual men. Ann Intern Med 105:679-682, 1986.

220. Jiminez-Acosta F, Fonseca E, Magallón M: Response to tetracycline of telangiectasias in a male hemophiliac with human immunodeficiency virus infection. J Am Acad Dermatol 19:369-370, 1988.

13

NEUROPATHOLOGY

Umberto De Girolami and Thomas W. Smith

Ten years ago several reports drew attention to a new disorder of cell-mediated immunity occurring in previously healthy homosexual men living in New York City and California.[1-5] Affected individuals were found to be susceptible to opportunistic infection of the lungs *(Pneumocystis carinii)*, oral candidiasis, and Kaposi's sarcoma of the skin and mucous membranes. The disease was named the acquired immune deficiency syndrome (AIDS), and soon thereafter the retrovirus, now called HIV-1, was demonstrated to be its cause.[6-8] Intravenous drug addicts, Haitians, hemophiliacs, and individuals transfused with blood or blood products were found to be especially at risk for HIV-1 infection. A relatively small number of AIDS cases in West Africa were later linked to a closely related virus, designated HIV-2.[9,10]

During the past decade AIDS has reached worldwide epidemic proportions. In the United States alone, 70,000 new cases are estimated to occur by the end of 1990. The virologic, epidemiologic, and extraneural clinicopathologic manifestations of AIDS are discussed elsewhere in the text. This chapter addresses the neurologic manifestations of the disease.

As patients with AIDS were carefully studied clinically in the months after the disease was recognized, the nervous system was recognized as a likely site of involvement by systemically disseminated opportunistic infectious agents.[11-14] In large series of AIDS patients from major medical centers in the United States and Europe, as many as 40% to 66% had neurologic dysfunction, including intel-

lectual, motor, sensory, and neuromuscular disturbances, during the course of their illness.[15-25] In some patients neurologic manifestations herald the infection and predominate throughout the duration of the illness. In recent surveys postmortem examination has shown neuropathologic abnormalities in up to 80% of AIDS patients.[26-43] The overview presented in this chapter is based on the cases published in the literature and on our analysis of a series of 172 AIDS patients who had a complete postmortem neuropathologic examination.[44]

The major neuropathologic manifestations of AIDS can be broadly divided into the following categories:

I. Primary or putative effect of HIV-1 on the nervous system

    A. HIV-1 meningoencephalitis

    B. Leukoencephalopathy

    C. Vacuolar myelopathy

    D. Neuropathy

    E. Myopathy

    F. Vascular lesions

    G. Other considerations

        1. AIDS-dementia complex

        2. Pediatric AIDS

II. Opportunistic infection of the CNS

    A. Parasitic infection: toxoplasmosis, amebiasis

    B. Fungal or bacterial infection: aspergillosis, candidiasis, cryptococcosis, tuberculosis, *M. avium-intracellulare* infection, syphilis

    C. Viral infection

1. Cytomegalovirus (CMV) meningoencephalitis
2. Progressive multifocal leukoencephalopathy (PML)
3. Herpes simplex meningoencephalitis
4. Herpes zoster meningoencephalitis

III. Neoplasia
    A. CNS lymphoma
    B. Metastatic disease

PRIMARY OR PUTATIVE EFFECTS OF HIV-1 ON THE NERVOUS SYSTEM

The clinicians who examined the first patients with AIDS suspected a primary direct infection of the nervous system by HIV-1 quite apart from the virus's attack on lymphoid cells. Within 1 week of seroconversion, and over the course of 1 to 2 weeks, a relatively small subgroup of patients come down with an acute neurologic illness suggesting aseptic meningitis or meningoencephalitis and characterized by headache, evidence of meningeal irritation, and generalized weakness.[45] Several research groups have found antibodies to HIV-1 in the cerebrospinal fluid (CSF) and have isolated the virus itself during this acute phase.[46-49] Neurodiagnostic studies have not been remarkable: the electroencephalogram sometimes demonstrates diffuse slowing, and radiographic imaging studies have largely shown no abnormalities. The majority of affected individuals, however, go through a phase of neurologically asymptomatic HIV-1 infection of the CNS, as evidenced by CSF screening studies of patients at risk.[23,24] Few neuropathologic studies have examined this early phase of symptomatic or asymptomatic HIV-1 invasion of the nervous system (HIV meningitis).[50] In one patient the meninges contained a greater than normal number of mononuclear cells, some lymphocytes, and polymorphonuclear leukocytes.[51] McArthur et al.[52] described a patient with early-onset HIV-related cognitive dysfunction who died suddenly. Postmortem examination showed slight pallor and astrocytosis of the cerebral white matter but no meningeal inflammation.

HIV-1 was also incriminated as a neurotropic virus when it was recovered from the brains of experimental animals who had received inoculations with CNS tissue from AIDS patients with neurologic disease.[53] Neuropathologic examination and virus localization studies in tissue sections have demonstrated a distinctive viral encephalitis (HIV encephalitis) and other unique clinicopathologic syndromes affecting the spinal cord and neuromuscular system that may also be caused by the virus.

HIV-1 Encephalitis

Well before HIV-1 was identified as the etiologic agent in AIDS, the earliest report of the neuropathologic findings in patients with the disease thoroughly described a new type of encephalitis.[15] Many other publications have added further details and elucidated the range of light microscopic abnormalities of this unique disorder.[26,28-32,34,35,37,54-59] These studies permit a tentative differentiation of the morphologic expressions of HIV-1 infection from those of other opportunistic viruses (such as CMV). HIV immunoperoxidase and in situ hybridization localization studies, as well as ultrastructural examination, have also greatly enhanced understanding of this encephalitis.

Macroscopic examination of the brain is usually unremarkable. The meninges are clear. Some ventricular dilatation and widening of the sylvian fissures and adjacent cortical sulci may be present. The cortical mantle is generally of normal thickness. In some cases the white matter is severely affected (see later discussion).

Microscopic examination shows an inflammatory reaction in the brain characterized by widely distributed infiltrates of microglial nodules, that is, aggregates of five or more microglial cells with or without small foci of tissue necrosis and surrounding slight pallor of myelin staining (Fig. 13–1). The nodules are often observed in the vicinity of small blood vessels and sometimes occur concurrently with sizable collections of perivascular foamy or pigment-laden macrophages. They resemble the "glial shrubs" of arbovirus infections or the Babès nodules of rickettsial diseases. In the affected areas the nuclei of capillary and venular endothelial cells may be numerous, large, and misshapen. Microglial nodules are ordinarily not accompanied by lymphocytic or plasma cellular infiltrates, either perivascularly or within the parenchyma. The degree of reactive astrocytosis varies with the severity of the lesion and can sometimes be extensive. Microglial nodules may be dis-

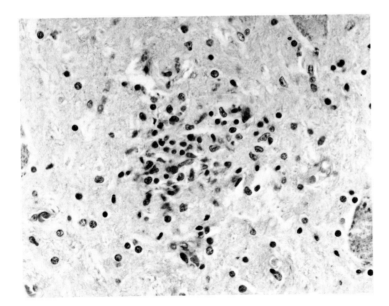

Figure 13–1. HIV encephalitis. Microglial nodule in anterior horn of spinal cord. (Hematoxylin and eosin, ×180.)

tributed diffusely throughout the neuraxis. In our experience they are most frequent in the subcortical white matter, followed by the diencephalon and brainstem gray or white matter.

An important although not invariable component of the microglial nodule is the multinucleated cell (Fig. 13–2A, B). These are macrophage-derived giant cells 15 to 25 μm in diameter as occur in the in situ and tissue culture cytopathic reaction to certain viral infections (for example, measles). They differ from foreign body or Langhans'-type giant cells because of their smaller size, scant cytoplasm, and haphazard arrangement of the nuclei.[33,57,60] They can occur admixed with other cells in the microglial nodule or appear in isolated clusters in the parenchyma or meninges (Fig. 13–2C). Some authors have considered their presence to be a hallmark of HIV infection of the brain,[28,32,57,61] whereas others find them infrequently.[42]

The identification of the type of cell infected by HIV-1 within the nervous system has been sought with viral cocultivation,[62] immunohistochemistry,[57,63-69] in situ hybridization,[57,67,70,71] and transmission electron microscopy.[57,72-74] The localization of HIV to the mononucleated and multinucleated macrophages and the activated microglial cells associated with microglial nodules in the brain, as well as to circulating monocytes and macrophages found elsewhere in the body, now appears well established (Fig. 13–3).[69,75] Furthermore, HIV-1 has been shown to have a selective tropism for the CD4 protein of

helper T-cells, which it uses as a binding site.[76] There seems to be no evidence of immunoreactivity to herpes simplex virus (HSV), CMV, and papovavirus antigens within microglial nodules containing HIV-1-positive mononuclear cells.[64] Wiley et al.[65] and Ward et al.[68] found HIV infection of endothelial cells; however, Kure et al.[69] have been unable to confirm this observation. Harouse et al.[77] were able to isolate HIV-1 in cultures of the choroid plexus from three patients who died of AIDS. Whether HIV-1 is capable of infecting neurons, astrocytes, or oligodendroglia at all has been difficult to ascertain.

Several explanations have been advanced for the sequence of events that leads to penetration of HIV-1 into CNS tissue and the mechanisms of injury that underlie the ensuing neurologic syndromes (see reviews by Dal Canto[41] and Rosenblum[39]). One postulate is that circulating monocytes latently infected with HIV are transported across the cerebral capillary endothelium as part of normal immunologic surveillance (Trojan horse hypothesis). Once the monocytes are in the brain, their maturation to macrophages permits viral replication, release of virions, and penetration of the virus into neighboring cells that express CD4 receptors on their surface (i.e., macrophages and microglial cells) through binding of the HIV envelope glycoprotein gp120 to the CD4 receptor. HIV-1 viremia could also seed the cerebral microcirculation, causing direct infection of endothelial cells. HIV-1 infection of the brain and the resulting HIV encephalitis could

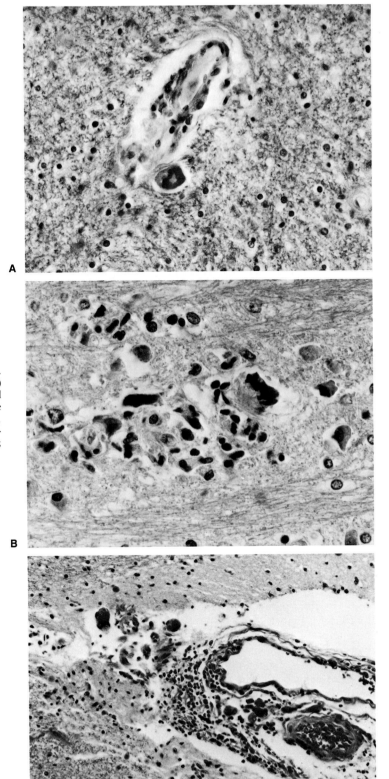

Figure 13–2. HIV encephalitis. *A,* Multinucleated giant cell (MNGC) adjacent to blood vessel in cerebral white matter. *B,* Microglial nodule with MNGCs in basis pontis. *C,* MNGCs in subarachnoid space. (Hematoxylin and eosin; *A* and *C,* ×120; *B,* ×180.)

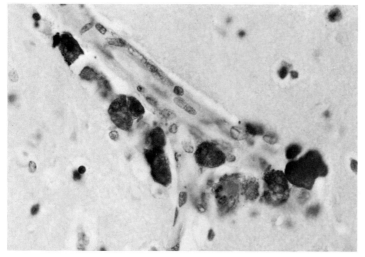

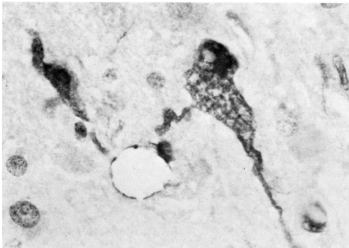

Figure 13–3. HIV encephalitis. *A,* Perivascular macrophages staining for HIV-1 antigen gp41. *B,* HIV-positive macrophages and microglial cells in brain parenchyma. (Perioxidase-antiperioxidase; *A,* ×180; *B,* ×300.)

cause brain injury by release of a macrophage-mediated monokine (e.g., tumor necrosis factor) or proteolytic enzymes that could be toxic to neurons or glia. Yet another hypothetical mechanism is that the HIV envelope glycoprotein competes with the neurotropic factor neuroleukin for binding to certain neurons, shortening the survival of affected cells.[78] Altered vascular permeability resulting from direct HIV infection of the endothelium[65] or possibly as an indirect effect of perivascular HIV-infected monocytes on the endothelium could cause accumulation of edema fluid within the extracellular space and allow various circulating macromolecules to enter the cerebral parenchyma. Last, the HIV-1 coat protein gp120 may cause neurologic damage by increasing intraneuronal free calcium.[79]

Leukoencephalopathy

Apart from the attack on oligodendroglial cells by opportunistic viruses (as in PML) and the white matter vacuolar myelopathy discussed later in the chapter, evidence from various laboratories[26,28,59] suggests that HIV might give rise to a primary attack on the central myelin comparable to other human demyelinating diseases (e.g., multiple sclerosis). The most remarkable examples of a diffuse "demyelinating" lesion involving large portions of the cerebral white matter are those reported by Nielsen et al.,[56] Horoupian et al.,[80] and Kleihues et al.[81] In our experience with three cases of this type,[82] whole brain sections stained for myelin showed a remarkable pallor of the centrum semiovale and the deep cerebellar white matter (Fig. 13–4). Microscopic examination of sections shows diffuse loss of myelin and gliosis, relative sparing of axons, and a paucity of inflammatory cells (Fig. 13–5A). Microglial nodules and giant cells may be seen within the lesion. Less severe forms of this process are characterized by focal, often angiocentric regions of myelin loss, sometimes related to aggregates of microglial nodules (Fig. 13–5B). Transitions between the focal and more diffuse white matter lesions may be present. One of our patients also had conspicuous axonal damage with axonal spheroids in the centrum semiovale and in long fiber tracts (Fig. 13–6). We found prominent changes of the microvasculature in the white matter, including mural thickening, increased cellularity, and enlargement and pleomorphism of endothelial cells (Fig. 13–7). These vascular abnormalities were usually associated with prominent perivascular aggregates of HIV-positive monocytes and multinucleated cells, which often contained hemosiderin pigment (Fig. 13–8). These observations suggested a role for altered vascular permeability in the pathogenesis of HIV-associated leukoencephalopathy, as discussed previously. Other possible causes

for the white matter degeneration include destruction of myelin and axons by soluble substances elaborated by HIV-infected monocytes,[83] autoimmune-associated demyelination,[41] and direct attack of HIV on the myelin-forming oligodendrocytes. Some investigators[30,43] have noted alterations in the number and size of oligodendrocytic nuclei within areas of myelin pallor, but the presence of HIV within oligodendroglial cells has not yet been conclusively demonstrated.

Vacuolar Myelopathy

In early 1985 two separate groups of investigators[84,85] described the clinical and pathologic aspects of a previously unrecognized spinal cord disorder in AIDS patients. The disease, named vacuolar myelopathy by Petito et al., was characterized by multiple 10 to 100 μm vacuoles within the white matter of the posterior and lateral columns of the lower thoracic cord (Fig. 13–9). They also stressed the importance of finding foamy macrophages in association with these vacuolar lesions to rule out artifactual changes. In the 20 cases recorded, the severity of the lesions was

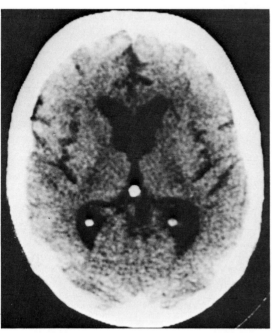 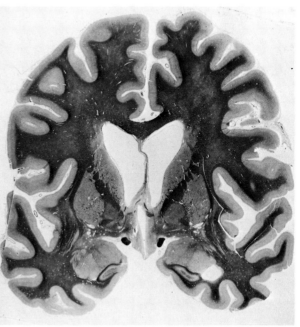

A **B**

Figure 13–4. HIV leukoencephalopathy. *A*, computed tomographic scan of head showing widening of cortical sulci, ventricular dilatation, and diffuse hypodensity of centrum semiovale. *B*, Whole mount (paraffin) of cerebrum showing patchiness and diffuse pallor of myelin staining throughout centrum semiovale. (Luxo-fast-blue and hematoxylin and eosin.) (From Smith TW, De Girolami U, Hénin D, et al: Human immunodeficiency virus [HIV] leukoencephalopathy and the microcirculation. J Neuropathol Exp Neurol 49:357-370, 1990, by permission of the authors and publishers.)

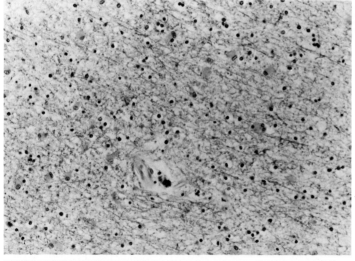

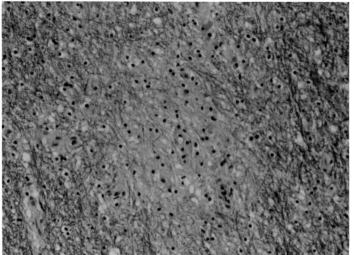

Figure 13–5. HIV leukoencephalopathy. *A,* Decreased density of myelinated fibers and gliosis in cerebral white matter. *B,* Perivascular myelin pallor. Macrophages are scattered around central capillary. Oligodendrocytes are well preserved. (*A* and *B,* Luxol-fast-blue and hematoxylin and eosin, ×60.) (From Smith TW, De Girolami U, Hénin D, et al: Human immunodeficiency virus [HIV] leukoencephalopathy and the microcirculation. J Neuropathol Exp Neurol 49:357-370, 1990, by permission of the authors and publishers.)

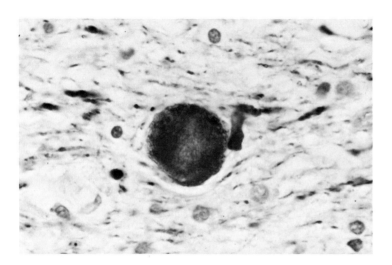

Figure 13–6. HIV leukoencephalopathy. Axonal spheroid in internal capsule stained with antibody to phosphorylated neurofilaments. (Peroxidase-antiperoxidase, ×300.) (From Smith TW, De Girolami U, Hénin D, et al: Human immunodefieciency virus [HIV] leukoencephalopathy and the microcirculation. J Neuropathol Exp neurol 49:357-370, 1990, by permission of the authors and publishers.)

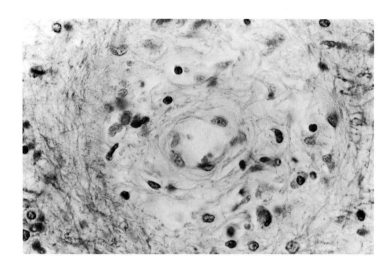

Figure 13–7. HIV leukoencephalopathy. Connective tissue proliferation is present around small blood vessel in centrum semiovale. (Luxol-fast-blue and hematoxylin and eosin, ×180.) (From Smith TW, De Girolami U, Hénin D, et al: Human immunodeficiency virus [HIV] leukoencephalopathy and the microcirculation. J Neuropathol Exp Neurol 49:357-370, 1990, by permission of the authors and publishers.)

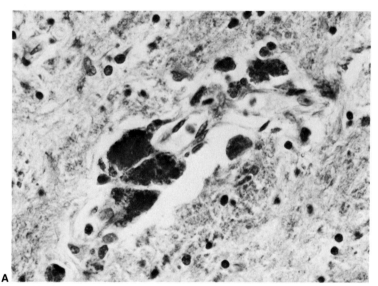

Figure 13–8. HIV leukoencephalopathy. Iron deposits within multinucleated giant cells and macrophages around and within vessel wall. (*A*, Hematoxylin and eosin, ×180; *B*, Prussian blue, ×180.) (From Smith TW, De Girolami U, Hénin D, et al: Human immunodeficiency virus [HIV] leukoencephalopathy and the microcirculation. J Neuropathol Exp Neurol 49:357-370, 1990, by permission of the authors and publishers.)

A

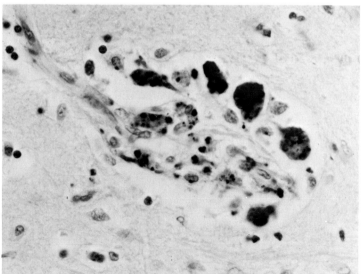

B

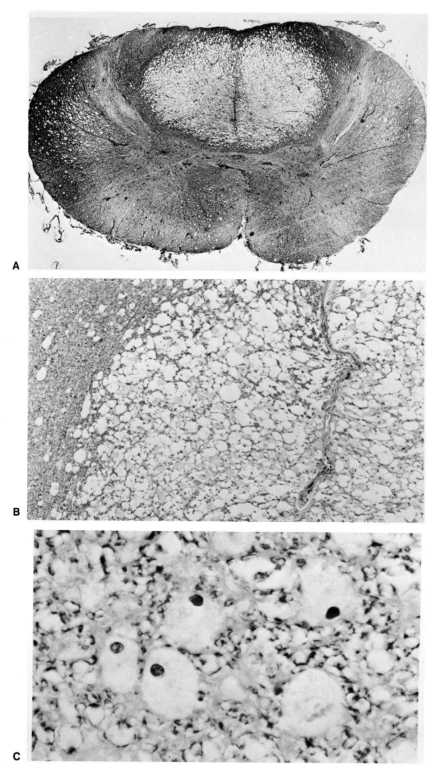

Figure 13–9. Vacuolar myelopathy. *A,* Upper thoracic spinal cord showing severe vacuolar degeneration in posterior columns and, to lesser extent, in lateral columns. *B,* Vacuolar change and macrophages in dorsal columns. *C,* Vacuoles containing lipid-laden macrohages. (Luxol-fast-blue; *A,* ×12; *B,* ×30; *C,* ×300.)

graded (from I [mild] to III [severe]) and transition forms between the prototypes were common. In subsequent large studies from the United States[28,86,87] the disorder has been estimated to be demonstrable at postmortem examination in 20% to 30% of unselected patients with AIDS; it has been found less often in Europe.[42] Although extensive reactive gliosis is rare, microglial nodules and multinucleated giant cells are sometimes seen in cord regions away from the vacuolar myelopathy. Ultrastructural studies indicate both axonal and myelin injury.[88]

The cause and pathogenesis of vacuolar myelopathy are unknown. The early reports pointed out the striking resemblance of the cord lesions to those of vitamin B_{12} deficiency (subacute combined degeneration), but this possibility was discarded after appropriate serum assays.[85] The role of HIV-1 has been controversial. Ho et al.[46] isolated the virus from the CSF and postmortem spinal cord tissue in a patient with clinical manifestations of a myelopathy. Budka et al.,[89] Maier et al.,[90] and Eilbott et al.[91] have demonstrated by immunohistochemistry (in one patient) and in situ hybridization (in three patients) that the macrophages and multinucleated giant cells near the vacuoles are HIV positive, suggesting that HIV causes vacuolar myelopathy. However, strong evidence supports the opposite viewpoint. Kamin and Petito[92] reported vacuolar myelopathy in 12 immunosuppressed patients without AIDS. Rosenblum et al.,[87] in a comprehensive study (39 patients, 24 with vacuolar myelopathy) combining immunohistochemistry (p24), in situ DNA hybridization, and HIV isolation, showed that the presence of the virus correlated not with the presence of vacuolar myelopathy but with an inflammatory myelitis closely resembling the so-called subacute encephalitis of HIV infection described previously (i.e., microglial nodules, multinucleated giant cells, and perivascular collections of macrophages). Grafe and Wiley,[86] in a study of 26 patients, 8 with vacuolar myelopathy, also showed a lack of association between immunocytologic localization of HIV antigens and vacuolar myelopathy. Similarly, neuropathologic observations of the spinal cord in children with AIDS dispute the assertion that vacuolar myelopathy is caused by HIV-1.[93-95]

It can be tentatively concluded that AIDS-associated vacuolar myelopathy either is unrelated to HIV infection of the spinal cord and brain or is a remote or indirect effect of HIV or some other infectious agent. The spinal cord can also undergo degenerative changes limited to the corticospinal tracts or the posterior columns. Such changes have been attributed to secondary wallerian degeneration consequent to proximal injury in the pyramidal system or dorsal root ganglia.[80,96] Of related interest is tropical spastic paraparesis, which has been reported in the Caribbean, along the Indian Ocean, and in South America. Pathologic studies are scant, but two recently reported cases have shown a severe lymphocytic meningomyelitis quite unlike that seen in vacuolar myelopathy.[97] Virologic studies have implicated human T-lymphotropic virus type I (HTLV-I) infection in the pathogenesis of this disorder.[98]

Opportunistic infections of the spinal cord unassociated with vacuolar myelopathy have been the subject of special attention in several studies. CMV necrotizing myelitis especially affecting the periphery of the lower cord and the roots has been reported in 11 patients.[54,99-106] CMV antigen could not be demonstrated by immunocytochemical localization in any of seven patients with vacuolar myelopathy. Toxoplasmosis of the cord in AIDS patients is generally manifest as a destructive mass lesion caused by a well-circumscribed abscess in which free or encysted organisms may be found.[107-110] Britton et al.[111] described a patient with HSV-2 thoracic myelitis associated with cutaneous herpetic infection.

Neuropathy

Patients with AIDS are susceptible to a wide range of cranial and peripheral nerve disturbances.[15,16,59,112-119] (See also reviews by Möbius and Schlote,[120] Dalakas and Pezeshkpour,[121] and Parry.[122]) The most commonly reported clinical syndromes include acute and chronic inflammatory demyelinating polyneuropathy, distal symmetric polyneuropathy, polyradiculopathy, and mononeuritis multiplex. A sensory neuropathy caused by ganglioneuronitis has also been described.[96,123] Histopathologic findings in most of these cases include segmental demyelination, axonal degeneration, and epineurial and endoneurial mononuclear cell inflammation. The cause of these AIDS-associated neuropathies is undoubtedly multifactorial and often obscure. HIV has been cultured from the nerve in some cases of AIDS-associated neuropathy[46,64,115]; however, immunocytochemical tests could not demonstrate the virus within Schwann cells or elsewhere in a series of 24 cases.[86] In one patient described by Bailey et al.,[114] electron microscopy showed retrovirus-like particles within peripheral nerve axoplasm. Necrotizing arteritis has been reported in some cases of AIDS-associated neuropathy.[124,125] In the two patients described by Gherardi et al.,[125] in situ hybridization demonstrated HIV replication within mononuclear cells infiltrating the vessels. Other infectious agents may cause a neuropathy in some HIV-infected individuals. Bishopric et al.,[126] Eidelberg et al.,[100] and Behar et al.[103] reported a Guillain-Barré-like syndrome related to CMV. Lanska et al.[127] described an HIV-positive patient with syphilitic polyradiculopathy. Other possible causes for AIDS-related neuropathies include immune-mediated attack against peripheral nerve components triggered by HIV or other viruses or by the immunodeficiency state itself; various toxic, metabolic, and nutritional factors; and infiltration of nerves and nerve roots by neoplasm (e.g., lymphoma) (Fig. 13–10).

Myopathy

Inflammatory myopathy has been the most frequently described skeletal muscle disorder in patients with AIDS or ARC.[121,128-137] The disease is characterized by the subacute onset of proximal weakness, sometimes pain, and elevated serum creatine kinase levels. The histologic findings have included muscle fiber necrosis and phagocytosis, interstitial infiltration with HIV-positive macrophages, and in a few cases cytoplasmic bodies and nemaline rods (Fig. 13–11A).[121,132,134] Direct viral invasion of skeletal muscle cells has not been reported. An inflammatory myopathy has been described in simian AIDS.[138] Wiley et al.[139] recently reported that a patient with polymyositis was seropositive for both HTLV-I and HIV. Using in situ hybridization and immunocytochemical tests, they observed direct infection of muscle fibers by HTLV-1 but no evidence of HIV in muscle or inflammatory cells. The pathogenesis of the inflammatory myopathy is not clear. The hypothesis that skeletal muscle cells are a primary target of HIV has not been borne out by tissue culture, ultrastructural, or viral localization studies. An alternative possibility is that immune effector cells attack skeletal muscle cells or that an opportunistic infectious agent alters muscle membranes, rendering them the target of an autoimmune reaction akin to idiopathic polymyositis.[140] In a case of HIV-associated myopathy we studied, we suggested that the virus might localize to the vascular bed of skeletal muscle, whether or not skeletal muscle is itself a target cell.[141] We based this hypothesis on the presence of structural abnormalities of the microcirculation, immunocytochemical localization of the virus within monocytes around vessel walls, and evidence of altered vascular permeability (extravasation of red blood cells, iron pigment–laden macrophages) (Fig. 13–11B). Such regional distribution of viruses has been proposed as a possible mechanism of viral tropism.[142]

Recently an acute toxic myopathy with myoglobulinuria has been reported in AIDS patients treated with zidovudine (AZT).[143-145] These cases seem to illustrate a different pathologic process from the inflammatory myopathy described previously. In the series reported by Dalakas et al.,[145] muscle biopsy specimens contained numerous "ragged red" fibers (fibers containing abnormal mitochondria with paracrystalline inclusions), which suggested the presence of a toxic mitochondrial myopathy. Some patients with AIDS or ARC have proximal muscle weakness with normal creatine kinase levels and severe type II fiber atrophy seen on muscle biopsy.[121,146,147] This condition may be related to poor nutrition, rapid weight loss, prolonged bed rest, or remote effect of malignancy.

Vascular Lesions

Embolic cerebral infarction and hemorrhages have been noted in various sites (intraparenchymal, subarachnoid, epidural, and subdural),[15,148,149] and CNS vasculitis has been reported in several patients with AIDS or ARC. Yankner et al.[150] described a patient with CNS granulomatous vasculitis associated with HIV-1 isolation from brain tissue and CSF. Scaravilli et al.[151] published the study of an AIDS patient who had multiple cerebral infarcts in association with chronic basal meningitis and vasculitis. Vinters et al.[152] described a patient with ARC who had evidence of a systemic necrotizing vasculitis most severely affecting the CNS, with hemorrhagic necrosis of the spinal cord and cauda equina. Nonvasculitic proliferative lesions affecting smaller diameter vessels within the leptomeninges[153] and cerebral parenchyma[148] have been recorded. Calcific vasculopathy involving the basal ganglia is seen in children with

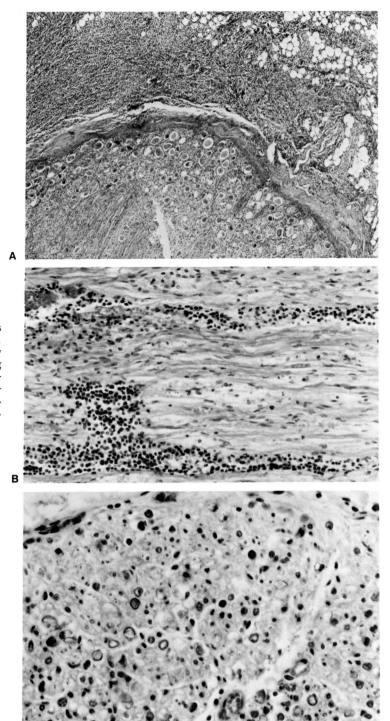

Figure 13–10. Lymphomatous infiltration of peripheral nerve. *A,* Dorsal root ganglion surrounded by tumor cells. *B,* Dorsal root showing lymphomatous infiltrates and wallerian degeneration. *C,* Loss of myelinated fibers in distal dorsal root. (Luxol-fast-blue; *A,* ×12; *B,* ×60; *C,* ×120.)

AIDS (see later discussion). We have observed abnormalities of the cerebral microvasculature with evidence of altered vascular permeability in patients with HIV meningoencephalitis and leukoencephalopathy (see previous discussion). As yet HIV has not been unequivocally demonstrated (by electron microscopy, in situ hybridization, or immunocytochemistry) within the walls of affected vessels in any of the AIDS-associated vasculopathies. Esiri et

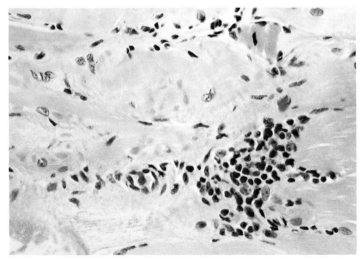

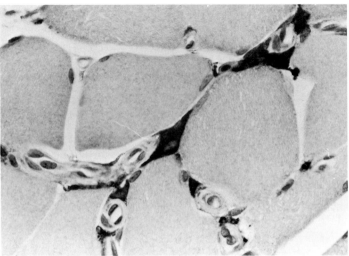

Figure 13–11. HIV myopathy. *A,* Skeletal muscle showing degenerating myofibers and mononuclear inflammatory cells in endomysium. *B,* Endomysial macrophages immunostaining for HIV-1 gp41. (*A,* Hematoxylin and eosin, ×300; *B,* avidin-biotin and hematoxylin, ×450.) (From Chad DA, Smith TW, Blumenfeld A, et al: Human immunodeficiency virus [HIV]-associated myopathy: Immunocytochemical identification of an HIV antigen (gp 41) in muscle macrophages. Ann Neurol 28:579-582, 1990, by permission of the authors and publishers.)

al.[36] have reported a high prevalence of recent and old intracranial hemorrhages in HIV-infected hemophiliacs as compared with AIDS patients without hemophilia.

Other Considerations

AIDS-Dementia Complex. Many clinical reports (see reviews by Price et al.[21,22]) refer to a progressive deterioration of intellectual function ("dementia") in AIDS patients. This dementia occurs well into the course of the disease and is rarely if ever the initial manifestation of AIDS.[20,154,155] The deterioration begins insidiously with mental slowing, memory loss, and mood disturbances such as apathy and depression. Motor abnormalities, ataxia, bladder and bowel incontinence, and seizures may also occur. Computed tomography of the brain has shown cortical atrophy and ventricular dilatation.[156,157] Diffuse or focal abnormalities of the cerebral white matter may be seen with magnetic resonance imaging.[158,159] The precise neuropathologic reason for these clinical and radiologic abnormalities is unknown, and the etiologic basis and pathogenesis of the dementia probably vary among affected individuals. Furthermore, the frequent occurrence of multiple opportunistic infections with or without HIV encephalitis makes the dementia difficult to understand. However, the more clinically advanced cognitive disorder seems to be correlated with neuropathologic features of HIV meningoencephalitis and leukoencephalopathy. Our studies have suggested that the brain "atrophy" and ventricular dilatation apparent on imaging studies may be largely due to loss of myelin and axons in the subcortical and central white matter rather than to degeneration of the cerebral cortex.[82]

Neuropathology of Pediatric AIDS. Neurologic disease is common in children with AIDS.[160] The virus is apparently transmitted in utero from an infected mother via the placenta. Clinical manifestations of neurologic dysfunction are evident in the first years of life and include microencephaly with mental retardation and delayed motor development with long tract signs.[161] The neuropathologic features of AIDS in children tend to differ from those in adults. They have been discussed in a few comprehensive reports and several recent reviews.[43,63,93,161] The most frequently reported abnormality is calcification of the basal ganglia and deep cerebral white matter. In some cases computed tomographic (CT) scans have demonstrated progressive calcification. Histopathologic studies of the lesion show a mineralizing angiopathy affecting both large and small vessels. Calcific deposits may also be found in ischemic neurons, microglial nodules, and large necrotic lesions associated with lymphoma or encephalomalacia.[63,93] The next most frequent finding is HIV meningoencephalitis and white matter degeneration, similar to those described in adults (see preceding discussion). The spinal cord in these patients may show pyramidal tract degeneration, but vacuolar myelopathy is extremely rare. Opportunistic infections of the CNS, including toxoplasmosis, CMV, PML, and cryptococcal meningitis, are rarer in infants and children with AIDS than in adults. The reason for this discrepancy may be that opportunistic infections in adults are most often due to reactivation of latent, previously acquired infection. The most common focal CNS abnormalities reported by Dickson et al.[93] were lymphomas and cerebrovascular lesions. Giangaspero et al.[162] described a patient with extensive destructive lesions of gray and white matter. Myopathy and peripheral neuropathy have not yet been described in children with AIDS.

OPPORTUNISTIC INFECTIONS

Parasitic Infections

Toxoplasmosis. Infection of the brain by *Toxoplasma gondii* is one of the most common causes of neurologic symptoms and morbidity in AIDS patients. The incidence of CNS infection in most clinical and autopsy series averages 10% to 15% and ranges from 4% to 30%.[163] The CNS infection tends to be more fulminant and destructive than in nonimmu-

nocompromised hosts.[107] The clinical symptoms are typically subacute, evolving during a 1- to 2-week period, and may be either focal or generalized.[38,107,163] The disorder is characterized by the formation of focal "abscesses" that are frequently multiple and most often involve the cerebral cortex (near the gray-white junction) and deep gray nuclei, less often the cerebellum and brainstem, and rarely the spinal cord.[107-109,163] In fact, toxoplasmosis is considered the most common cause of focal mass lesions of the brain in AIDS patients. CT and magnetic resonance imaging may show multiple ring-enhancing lesions, but this radiographic appearance is not pathognomonic, since similar findings may be associated with CNS lymphoma, tuberculosis, or fungal infections.[38,163]

Three phases of CNS toxoplasmosis have been identified: acute (necrotizing), organizing, and chronic.[107] Histologic examination of acute lesions shows central foci of necrosis with variable petechial hemorrhages surrounded by acute and chronic inflammation, macrophage infiltration, and vascular proliferation (Fig. 13–12*A*). Both free tachyzoites and encysted bradyzoites may be found at the periphery of the necrotic foci. The organisms are usually seen on routine hematoxylin and eosin or Giemsa stains (Fig. 13–12*B*) but in many instances can be more easily recognized by immunocytochemical staining of paraffin-embedded sections with commercially available anti-*Toxoplasma* antisera (Fig. 13–12*C*). The diagnosis of acute *Toxoplasma* infection requires the presence of free tachyzoites in the tissue; unruptured cysts alone are not sufficient.[163] Blood vessels near the lesions can also be invaded by the organisms and may show marked intimal proliferation or even frank vasculitis with fibrinoid necrosis and thrombosis.[38,164] The organizing lesions consist of large, well-demarcated areas of coagulation necrosis surrounded by lipid-laden macrophages. Cysts and free tachyzoites can also be found adjacent to these lesions but may be considerably reduced in number if therapy has been effective. Chronic lesions consist of small cystic spaces containing small numbers of lipid- and hemosiderin-laden macrophages with surrounding gliosis. Organisms may be difficult to detect near these lesions. In addition to the more typical presentation of CNS toxoplasmosis, a diffuse "encephalitic" form of cerebral toxoplasmosis characterized by widespread microglial nodules rather than focal necrotizing abscesses has been described.[165]

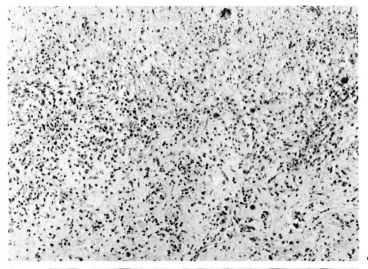

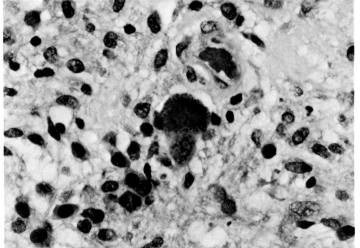

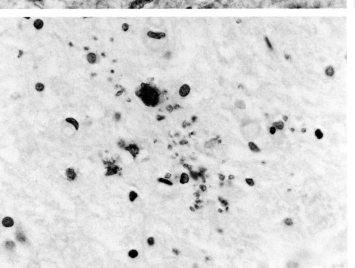

Figure 13–12. Cerebral toxoplasmosis. *A,* Wall of acute abscess showing acute and chronic inflammation, vascular proliferation, and scattered *Toxoplasma* cysts. *B, Toxoplasma* cysts containing bradyzoites. *C,* Cyst and free tachyzoites immunostained with anti-*Toxoplasma* antibody. (*A,* Hematoxylin and eosin, ×12; *B,* hematoxylin and eosin, ×180; *C,* peroxidase-antiperoxidase, ×180.) (From De Girolami U, Smith TW, Hénin D, et al: Neuropathology of the acquired immunodeficiency syndrome. Arch Pathol Lab Med 114:643-655, 1990, by permission of the authors and publishers.)

Amebiasis. CNS infection by *Acanthamoeba* species has been reported in several patients with AIDS.[38,166] Pathologic examination showed acute necrotizing meningoencephalitis with areas of extensive tissue necrosis containing *Acanthamoeba*. The amebae are sometimes difficult to distinguish from histiocytes.[38] Periodic acid–Schiff (PAS) or methenamine-silver stain is helpful in visualizing the organisms, although definitive identification may depend ultimately on combined immunofluorescence, morphologic, and culture studies.[163]

Fungal Infections

Cryptococcosis. *Cryptococcus neoformans* is the fungus most commonly infecting the CNS in AIDS patients and has been reported in 5% to 12% of patients in clinical and autopsy series.[38,163] The histopathologic characteristics of fungal meningoencephalitis caused by *Cryptococcus* and other fungi (see later discussion) are generally indistinguishable from those in immunocompromised individuals without AIDS except that in AIDS the lesions tend to be more extensive and destructive, with a less prominent inflammatory response.[38,163] Patients with cryptococcal infection of the CNS have chronic meningitis typically affecting the basal leptomeninges, which become thickened by reactive connective tissue. The latter may obstruct the outflow of CSF from the foramina of Luschka and Magendie, giving rise to hydrocephalus. Sections of the brain disclose a gelatinous material within the subarachnoid space and small cysts within the parenchyma, which are especially prominent in the basal ganglia in the distribution of the lenticulostriate arteries. Microscopic examination of the parenchymal lesions shows aggregates of organisms within expanded perivascular (Virchow-Robin) spaces associated with minimal or absent inflammation or gliosis (Fig. 13–13*A*). The meningeal infiltrates consist of chronic inflammatory cells and fibroblasts admixed with the cryptococcal organisms, whose capsules can be readily demonstrated with the mucicarmine and PAS stains (Fig. 13–13*B*). Well-formed granulomas are not seen.

Other Fungal Infections. CNS infection by *Candida albicans*, *Aspergillus fumigatus*, *Mucor* species, *Histoplasma capsulatum*, *Coccidiodes immitis*, *Blastomyces dermatitidis*, *Acremonium alabamensis*, and *Cladosporidium* has been reported in AIDS patients.[38,163]

Bacterial Infections

Mycobacterial Infections. CNS infection by *Mycobacterium avium-intracellulare* has been reported infrequently in AIDS patients.[26,42] It usually occurs in patients with disseminated infection by the organism. The disease may cause chronic meningitis, brain abscesses, and rarely diffuse encephalitis or cranial or peripheral neuropathy.[38,163] The inflammatory response tends to be less pronounced than with *Mycobacterium tuberculosis* and consists of foamy macrophages and mononuclear inflammatory cells without the formation of distinctive tubercles. Acid-fast mycobacteria are readily demonstrated by special stains. The response to antituberculous agents has been poor.

M. tuberculosis infection of the CNS is likewise relatively uncommon in patients with AIDS but is being reported with increasing frequency.[167] Intravenous drug users and Haitians have been most commonly affected.[168] In the CNS the organism may cause either focal cerebral masses (tuberculomas) or chronic meningitis. Unlike *M. avium–intracellulare* infection, the microscopic appearance of *M. tuberculosis* lesions resembles that in non-AIDS patients, with well-formed epithelioid granulomas.

Neurosyphilis. Patients with HIV infection are at increased risk for neurosyphilis.[169,170] The rate of progression and severity of the disease appear to be accelerated in AIDS patients, presumably because of their altered cell-mediated immunity.[169] CNS involvement by *Treponema pallidum* may be manifest as asymptomatic infection, acute syphilitic meningitis, meningovascular syphilis, and rarely direct parenchymal invasion of the brain. Standard CSF serologic tests for neurosyphilis (the Venereal Disease Research Laboratory and fluorescent treponemal antibody absorption tests) may be nonreactive in HIV-seropositive individuals in the presence of viable *T. pallidum* in the CSF.[171] An exceptionally severe necrotizing encephalitis with massive treponemal invasion of the brain ("quaternary" neurosyphilis) has been reported in a patient with HIV infection.[172,173] The more classic forms of parenchymal involvement in neurosyphilis, general paresis and tabes dorsalis, have not yet been reported in HIV-infected individuals, possibly because the disease has a shorter latency period and more severe course in these patients.[38]

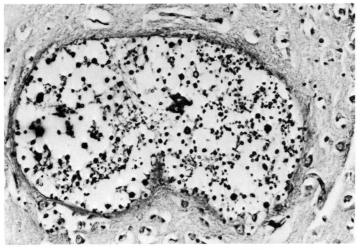

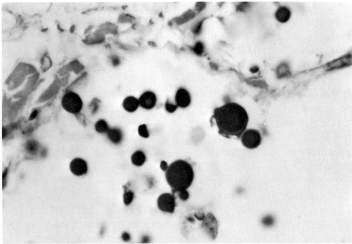

Figure 13–13. Cryptococcal meningitis. *A*, Enlarged perivascular space containing numerous cryptococcal organisms. *B*, Cryptococci in subarachnoid space. (Periodic acid–Schiff; *A*, ×60; *B*, ×300).

Viral Infections

Cytomegalovirus Encephalitis. CMV is the most common opportunistic viral pathogen affecting the CNS in AIDS patients.[105,174] Evidence of CMV infection has been found at autopsy in the CNS in 15% to 20% of AIDS patients.[105] CNS infection can have several different manifestations.[38,105,174] Probably the most common pattern of involvement is a subacute encephalitis with the formation of microglial nodules primarily within gray matter, which may or may not be associated with CMV inclusion-bearing cells. This histologic pattern of diffuse MGN encephalitis is similar to that in HIV encephalitis, and indeed some patients with AIDS have been found to have brain infection with both HIV and CMV.[175] Although virtually any type of cell within the CNS (neurons, glia, ependyma, endothelium) can be infected by CMV, the virus tends to localize in the ependyma and subependymal regions of the brain. This can result in a severe necrotizing ventriculoencephalitis with massive necrosis, hemorrhage, ventriculitis, and choroid plexitis. Prominent cytomegalic cells with intranuclear and intracytoplasmic CMV inclusions can be readily identified both by conventional light microscopy (Fig. 13–14*A*) and by immunocytochemistry (Fig. 13–14*B*) and in situ hybridization. The latter techniques have also shown that normal-appearing, noncytomegalic cells at the edges of the lesions may contain virus.[176] Somewhat less frequently encountered are isolated inclusion-bearing cells, unassociated with tissue reaction,[174] and a necrotizing radiculomyelitis.[100,103,105,126,174]

Herpes Simplex and Zoster Infections. In AIDS patients HSV may rarely cause acute encephalitis whose clinical presentation and pathologic features are essentially identi-

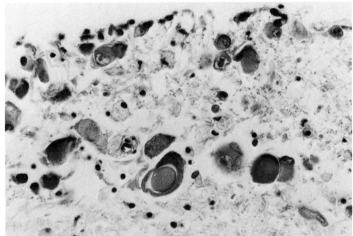

A

Figure 13–14. Cytomegalovirus (CMV) encephalitis. *A,* Section from periventricular region shows enlarged glial cells with typical CMV intranuclear inclusions. *B,* Intranuclear and intracytoplasmic inclusions immunostained with anti-CMV antibody. (*A,* Hematoxylin and eosin, ×180; *B,* peroxidase-antiperoxidase, ×300.)

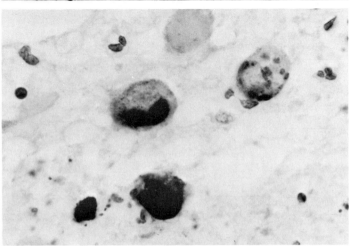

B

cal to those in immunocompetent individuals.[177] Interestingly, HSV-2 has been cultured from the brains of these patients. HSV-1 may cause subacute encephalitis with clinical manifestations (weakness, lethargy, ataxia, and seizures) developing over a more protracted period (4 to 6 weeks) and with more diffuse involvement of the brain rather than restriction to the temporal lobes.[177] Combined HSV and CMV ventriculoencephalitis[174] and HSV-2 necrotizing myelitis[99,111,178,179] have been reported in AIDS patients.

Varicella-zoster virus (VZV) infection accounts for about 12% of herpesvirus infections in AIDS patients.[178] VZV-associated disorders involving the CNS in AIDS include encephalomyelitis,[28,180,181] herpes zoster ophthalmicus,[182,183] trigeminal encephalitis,[184] leukoencephalitis[185] and cerebral vasculopathy.[185]

Progressive Multifocal Leukoencephalopathy. PML, or Richardson's disease, was initially described by Aström et al.[186] and Rich-

ardson[187] as a disorder of the white matter in patients with defective immune responses. The most commonly observed predisposing conditions have been chronic lymphoproliferative, myeloproliferative, or granulomatous diseases. From the outset the disorder was suspected to result from an atypical viral infection, and in 1965 Zu Rhein and Chou[188] published the first ultrastructural images of oligodendroglial nuclei containing profiles resembling papovavirus.[188] Virus isolation followed in 1971[189]; over the years the virus has almost always been identified as the JC papovavirus.

Pathologic examination of the lesions shows patches of irregular, ill-defined granular destruction of the white matter ranging in size from a few millimeters to involvement of an entire lobe of the brain or cerebellar hemisphere. In whole brain histologic sections stained for myelin the multifocal lesions have a star-burst appearance reminiscent of astronomic images of galaxies. On microscopic examination the typical PML lesion consists of a patch of demyelination in the center of which are many lipid-laden macrophages and a few axons (Fig. 13–15A, B). At the edge of the lesion are greatly enlarged oligodendroglial nuclei whose chromatin is replaced by glassy, amphophilic viral inclusion material (Fig. 13–15C). The immunoperoxidase method (Fig. 13–15D) and in situ hybridization show viral infection in these oligodendrocytes.[190] Additional characteristics include the presence of

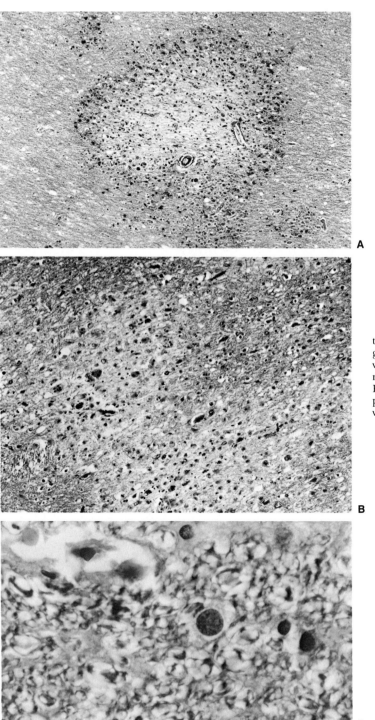

Figure 13–15. Progressive multifocal leukoencephalopathy. *A,* Region of demyelination with enlarged virus-infected oligodendrocytes primarily at periphery of lesion. *B,* Foci of demyelination with macrophages and gliosis. *C,* Enlarged virus-infected oligodendrocyte.

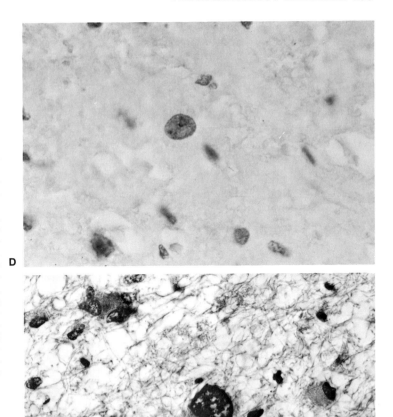

Figure 13–15. *Continued D,* Infected oligodendrocyte immunostained for papovavirus. (Immunostained with antipapovavirus antibody, gift of D.L. Walker, Ph.D., University of Wisconsin Medical School, Madison.) *E,* Lesion with bizarre giant astrocyte. (*A,* Peroxidase-antiperoxidase and Luxol-fast-blue; *B, C,* and *E,* Luxol-fast-blue and hematoxylin and eosin; *D,* peroxidase-antiperoxidase. *A, B,* and *E,* ×180; *C* and *D,* ×300.) (From De Girolami U, Smith TW, Hénin D, et al: Neuropathology of the acquired immunodeficiency syndrome. Arch Pathol Lab Med 114:643-655, 1990, by permission of the authors and publishers. Copyright 1990, American Medical Association.)

bizarre, giant astrocytic nuclei (Fig. 13–15E) and occasional perivascular and subarachnoid infiltrates with lymphocytes and plasma cells.

PML has been reported with increasing frequency in patients with AIDS.[191-197] The incidence of PML in these patients may range from 1% to 6%.[38,163] The neuropathologic features of PML in AIDS patients are essentially identical to those in immunocompromised individuals without AIDS except that the extent and severity of the lesions may be greater, with an increased tendency toward necrosis and a higher density of papovavirus-infected cells.[198] Simultaneous HIV and papovavirus infection of the brain has been described in several patients.[196,197,199,200] Wiley et al.[197] demonstrated that macrophages infiltrating the demyelinating PML lesions in these patients may also be infected by HIV. The clinical course of PML in AIDS patients has been uniformly dis-

mal, with a mean survival of only 4 months in one study.[195] However, several AIDS patients with PML have had exceptionally long survivals (more than 2 years) and clinical improvement without therapy; brain biopsy in these cases has shown an unusually prominent inflammatory response.[201]

NEOPLASMS

Lymphomas

Lymphoma in AIDS patients is discussed in detail in Chapter 7. Primary CNS lymphoma is being reported with increasing frequency in AIDS patients.[202-208] It is second only to toxoplasmosis as a cause of focal cerebral masses in AIDS.[209] Spread of systemic lymphoma to the CNS has been recorded with greater frequency in the AIDS population.[210-212] These systemic lymphomas have demonstrated an unusually high prevalence of high-grade neoplasia and a poor response to therapy.

Kaposi's Sarcoma

Kaposi's sarcoma infrequently metastasizes to the CNS. This subject has been reviewed by Gorin et al.[213]

REFERENCES

1. Centers for Disease Control: *Pneumocystis* pneumonia. MMWR 30:250-252, 1981.
2. Centers for Disease Control: Kaposi's sarcoma and *Pneumocystis* pneumonia among homosexual men—New York City and California. MMWR 30:305-308, 1981.
3. Gottlieb MS, Schroff R, Schanker HM, et al: *Pneumocystis carinii* pneumonia and mucosal candidiasis in previously healthy homosexual men: Evidence of a new acquired cellular immunodeficiency. N Engl J Med 305:1425-1431, 1981.
4. Masur H, Michelis MA, Greene JB, et al: An outbreak of community-acquired *Pneumocystis carinii* pneumonia: Initial manifestations of cellular immune dysfunction. N Engl J Med 305:1431-1438, 1981.
5. Centers for Disease Control: Update on acquired immune deficiency syndrome (AIDS)—United States. MMWR 31:507-514, 1982.
6. Barré-Sinoussi F, Chermann JC, Rey F, et al: Isolation of a T-lymphotropic retrovirus from a patient at risk for acquired immune deficiency syndrome (AIDS). Science 220:868-871, 1983.
7. Gallo RC, Salahuddin SZ, Popovic M, et al: Frequent detection and isolation of cytopathic retroviruses (HTLV-III) from patients with AIDS and at risk for AIDS. Science 224:500-503, 1984.
8. Richman DD: HIV and other human retroviruses. In Galasso GJ, Whitley RJ, Merigan TC (eds): Antiviral Agents and Viral Diseases of Man, ed 3. New York, Raven Press, 1990, pp 581-646.
9. Clavel F, Guetard D, Brun-Vezinet F, et al: Isolation of a new human retrovirus from West African patients with AIDS. Science 233:343-346, 1986.
10. Clavel F, Mansinho D, Chamaret S, et al: Human immunodeficiency virus type 2 infection associated with AIDS in West Africa. N Engl J Med 316:1180-1185, 1987.
11. Horowitz SL, Benson DF, Gottlieb MS, et al: Neurological complications of gay-related immunodeficiency disorder. Ann Neurol 12:80, 1982.
12. Horowitz SL, Bentson JR, Benson F, et al: CNS toxoplasmosis in acquired immunodeficiency syndrome. Arch Neurol 40:649-652, 1983.
13. Britton CB, Marquardt MD, Koppel B, et al: Neurological complications of the gay immunosuppressed syndrome: Clinical and pathological features. Ann Neurol 12:80, 1982.
14. Britton CB, Miller JB: Neurologic complications in acquired immunodeficiency syndrome (AIDS). Neurol Clin 2:315-339, 1984.
15. Snider WD, Simpson DM, Nielsen S, et al: Neurological complications of acquired immune deficiency syndrome: Analysis of 50 patients. Ann Neurol 14:403-418, 1983.
16. Levy RM, Bredesen DE, Rosenblum ML: Neurological manifestations of the acquired immunodeficiency syndrome (AIDS): Experience at UCSF and review of the literature. J Neurosurg 62:475-495, 1985.
17. Fenelon G, Bolgert F, Dehen H: Les manifestations neurologiques du syndrome d'immunodépression acquise (SIDA). Rev Neurol 142:97-106, 1986.
18. Helweg-Larsen S, Jakobsen J, Boesen F, et al: Neurological complications and concomitants of AIDS. Acta Neurol Scand 74:467-474, 1986.
19. McArthur JC: Neurologic manifestations of AIDS. Medicine 66:407-437, 1987.
20. Navia BA, Price RW: The acquired immunodeficiency syndrome dementia complex as the presenting or sole manifestation of human immunodeficiency virus infection. Arch Neurol 44:65-69, 1987.
21. Price RW, Brew B, Sidtis J, et al: The brain in AIDS: Central nervous system HIV-1 infection and AIDS dementia complex. Science 239:586-592, 1988.
22. Price RW, Sidtis JJ, Navia BA, et al: The AIDS dementia complex. In Rosenblum ML, Levy RM, Bredesen DE (eds): AIDS and the Nervous System. New York, Raven Press, 1988, pp 203-219.
23. Brew BJ, Sidtis JJ, Petito CK, et al: The neurologic complications of AIDS and human immunodeficiency virus infection. In Plum F (ed): Advances in Contemporary Neurology. Philadelphia, FA Davis, 1988, pp 1-49.
24. de Gans J, Portegies P: Neurological complications of infection with human immunodeficiency virus type 1: A review of literature and 241 cases. Clin Neurol Neurosurg 91:199-219, 1989.
25. Freeman R, Roberts MS, Friedman LS, et al: Autonomic function and human immunodeficiency virus infection. Neurology 40:575-580, 1990.
26. Anders KH, Guerra WF, Tomiyasu U, et al: The neuropathology of AIDS: UCLA experience and review. Am J Pathol 124:537-558, 1986.
27. Moskowitz LB, Hensley GT, Chan JC, et al: The neuropathology of acquired immune deficiency syndrome. Arch Pathol Lab Med 108:867-872, 1984.
28. Petito CK, Cho E-S, Lemann W, et al: Neuropathology of acquired immunodeficiency syndrome (AIDS): An autopsy review. J Neuropathol Exp Neurol 45:635-646, 1986.
29. Budka H, Costanzi G, Cristina S, et al: Brain pathology induced by infection with the human immunodeficiency virus (HIV): A histological, immunocytochemical, and electron microscopical study of 100 autopsy cases. Acta Neuropathol 75:185-198, 1987.
30. de la Monte SM, Ho DD, Schooley RT, et al: Subacute encephalomyelitis of AIDS and its relation to HTLV-III infection. Neurology 37:562-569, 1987.
31. Hénin D, Duyckaerts C, Chaunu M-P, et al: Etude neuropathologique de 31 cas de syndrome d'immuno-dépression acquise. Rev Neurol 143:631-642, 1987.
32. Kato T, Hirano A, Llena JF, et al: Neuropathology of acquired immune deficiency syndrome (AIDS)

in 53 autopsy cases with particular emphasis on microglial nodules and multinucleated giant cells. Acta Neuropathol 73:287-294, 1987.

33. Rhodes RH: Histopathology of the central nervous system in the acquired immunodeficiency syndrome. Hum Pathol 18:636-643, 1987.

34. Gonzales MF, Davis RL: Neuropathology of acquired immunodeficiency syndrome. Neuropathol Appl Neurobiol 14:345-363, 1988.

35. Gray F, Gherardi R, Scaravilli F: The neuropathology of the acquired immune deficiency syndrome (AIDS). Brain 111:245-266, 1988.

36. Esiri MM, Scaravilli F, Millard PR, et al: Neuropathology of HIV infection in haemophiliacs: Comparative necropsy study. Br Med J 299:1312-1315, 1989.

37. Lantos PL, McLaughlin JE, Scholtz CL, et al: Neuropathology of the brain in HIV infection. Lancet 1:309-311, 1989.

38. Kanzer MD: Neuropathology of AIDS. CRC Crit Rev Neurobiol 5:313-362, 1990.

39. Rosenblum MK: Infection of the central nervous system by the human immunodeficiency virus type 1: Morphology and relation to syndromes of progressive encephalopathy and myelopathy in patients with AIDS. Pathol Annu 25:117-169, 1990.

40. Nielsen SL, Davis RL: Neuropathology of acquired immunodeficiency syndrome. In Rosenblum ML, Levy BM, Bredesen DE (eds): AIDS and the Nervous System. New York, Raven Press, 1988, pp 155-181.

41. Dal Canto MC: AIDS and the nervous system: Current status and future perspectives. Hum Pathol 20:410-418, 1989.

42. Hénin D, Hauw J-J: The neuropathology of AIDS. In McKendall RR (ed): Handbook of Clinical Neurology. Amsterdam, Elsevier, 1989, pp 507-524.

43. Sotrel A: The nervous system. In Harawi SJ, O'Hara CJ (eds): Pathology and Pathophysiology of AIDS and HIV-Related Diseases. St Louis, Mosby, 1989, pp 201-268.

44. De Girolami U, Smith TW, Hénin D, et al: Neuropathology of the acquired immunodeficiency syndrome. Arch Pathol Lab Med 114:643-655, 1990.

45. Carne CA, Smith A, Elkington SG, et al: Acute encephalopathy coincident with seroconversion for anti-HTLV-III. Lancet 2:1206-1208, 1985.

46. Ho DD, Rota TR, Schooley RT, et al: Isolation of HTLV-III from cerebrospinal fluid and neural tissues of patients with neurologic syndromes related to the acquired immunodeficiency syndrome. N Engl J Med 313:1493-1497, 1985.

47. Levy JA, Shimabukuro J, Hollander H, et al: Isolation of AIDS-associated retroviruses from cerebrospinal fluid and brain of patients with neurological symptoms. Lancet 2:586-588, 1985.

48. Resnick L, diMarzo-Veronese F, Schüpbach J, et al: Intra-blood-brain-barrier synthesis of HTLV-III-specific IgG in patients with neurologic symptoms associated with AIDS or AIDS-related complex. N Engl J Med 313:1498-1504, 1985.

49. Hollander H, Levy JA: Neurologic abnormalities and recovery of human immunodeficiency virus from cerebrospinal fluid. Ann Intern Med 106:692-695, 1987.

50. Levy JA, Bredesen DE: Neurologic disorders associated with AIDS retroviral infection. AIDS 1:41-64, 1988.

51. Lenhardt TM, Super MA, Wiley CA: Neuropathological changes in an asymptomatic HIV seropositive man. Ann Neurol 23:209-210, 1988.

52. McArthur JC, Becker PS, Parisi JE, et al: Neuropathological changes in early HIV-1 dementia. Ann Neurol 26:681-684, 1989.

53. Gajdusek DC, Amyx HL, Gibbs CJ Jr, et al: Infection of chimpanzees by human T-lymphotropic retroviruses in brain and other tissues from AIDS patients. Lancet 1:55-56, 1985.

54. Moskowitz LB, Gregorios JB, Hensley GT, et al: Cytomegalovirus: Induced demyelination associated with acquired immune deficiency syndrome. Arch Pathol Lab Med 108:873-877, 1984.

55. Moskowitz LB, Hensley GT, Chan JC, et al: Brain biopsies in patients with acquired immune deficiency syndrome. Arch Pathol Lab Med 108:368-371, 1984.

56. Nielsen SL, Petito CK, Urmacher CD, et al: Subacute encephalitis in acquired immune deficiency syndrome: A postmortem study. Am J Clin Pathol 82:678-682, 1984.

57. Sharer LR, Cho E-S, Epstein LG: Multinucleated giant cells and HTLV-III in AIDS encephalopathy. Hum Pathol 16:760, 1985.

58. Sharer LR, Kapila R: Neuropathologic observations in acquired immunodeficiency syndrome (AIDS). Acta Neuropathol 66:188-198, 1985.

59. Navia BA, Cho E-S, Petito CK, et al: The AIDS dementia complex. II. Neuropathology. Ann Neurol 19:525-535, 1986.

60. Dickson DW: Multinucleated giant cells in acquired immunodeficiency syndrome encephalopathy: Origin from endogenous microglia? Arch Pathol Lab Med 110:967-968, 1986.

61. Budka H: Multinucleated giant cells in brain: A hallmark of the acquired immune deficiency syndrome (AIDS). Acta Neuropathol 69:253-258, 1986.

62. Koenig S, Gendelman HE, Orenstein JM, et al: Detection of AIDS virus in macrophages in brain tissue from AIDS patients with encephalopathy. Science 233:1089-1093, 1986.

63. Sharer LR, Epstein LG, Cho E-S, et al: Pathologic features of AIDS encephalopathy in children: Evidence for LAV/HTLV-III infection of brain. Hum Pathol 17:271-284, 1986.

64. Gabuzda DH, Ho DD, de la Monte S, et al: Immunohistochemical identification of HTLV-III antigen in brains of patients with AIDS. Ann Neurol 20:289-295, 1986.

65. Wiley CA, Schrier RD, Nelson JA, et al: Cellular localization of human immunodeficiency virus infection within the brains of acquired immune deficiency syndrome patients. Proc Natl Acad Sci USA 83:7089-7093, 1986.

66. Pumarola-Sune T, Navia BA, Cordon-Cardo C, et al: HIV antigen in the brains of patients with the AIDS dementia complex. Ann Neurol 21:490-496, 1987.

67. Vazeux R, Brousse N, Jarry A, et al: AIDS subacute encephalitis: Identification of HIV-infected cells. Am J Pathol 126:403-410, 1987.

68. Ward JM, O'Leary TJ, Baskin GB, et al: Immunohistochemical localization of human and simian immunodeficiency viral antigens in fixed tissue sections. Am J Pathol 127:199-205, 1987.

69. Kure K, Lyman WD, Weidenheim KM, et al: Cellular localization of an HIV-1 antigen in subacute AIDS encephalitis using an improved double-

labeling immunohistochemical method. Am J Pathol 136:1085-1092, 1990.

70. Shaw GM, Harper ME, Hahn BH, et al: HTLV-III infection in brains of children and adults with AIDS encephalopathy. Science 227:177-182, 1985.

71. Stoler MH, Eskin TA, Benn S, et al: Human T-cell lymphotropic virus type III infection of the central nervous system: A preliminary in situ analysis. JAMA 256:2360-2364, 1986.

72. Epstein LG, Sharer LR, Cho E-S, et al: HTLV-III/LAV-like retrovirus particles in the brains of patients with AIDS encephalopathy. AIDS Res 1:447-454, 1984-1985.

73. Meyenhofer MF, Epstein LG, Cho E-S, et al: Ultrastructural morphology and intracellular production of human immunodeficiency virus (HIV) in brain. J Neuropathol Exp Neurol 46:474-484, 1987.

74. Mirra SS, del Rio C: The fine structure of acquired immunodeficiency syndrome encephalopathy. Arch Pathol Lab Med 113:858-865, 1989.

75. Watkins BA, Dorn HH, Kelly WB, et al: Specific tropism of HIV-1 for microglial cells in primary human brain cultures. Science 249:549-553, 1990.

76. Bradford BA, Rao PE, Kong LI, et al: Location and chemical synthesis of a binding site for HIV-1 on the CD4 protein. Science 240:1335-1341, 1988.

77. Harouse JM, Wroblewska Z, Laughlin MA, et al: Human choroid plexus cells can be latently infected with human immunodeficiency virus. Ann Neurol 25:406-411, 1989.

78. Lee MR, Ho DD, Gurney ME: Functional interaction and partial homology between human immunodeficiency virus and neuroleukin. Science 237:1047-1051, 1987.

79. Dreyer EB, Kaiser PK, Offermann JT, et al: HIV-1 coat protein neurotoxicity prevented by calcium channel antagonists. Science 248:364-367, 1990.

80. Horoupian DS, Pick P, Spigland I, et al: Acquired immune deficiency syndrome and multiple tract degeneration in a homosexual man. Ann Neurol 15:502-505, 1984.

81. Kleihues P, Lang W, Burger PC, et al: Progressive diffuse leukoencephalopathy in patients with acquired immune deficiency syndrome (AIDS). Acta Neuropathol 68:333-339, 1985.

82. Smith TW, De Girolami U, Hénin D, et al: HIV leukoencephalopathy and the microcirculation. J Neuropathol Exp Neurol 49:357-370, 1990.

83. Selmaj KW, Raine CS: Tumor necrosis factor mediates myelin and oligodendrocyte damage in vitro. Ann Neurol 23:339-346, 1988.

84. Goldstick L, Mandybur TI, Bode R: Spinal cord degeneration in AIDS. Neurology 35:103-106, 1985.

85. Petito CK, Navia BA, Cho E-S, et al: Vacuolar myelopathy pathologically resembling subacute combined degeneration in patients with the acquired immunodeficiency syndrome. N Engl J Med 312:874-879, 1985.

86. Grafe MR, Wiley CA: Spinal cord and peripheral nerve pathology in AIDS: The roles of cytomegalovirus and human immunodeficiency virus. Ann Neurol 25:561-566, 1989.

87. Rosenblum M, Scheck AC, Cronin K, et al: Dissociation of AIDS-related vacuolar myelopathy and productive HIV-1 infection of the spinal cord. Neurology 39:892-896, 1989.

88. Artigas J, Grosse G, Niedobitek F: Vacuolar myelopathy in AIDS: A morphological analysis. Pathol Res Pract 186:228-237, 1990.

89. Budka H, Maier H, Pohl P: Human immunodeficiency virus in vacuolar myelopathy of the acquired immunodeficiency syndrome. N Engl J Med 319:1667-1668, 1988.

90. Maier H, Budka H, Lassmann H, et al: Vacuolar myelopathy with multinucleated giant cells in the acquired immune deficiency syndrome (AIDS): Light and electron microscopic distribution of human immunodeficiency virus (HIV) antigens. Acta Neuropathol 78:497-503, 1989.

91. Eilbott DJ, Peress N, Burger H, et al: Human immunodeficiency virus type 1 in spinal cords of acquired immunodeficiency syndrome patients with myelopathy: Expression and replication in macrophages. Proc Natl Acad Sci USA 86:3337-3341, 1989.

92. Kamin SS, Petito CK: Vacuolar myelopathy in immunocompromised non AIDS patients. J Neuropathol Exp Neurol 47:385, 1988.

93. Dickson DW, Belman AL, Park YD, et al: Central nervous system pathology in pediatric AIDS: An autopsy study. Acta Pathol Microbiol Immunol Scand [Suppl] 8:40-57, 1989.

94. Sharer LR, Epstein LG, Blumberg BM, et al: Histological and molecular probe analysis of spinal cords from children with HIV infection and AIDS. J Neuropathol Exp Neurol 47:347, 1988.

95. Sharer LR, Dowling PC, Michaels J, et al: Spinal cord disease in children with HIV-1 infection: A combined molecular biological and neuropathological study. Neuropathol Appl Neurobiol 16:317-331, 1990.

96. Rance NE, McArthur JC, Cornblath DR, et al: Gracile tract degeneration in patients with sensory neuropathy and AIDS. Neurology 38:265-271, 1988.

97. Piccardo P, Ceroni M, Rodgers-Johnson P, et al: Pathological and immunological observations on tropical spastic paraparesis in patients from Jamaica. Ann Neurol 23(suppl):S156-S160, 1988.

98. Brew BJ, Hardy W, Zuckerman E, et al: AIDS-related vacuolar myelopathy is not associated with coinfection by human T-lymphotropic virus type I. Ann Neurol 26:679-681, 1989.

99. Tucker T, Dix RD, Katzen C, et al: Cytomegalovirus and herpes simplex virus ascending myelitis in a patient with acquired immune deficiency syndrome. Ann Neurol 18:74-79, 1985.

100. Eidelberg D, Sotrel A, Vogel H, et al: Progressive polyradiculopathy in acquired immune deficiency syndrome. Neurology 36:912-916, 1986.

101. Jeantils V, Lemaitre M-O, Robert J, et al: Subacute polyneuropathy with encephalopathy in AIDS with human cytomegalovirus pathogenicity? Lancet 2:1039, 1986.

102. Singh BM, Levine S, Yarrish RL, et al: Spinal cord syndromes in the acquired immune deficiency syndrome. Acta Neurol Scand 73:590-598, 1986.

103. Behar R, Wiley C, McCutchan JA: Cytomegalovirus polyradiculoneuropathy in acquired immune deficiency syndrome. Neurology 37:557-561, 1987.

104. Mahieux F, Gray F, Fenelon G, et al: Acute myeloradiculitis due to cytomegalovirus as the initial manifestation of AIDS. J Neurol Neurosurg Psychiatry 52:270-274, 1989.

105. Vinters HV, Kwok MK, Ho HW, et al: Cytomegalovirus in the nervous system of patients with the

acquired immune deficiency syndrome. Brain 112:245-268, 1989.

106. Chimelli L, de Freitas MRG, Bazin AR, et al: Encéphalomyélo-radiculite à cytomégalovirus au cours du syndrome d'immuno-déficience acquise. Rev Neurol 146:354-360, 1990.

107. Navia BA, Petito CK, Gold JWM, et al: Cerebral toxoplasmosis complicating the acquired immune deficiency syndrome: Clinical and neuropathological findings in 27 patients. Ann Neurol 19:224-238, 1986.

108. Mehren M, Burns PJ, Mamani F, et al: Toxoplasmic myelitis mimicking intramedullary spinal cord tumor. Neurology 38:1648-1650, 1988.

109. Herskovitz S, Siegel SE, Schneider AT, et al: Spinal cord toxoplasmosis in AIDS. Neurology 39:1552-1553, 1989.

110. Nag S, Jackson AC: Myelopathy: An unusual presentation of toxoplasmosis. Can J Neurol Sci 16:422-425, 1989.

111. Britton CB, Mesa-Tejada R, Fenoglio CM, et al: A new complication of AIDS: Thoracic myelitis caused by herpes simplex virus. Neurology 35:1071-1074, 1985.

112. Lipkin WI, Parry G, Kiprov D, et al: Inflammatory neuropathy in homosexual men with lymphadenopathy. Neurology 35:1479-1483, 1985.

113. Cornblath DR, McArthur JC, Kennedy PGE, et al: Inflammatory demyelinating peripheral neuropathies associated with human T-cell lymphotropic virus type III infection. Ann Neurol 21:32-40, 1987.

114. Bailey RO, Baltch AL, Venkatesh R, et al: Sensory motor neuropathy associated with AIDS. Neurology 38:886-891, 1988.

115. de la Monte SM, Gabuzda DH, Ho DD, et al: Peripheral neuropathy in the acquired immunodeficiency syndrome. Ann Neurol 23:485-492, 1988.

116. Miller RG, Parry GJ, Pfaeffl W, et al: The spectrum of peripheral neuropathy associated with ARC and AIDS. Muscle Nerve 11:857-863, 1988.

117. Chaunu M-P, Ratinahirana H, Raphael M, et al: The spectrum of changes on 20 nerve biopsies in patients with HIV infection. Muscle Nerve 12:452-459, 1989.

118. Gastaut JL, Gastaut JA, Pellissier JF, et al: Neuropathies périphériques au cours de l'infection par le virus de l'immunodéficience humaine. Rev Neurol 145:451-459, 1989.

119. Léger JM, Bouche P, Bolgert F, et al: The spectrum of polyneuropathies in patients infected with HIV. J Neurol Neurosurg Psychiatry 52:1369-1374, 1989.

120. Möbius HJ, Schlote W, Enzensberger W: Peripheres Nervensystem und AIDS. In Fischer P-A, Schlote W (eds): AIDS und Nervensystem. Berlin, Springer-Verlag, 1987, pp 73-84.

121. Dalakas MC, Pezeshkpour GH: Neuromuscular diseases associated with human immunodeficiency virus infection. Ann Neurol 23(suppl):S38-S48, 1988.

122. Parry GJ: Peripheral neuropathies associated with human immunodeficiency virus infection. Ann Neurol 23(suppl):S49-S53, 1988.

123. Elder G, Dalakas M, Pezeshkpour G, et al: Ataxic neuropathy due to ganglioneuronitis after probable acute human immunodeficiency virus infection. Lancet 2:1275-1276, 1986.

124. Said G, Lacroix-Ciaudo C, Fujimura H, et al: The peripheral neuropathy of necrotizing arteritis: A clinicopathologic study. Ann Neurol 23:461-465, 1988.

125. Gherardi R, Lebargy F, Gaulard P, et al: Necrotizing vasculitis and HIV replication in peripheral nerves. N Engl J Med 321:685-686, 1989.

126. Bishopric G, Bruner J, Butler J: Guillain-Barré syndrome with cytomegalovirus infection of peripheral nerves. Arch Pathol Lab Med 109:1106-1108, 1985.

127. Lanska MJ, Lanska DJ, Schmidley JW: Syphilitic polyradiculopathy in an HIV-positive man. Neurology 38:1297-1301, 1988.

128. Dalakas MC, Pezeshkpour GH, Gravell M, et al: Polymyositis associated with AIDS retrovirus. JAMA 256:2381-2383, 1986.

129. Bailey O, Turok DI, Jaufmann BP, et al: Myositis and acquired immunodeficiency syndrome. Hum Pathol 18:749-751, 1987.

130. Stern R, Gold J, DiCarlo EF: Myopathy complicating the acquired immune deficiency syndrome. Muscle Nerve 10:318-322, 1987.

131. Berman A, Espinoza LR, Diaz JD, et al: Rheumatic manifestations of human immunodeficiency virus infection. Am J Med 85:59-64, 1988.

132. Gonzales MF, Olney RK, So YT, et al: Subacute structural myopathy associated with human immunodeficiency virus infection. Arch Neurol 45:585-587, 1988.

133. Lange DJ, Britton CB, Younger DS, et al: The neuromuscular manifestations of human immunodeficiency virus infections. Arch Neurol 45:1084-1088, 1988.

134. Simpson DM, Bender AN: Human immunodeficiency virus–associated myopathy: Analysis of 11 patients. Ann Neurol 24:79-84, 1988.

135. Marolda M, De Mercato R, Camporeale FS, et al: Myopathy associated with AIDS. Ital J Neurol Sci 10:423-427, 1989.

136. Nordstrom DM, Petropolis AA, Giorno R, et al: Inflammatory myopathy and acquired immunodeficiency syndrome. Arthritis Rheum 32:475-479, 1989.

137. Gabbai AA, Schmidt B, Castelo A, et al: Muscle biopsy in AIDS and ARC: Analysis of 50 patients. Muscle Nerve 13:541-544, 1990.

138. Dalakas MC, Gravell M, London WT, et al: Morphological changes of an inflammatory myopathy in rhesus monkeys with simian acquired immunodeficiency syndrome. Proc Soc Exp Biol Med 185:368-376, 1987.

139. Wiley CA, Nerenberg M, Cros D, et al: HTLV-1 polymyositis in a patient also infected with the human immunodeficiency virus. N Engl J Med 320:992-995, 1989.

140. Plotz PH, Dalakas M, Leff RL, et al: Current concepts in the idiopathic inflammatory myopathies: Polymyositis, dermatomyositis, and related disorders. Ann Intern Med 111:143-157, 1989.

141. Chad DA, Smith TW, Blumenfeld A, et al: Human immunodeficiency virus (HIV)-associated myopathy: Immunocytochemical identification of an HIV antigen (gp 41) in muscle macrophages. Ann Neurol 28:579-582, 1990.

142. Mims CA: The pathogenetic basis of viral tropism. Am J Pathol 135:447-455, 1989.

143. Bessen LJ, Greene JB, Louie E, et al: Severe polymyositis-like syndrome associated with zidovudine therapy of AIDS and ARC. N Engl J Med 318:708, 1988.

144. Curtis M, Gill MJ, Brownell AKW: Polymyositislike syndromes in the acquired immunodeficiency syndrome. Arch Neurol 46:841, 1989.

145. Dalakas MC, Illa I, Pezeshkpour GH, et al: Mitochondrial myopathy caused by long-term zidovudine therapy. N Engl J Med 322:1098-1105, 1990.

146. Verma RD, Ziegler DK, Kepes JJ: HIV-related neuromuscular syndrome simulating motor neuron disease. Neurology 40:544-546, 1990.

147. Simpson DM, Bender AN, Farraye J, et al: Human immunodeficiency virus wasting syndrome may represent a treatable myopathy. Neurology 40: 535-538, 1990.

148. Mizusawa H, Hirano A, Llena JF, et al: Cerebrovascular lesions in acquired immune deficiency syndrome (AIDS). Acta Neuropathol 76:451-457, 1988.

149. Berger JR, Harris JO, Gregorios J, et al: Cerebrovascular disease in AIDS: A case-control study. AIDS 4:239-244, 1990.

150. Yankner BA, Skolnik PR, Shoumikas GM, et al: Cerebral granulomatous angiitis associated with isolation of human T-lymphotropic virus type III from the central nervous system. Ann Neurol 20:362-364, 1986.

151. Scaravilli F, Daniel SE, Harcourt-Webster N, et al: Chronic basal meningitis and vasculitis in acquired immunodeficiency syndrome. Arch Pathol Lab Med 113:192-195, 1989.

152. Vinters HV, Guerra WF, Eppolito L, et al: Necrotizing vasculitis of the nervous system in a patient with AIDS-related complex. Neuropathol Appl Neurobiol 14:417-424, 1988.

153. Cho E-S, Sharer LR, Peress NS, et al: Intimal proliferation of leptomeningeal arteries and brain infarcts in subjects with AIDS. J Neuropathol Exp Neurol 46:385, 1987.

154. Selnes OA, Miller E, McArthur J, et al: HIV-1 infection: No evidence of cognitive decline during the asymptomatic stages. Neurology 40: 204-208, 1990.

155. Sidtis JJ, Price RW: Early HIV-1 infection and the AIDS dementia complex. Neurology 40:323-326, 1990.

156. Balakrishnan J, Becker PS, Kumar AJ, et al: Acquired immunodeficiency syndrome: Correlation of radiologic and pathologic findings in the brain. Radiographics 10:201-215, 1990.

157. Chrysikopoulos HS, Press GA, Grafe MR, et al: Encephalitis caused by human immunodeficiency virus: CT and MR imaging manifestations with clinical and pathologic correlation. Radiology 175:185-191, 1990.

158. De La Paz R, Enzmann D: Neuroradiology of acquired immunodeficiency syndrome. In Rosenblum ML, Levy RM, Bredesen DE (eds): AIDS and the Nervous System. New York, Raven Press, 1988, pp 121-153.

159. McArthur JC, Kumar AJ, Johnson DW, et al: Incidental white matter hyperintensities on magnetic resonance imaging in HIV-1 infection. J AIDS 3:252-259, 1990.

160. Belman AL, Diamond G, Dickson D, et al: Pediatric acquired immunodeficiency syndrome: Neurologic syndromes. Am J Dis Child 142:29-35, 1988.

161. Epstein LG, Sharer LR: Neurology of human immunodeficiency virus infection in children. In Rosenblum ML, Levy RM, Bredesen DE (eds): AIDS and the Nervous System. New York, Raven Press, 1988, pp 79-101.

162. Giangaspero F, Scanabissi E, Baldacci MC, et al: Massive neuronal destruction in human immunodeficiency virus (HIV) encephalitis: A clinicopathological study of a pediatric case. Acta Neuropathol 78:662-665, 1989.

163. Vinters HV, Anders KH: Neuropathology of AIDS. Boca Raton, Fla, CRC Press, 1990.

164. Huang TE, Chou SM: Occlusive hypertrophic arteritis as the cause of discrete necrosis in CNS toxoplasmosis in the acquired immunodeficiency syndrome. Hum Pathol 19:1210-1214, 1988.

165. Gray F, Gherardi R, Wingate E, et al: Diffuse "encephalitic" cerebral toxoplasmosis in AIDS: Report of four cases. J Neurol 236:273-277, 1989.

166. Wiley CA, Safrin RE, Davis CE, et al: Acanthamoeba meningoencephalitis in a patient with AIDS. J Infect Dis 155:130-133, 1987.

167. Centers for Disease Control: Diagnosis and management of mycobacterial infection and disease in persons with human immunodeficiency virus infection. Ann Intern Med 106:254-256, 1987.

168. Bishburg E, Sunderam G, Reichman LB, et al: Central nervous system tuberculosis with the acquired immunodeficiency syndrome and its related complex. Ann Intern Med 105:210-213, 1986.

169. Johns DR, Tierney M, Felsenstein D: Alteration in the natural history of neurosyphilis by concurrent infection with the human immunodeficiency virus. N Engl J Med 316:1569-1572, 1987.

170. Katz DA, Berger JR: Neurosyphilis in acquired immunodeficiency syndrome. Arch Neurol 46:895-898, 1989.

171. Lukehart SA, Hook EW III, Baker-Zander SA, et al: Invasion of the central nervous system by *Treponema pallidum:* Implications for diagnosis and treatment. Ann Intern Med 109:855-862, 1988.

172. Morgello S, Laufer H: Quaternary neurosyphilis. N Engl J Med 319:1549-1550, 1988.

173. Morgello S, Laufer H: Quaternary neurosyphilis in a Haitian man with human immunodeficiency virus infection. Hum Pathol 20:808-811, 1989.

174. Morgello S, Cho E-S, Nielsen S, et al: Cytomegalovirus encephalitis in patients with acquired immunodeficiency syndrome: An autopsy study of 30 cases and a review of the literature. Hum Pathol 18:289-297, 1987.

175. Wiley CA, Nelson JA: Role of human immunodeficiency virus and cytomegalovirus in AIDS encephalitis. Am J Pathol 133:73-81, 1988.

176. Wiley CA, Schrier RD, Denaro FJ, et al: Localization of cytomegalovirus proteins and genome during fulminant central nervous system infection in an AIDS patient. J Neuropathol Exp Neurol 45:127-139, 1986.

177. Dix RD, Bredesen DE: Opportunistic viral infections in acquired immunodeficiency syndrome. In Rosenblum ML, Levy RM, Bredesen DE (eds): AIDS and the Nervous System. New York, Raven Press, 1988, pp 221-261.

178. Quinnan GV Jr, Masur H, Rook AH, et al: Herpesvirus infections in the acquired immune deficiency syndrome. JAMA 252:72-77, 1984.

179. Dix RD, Waitzman DM, Follansbee S, et al: Herpes simplex virus type 2 encephalitis in two homo-

sexual men with persistent lymphadenopathy. Ann Neurol 17:203-206, 1985.

180. Ryder JW, Croen K, Kleinschmidt-DeMasters BK, et al: Progressive encephalitis three months after resolution of cutaneous zoster in a patient with AIDS. Ann Neurol 19:182-188, 1986.

181. Gilden DH, Murray RS, Wellish M, et al: Chronic progressive varicella-zoster virus encephalitis in an AIDS patient. Neurology 38:1150-1153, 1988.

182. Sandor E, Croxson TS, Millman A, et al: Herpes zoster ophthalmicus in patients at risk for AIDS. N Engl J Med 310:1118-1119, 1984.

183. Rostad SW, Olson K, McDougall J, et al: Transsynaptic spread of varicella zoster virus through the visual system: A mechanism of viral dissemination in the central nervous system. Hum Pathol 20:174-179, 1989.

184. Rosenblum MK: Bulbar encephalitis complicating trigeminal zoster in the acquired immune deficiency syndrome. Hum Pathol 20:292-295, 1989.

185. Morgello S, Block GA, Price RW, et al: Varicella-zoster virus leukoencephalitis and cerebral vasculopathy. Arch Pathol Lab Med 112:173-177, 1988.

186. Aström K-E, Mancall EL, Richardson EP Jr: Progressive multifocal leuko-encephalopathy. Brain 81:93-111, 1958.

187. Richardson EP Jr: Progressive multifocal leukoencephalopathy. N Engl J Med 265:815-823, 1961.

188. Zu Rhein GM, Chou S-M: Particles resembling papova viruses in human cerebral demyelinating disease. Science 148:1477-1479, 1965.

189. Padgett BL, Walker DL, Zu Rhein GM, et al: Cultivation of papova-like virus from human brain with progressive multifocal leucoencephalopathy. Lancet 1:1257-1260, 1971.

190. Aksamit AJ, Major EO, Ghatak NR, et al: Diagnosis of progressive multifocal leukoencephalopathy by brain biopsy with biotin labeled DNA: DNA in situ hybridization. J Neuropathol Exp Neurol 46:556-566, 1987.

191. Miller JR, Barrett RE, Britton CB, et al: Progressive multifocal leukoencephalopathy in a male homosexual with T-cell immune deficiency. N Engl J Med 307:1436-1438, 1982.

192. Bedri J, Weinstein W, DeGregorio P, et al: Progressive multifocal leukoencephalopathy in acquired immunodeficiency syndrome. N Engl J Med 309:492-493, 1983.

193. Bernick C, Gregorios JB: Progressive multifocal leukoencephalopathy in a patient with acquired immune deficiency syndrome. Arch Neurol 41:780-782, 1984.

194. Blum LW, Chambers RA, Schwartzman RJ, et al: Progressive multifocal leukoencephalopathy in acquired immune deficiency syndrome. Arch Neurol 42:137-139, 1985.

195. Berger JR, Kaszovitz B, Post MJD, et al: Progressive multifocal leukoencephalopathy associated with human immunodeficiency virus infection: A review of the literature with a report of sixteen cases. Ann Intern Med 107:78-87, 1987.

196. Rhodes RH, Ward JM, Walker DL: Progressive multifocal leukoencephalopathy and retroviral encephalitis in acquired immunodeficiency syndrome. Arch Pathol Lab Med 112:1207-1213, 1988.

197. Wiley CA, Grafe M, Kennedy C, et al: Human immunodeficiency virus (HIV) and JC virus in acquired immune deficiency syndrome (AIDS) patients with progressive multifocal leukoencephalopathy. Acta Neuropathol 76:338-346, 1988.

198. Aksamit AJ, Gendelman HE, Orenstein JM, et al: AIDS-associated progressive multifocal leukoencephalopathy (PML): Comparison to non-AIDS PML with in situ hybridization and immunohistochemistry. Neurology 40:1073-1078, 1990.

199. Orenstein JM, Jannotta F: Human immunodeficiency virus and papovavirus infections in acquired immunodeficiency syndrome: An ultrastructural study of three cases. Hum Pathol 19:350-361, 1988.

200. Scaravilli F, Ellis DS, Tovey G, et al: Unusual development of polyoma virus in the brains of two patients with the acquired immune deficiency syndrome (AIDS). Neuropathol Appl Neurobiol 15:407-418, 1989.

201. Berger JR, Mucke L: Prolonged survival and partial recovery in AIDS-associated progressive multifocal leukoencephalopathy. Neurology 38:1060-1065, 1988.

202. Case records of the Massachusetts General Hospital: Case 32-1983. N Engl J Med 309:359-369, 1983.

203. Case records of the Massachusetts General Hospital: Case 22-1986. N Engl J Med 314:1498-1507, 1986.

204. Hochberg FH, Miller G, Schooley RT, et al: Central-nervous-system lymphoma related to Epstein-Barr virus. N Engl J Med 309:745-748, 1983.

205. Snider WD, Simpson DM, Aronyk KE, et al: Primary lymphoma of the nervous system associated with acquired immune-deficiency syndrome. N Engl J Med 308:45, 1983.

206. Gill PS, Levine AM, Meyer PR, et al: Primary central nervous system lymphoma in homosexual men: Clinical, immunologic, and pathologic features. Am J Med 78:742-748, 1985.

207. Freeman CR, Shustik C, Brisson M-L, et al: Primary malignant lymphoma of the central nervous system. Cancer 58:1106-1111, 1986.

208. So YT, Beckstead JH, Davis RL: Primary central nervous system lymphoma in acquired immune deficiency syndrome: A clinical and pathological study. Ann Neurol 20:566-572, 1986.

209. Levy RM, Pons VG, Rosenblum ML: Central nervous system mass lesions in the acquired immunodeficiency syndrome (AIDS). J Neurosurg 61:9-16, 1984.

210. Levine AM, Meyer PR, Begandy MK, et al: Development of B-cell lymphoma in homosexual men: Clinical and immunologic findings. Ann Intern Med 100:7-13, 1984.

211. Ziegler JL, Beckstead JA, Volberding PA, et al: Non-Hodgkin's lymphoma in 90 homosexual men. N Engl J Med 311:565-570, 1984.

212. Ioachim HL, Cooper MC, Hellman GC: Lymphomas in men at high risk for acquired immune deficiency syndrome (AIDS): A study of 21 cases. Cancer 56:2831-2842, 1985.

213. Gorin FA, Bale JF, Halks-Miller M, et al: Kaposi's sarcoma metastatic to the CNS. Arch Neurol 42:162-165, 1985.

14

OCULAR PATHOLOGY

Umberto De Girolami, Dominique Hénin, and Jean-Jacques Hauw

Since the initial recognition of AIDS there has been increasing awareness throughout the world that the disease could be associated with visual impairment.[1] During the past 10 years many original studies and reviews have described in detail the range of clinical ophthalmalogic manifestations in adults and children with AIDS from North America, Europe, and Africa.[2-19] Although ocular lesions develop in up to 70% of adults with AIDS during the course of the disease, perhaps no more than 200 reports in the literature give a detailed account of the histopathology of the eye at autopsy. We reported a series of 25 cases at the R. Escourolle Laboratory at the Hôpital de La Salpêtrière in Paris.[20,21] These patients had been extensively studied clinically and had a complete autopsy examination including a study of the eyes. We have subsequently studied a total of 40 cases.

The principal ophthalmologic disturbances in AIDS patients can be divided into four general categories:

I.   Retinal microvascular disorders (including cotton-wool spots)
II. Infectious diseases of the eye
   A.   Viral
      1.   Cytomegalovirus (CMV) retinitis
      2.   HIV-1
      3.   Herpes simplex and zoster viral infections
   B.   Parasitic
      1.   Toxoplasmosis
      2.   *Pneumocystic carinii* choroiditis
   C.   Other infrequent infections
III. Neoplasms
   A.   Kaposi's sarcoma of the eyelid, conjunctiva, or orbit
   B.   Lymphoma of the globe or orbit
IV. Neuroophthalmologic disorders
   A.   Disorders of the optic nerve (including optic neuritis and optic nerve atrophy)
   B.   Disturbances of ocular motility
   C.   Disturbances of vision

RETINAL MICROVASCULAR DISORDERS

The most commonly observed ophthalmologic abnormality in AIDS patients is cotton-wool spots, which occur in 50% to 90% of cases.[8,11,14,22,23] On funduscopic examination cotton-wool spots are whitish, superficial, flocculent retinal blotches ranging from one-eighth to one-half papillary diameter, most often seen along the temporal side of the posterior pole (Fig. 14–1). Characteristically they are transient (regression often occurs after 4 to 6 weeks) and recurrent, leaving no residual scar on funduscopic or angiographic examination when studied over a period of time. In both AIDS and non-AIDS patients, correlative funduscopic-histologic studies[4,24] have shown that the ophthalmoscopic cotton-wool spots correspond to light microscopic foci of retinal thickening of the nerve fiber layer containing "cytoid bodies," eosinophilic hyaline structures averaging 50 μm in diameter with a

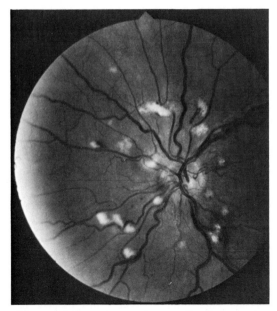

Figure 14–1. Cotton-wool spots. Funduscopic view. (Courtesy Dr. B. Girard, Paris.)

poorly defined dense core (Fig. 14–2). Cytoid bodies can be demonstrated to be axonal swellings by silver impregnation, immunocytochemistry, and electron microscopy.

The pathogenesis of cotton-wool spots is not completely understood (see discussion by McLeod[25]). They are observed in many diseases associated with an underlying disturbance of the retinal microcirculation: hypertension, diabetes mellitus, systemic lupus erythematosus, leukemia, and Waldenström's macroglobulinemia.[24,26] McLeod et al.[27] have reproduced the lesion experimentally with laser photocoagulation of retinal arterioles. Furthermore, they demonstrated that the axonal swelling is brought about by an arrest of retrograde or anterograde axoplasmic transport, presumably on an ischemic basis. The basis for reversibility of the lesion and temporal relationship between the vascular insult and the structural changes are unknown.[27-29] Several studies have investigated the pathogenesis of the cotton-wool spots in AIDS patients. Hypothetical mechanisms of injury include infection of the vessel wall or perivascular cells by viruses (CMV, HIV-1), microthrombosis or embolization, and altered vascular permeability.[30] A single unconfirmed report attributes the formation of cotton-wool spots to retinal infection by *P. carinii*.[31] Tanenbaum et al.[32] indicated that the cytoid bodies encountered in the AIDS patient can

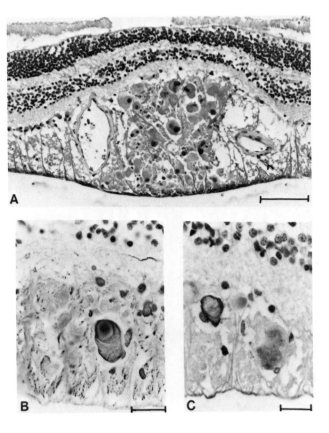

Figure 14–2. Cotton-wool spots. Histologic section of retina. *A*, Nerve fiber layer (bottom layer) is thickened with cytoid bodies between two normally patent blood vessels. *B*, Close-up view of cytoid body showing silver impregnation of swollen axon with central dense core. *C*, Swollen axon reacts to phosphorylated neurofilament antiserum (PNA). (*A*, Hematoxylin and eosin, bar = 100 µm; *B*, Bodian's stain, bar = 20 µm; *C*, peroxidase-antiperoxidase, bar = 20µm.)

undergo calcification, possibly secondary to alterations in the blood-retinal barrier. Indeed, evidence suggests altered retinal microcirculation. Immune complex deposits on the microvasculature and luminal compromise or occlusion have been observed.[4,33] Johnson[34] noted that the axonal swellings seen in the cytoid bodies are comparable to the axonal swellings in the microinfarcts of the brainstem and spinal cord observed in AIDS patients.[35]

Other ophthalmoscopic findings indicative of vascular disease have included retinal hemorrhages and ischemic maculopathy.[5,6,8,36,37] Kestelyn et al.[37] described a clinical "perivasculitis" in African children with AIDS-related complex. Microaneurysms have been noted on funduscopic and angiographic examinations. Trypsin digestion preparations of the retina viewed en-face demonstrate many more microaneurysms than anticipated from angiographic examination.[4,30]

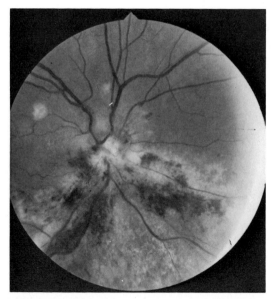

Figure 14–3. Acute cytomegalovirus infection. Funduscopic view. (Courtesy Dr. B. Girard, Paris.)

INFECTIOUS DISEASES OF THE EYE

Viral Infections

A variety of infectious agents have been reported to infect the retina and choroid in AIDS patients.[12,38] CMV retinitis is the second most frequently observed ophthalmologic abnormality in AIDS patients and the most common ocular infectious pathogen, found in 15% to 40%.[5,6,8,23,39-46] The funduscopic appearance of early CMV retinitis is an irregular, fairly well-demarcated, yellowish, flat lesion that occurs along the vascular arcades and generally begins at the posterior pole.[40,47] As the infection progresses, foci of hemorrhage are often observed (Fig. 14–3). The histologic appearance of CMV retinitis in AIDS patients is similar to that in patients receiving immunosuppressive drugs and in newborns with disseminated cytomegalovirus inclusion disease.[48-50] The early lesion consists of single greatly enlarged cells with large viral intranuclear inclusions. Intranuclear inclusions have a homogeneous amphophilic hue on hematoxylin and eosin stain and may vary considerably in diameter (from less than 1 to 10 μm). A clear zone may be present between the nuclear chromatin aggregated along the nuclear envelope and the intranuclear inclusions—the so-called owl's-eye effect (Fig. 14–4). Also frequently observed are intracytoplasmic granular inclusions of viral material, which are best demonstrated with im-

munocytochemical reactions. The acute florid lesion has multiple discrete foci of hemorrhagic necrosis in all layers of the retina, the retinal pigment epithelium, the optic nerve, and the vitreous. Light microscopic examination does not always permit identification of the precise type of retinal cell that harbors the infection. At times inclusions are seen clearly in ganglion cells or cells having cytoplasmic extensions suggestive of glia. Often infected cells form syncytia, giving the appearance of a multinucleated macrophage. Ultrastructural and immunocytochemical investigations of CMV retinitis and CMV encephalitis have conclusively demonstrated that glia, neurons, and macrophages are capable of harboring the virus.[3,51-55] In a recent study infection of retinal endothelial cells was demonstrated by in situ hybridization and electron microscopy.[46] Remarkably little inflammatory response is present despite the remarkable extent of tissue destruction. We have observed a fairly constant, mild to moderate, chronic inflammatory response in the choroid. Older or treated lesions typically consist of foci of retina so thinned out that the normal layers are no longer recognizable.[56] A plate of glial-fibrous tissue that may be heavily calcified remains. A recent study has shown that even after clinically successful intravenous treatment with ganciclovir, widespread CMV infection of the sclera and uveal tract may be found at autopsy by ultrastructural and immunocytochemical methods.[57] Intravitreal treatment with ganci-

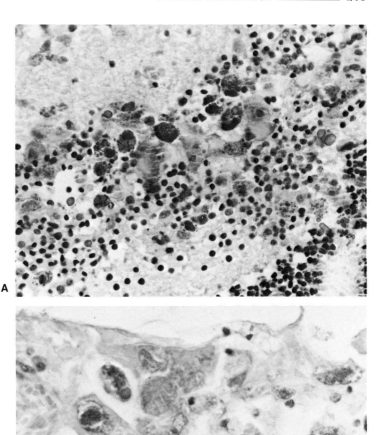

Figure 14–4. Cytomegalovirus (CMV). Histologic section of retina. *A,* Complete destruction of all layers of retina. Infected cells have large intranuclear inclusions (owl's-eye) and intracytoplasmic granular inclusions. *B,* Anti-CMV immunoperoxidase reaction demonstrates immunoreactivity of intranuclear inclusion. (*A,* Hematoxylin and eosin, ×570; *B,* anti-CMV immunoperoxidase, ×1000.)

clovir may prove a more effective treatment method.[42,45]

Retinal infection with HIV-1 has been documented in four recent reports. Pomerantz et al.[58] found no retinal abnormality in two patients examined by routine histologic methods. However, they were able to demonstrate the virus when they performed immunoperoxidase studies (gp120, p15/17, and p24 HIV-1 antigens) on frozen retinal tissue and virologic studies on retinal homogenates (enzyme-linked immunosorbent assay [ELISA] on cultured leukocytes). Double labeling studies could not conclusively identify the infected cells observed in the retina and perivascular tissue. In a second study by Cantrill et al.,[59] HIV-1 was detected by tissue culture methods

and ELISA in the retina, iris, conjunctiva, and cornea of one patient with AIDS. In one of three patients, it was shown in the retina by immunofluorescence methods (monoclonal antibody to HIV p24). Qavi et al.[60] demonstrated HIV-1 in retinal inflammatory lesions by immunofluorescence techniques in two patients and in total retinal tissue by the polymerase chain reaction to detect HIV-1 DNA sequences (four cases including two of the ones positive by immunofluorescence). Schmitt-Gräff et al.[46] reported the immunoperoxidase reactivity to p24 HIV-1 antigen in the retinal glial cells of a patient with bilateral CMV retinitis and CNS toxoplasmosis. HIV-1 has been shown to infect human glial cells in tissue culture.[61] The virus has also been identified in the

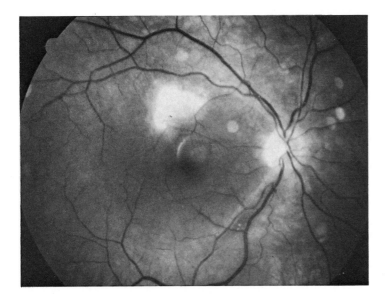

Figure 14–5. Toxoplasmosis. Funduscopic view. (Courtesy Dr. B. Girard, Paris.)

tears,[62] conjunctival epithelium,[63] cornea,[64,65] and aqueous humor[66] of affected individuals.

Herpetic infections have infrequently been reported to infect the eyes of AIDS patients. Culbertson et al.[67] described two cases of necrotizing retinitis proved to be due to varicella-zoster virus by immunoperoxidase methods using a monoclonal antibody directed against glycoprotein viral antigens. The virus was also cultured from the vitreous of one patient. Similar cases of necrotizing retinitis were recorded by Forster et al.[68] A dual retinal infection with CMV and HSV was observed in a patient who was also shown to have HSV and CMV in the brain by immunocytochemistry.[69] Herpes zoster ophthalmicus in the distribution of the first division of the trigeminal nerve has been noted clinically as an important and perhaps early manifestation of AIDS, especially in Africa.[19,70,71]

Parasitic Infestations

Although toxoplasmosis is the most common nonviral intracranial infection in AIDS patients,[72,73] only a few cases of AIDS-related ocular toxoplasmosis have been documented histopathologically.[74-78] The organism can involve the retina and cause necrotizing retinitis, chronic choroiditis, and optic neuritis. In the eight patients with ocular toxoplasmosis studied by Holland et al.,[76] five had coexistent intracranial toxoplasmosis. In two case series from Paris and Copenhagen, where complete postmorten examinations of the brain and eye were carried out in 68 patients, only one had toxoplasmosis in both brain and eye.[15,20] Our

patient had optic neuritis with encysted bradyzoites in the optic nerve and CMV retinitis (Figs. 14–5 and 14–6).

P. carinii choroiditis has been documented in a few cases.[79-82]

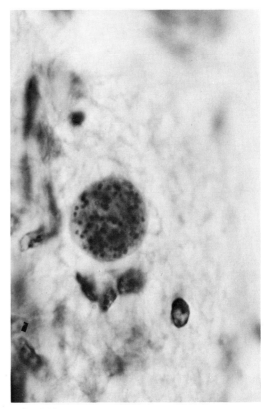

Figure 14–6. Toxoplasmosis. Histologic section of optic nerve. Note encysted bradyzoites. (Hematoxylin and eosin, ×570.)

Other Infrequent Infections

Infectious agents that have been described to affect the eye in single case studies include *Cryptococcus neoformans*,[4,51,83] *Histoplasma capsulatum*,[84] *Sporothrix schenckii*,[85] *Candida albicans*,[74] *Microsporidium*,[86] *Mycobac-* *terium tuberculosis*,[87,88] *Mycobacterium avium-intracellulare*,[4] and *Treponema pallidum*.[89,90] Bacterial retinitis occurs rarely in the context of sustained immunosuppression with or without septicemia.[91] Severe morbidity has also been reported with bacterial external ocular disease.[92]

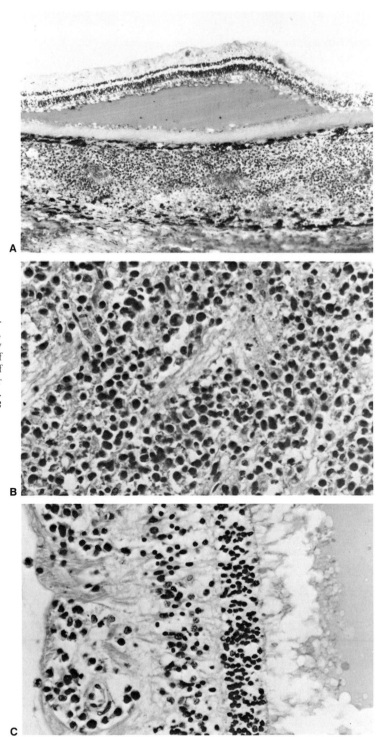

Figure 14–7. Large cell lymphoma. Histologic sections of retina. *A,* Retinal detachment characterized by elevation of retina over collection of proteinaceous fluid. *B,* Extension of tumor to optic nerve. *C,* Perivascular collection of lymphoma cells in retina. (Hematoxylin and eosin; *A,* ×63; *B* and *C,* ×570.)

NEOPLASMS

Kaposi's sarcoma is the most common AIDS-associated tumor, and ophthalmic involvement occurs in 15% to 24% of AIDS patients with this neoplasm.[14,93,94] We have found the histologic appearance of the lesion in the conjunctiva, eyelid, and orbit to be identical to that elsewhere in the body.

Orbital Burkitt's lymphoma has been reported in a patient with AIDS.[95] We have observed a large cell lymphoma involving the retina, optic nerve, and uveal tract in a patient with a central nervous system lymphoma (Fig. 14–7). Similar cases are described by Lauer et al.[96] and Jensen and Klinken.[15]

NEUROOPHTHALMOLOGY

Neuroophthalmic disturbances occur in about 8% of AIDS patients.[1,8,14] They may be secondary to cranial nerve, nuclear, or supranuclear involvement.[97] Zaidman[98] reported syphilitic retrobulbar neuritis in a patient with AIDS. Severe optic atrophy may occur in patients with long-standing CMV retinitis[3] or arachnoiditis.[99] Supratentorial lesions (infectious or neoplastic) that interrupt the course of visual tracts may of course give rise to visual field disturbances.

REFERENCES

1. Le Hoang P, Girard B, Rousselie F: Oeil et SIDA. Paris, Doin, 1989.
2. Khadem M, Kalish SB, Goldsmith J-A, et al: Ophthalmologic findings in acquired immune deficiency syndrome (AIDS). Arch Ophthalmol 102: 201-206, 1984.
3. Palestine AG, Rodrigues MM, Macher AM, et al: Ophthalmic involvement in acquired immunodeficiency syndrome. Ophthalmology 91:1092-1099, 1984.
4. Pepose JS, Holland GN, Nestor MS, et al: Acquired immune deficiency syndrome: Pathogenic mechanisms of ocular disease. Ophthalmology 92: 472-484, 1985.
5. Mines JA, Kaplan HJ: Acquired immunodeficiency syndrome (AIDS): The disease and its ocular manifestations. Int Ophthalmol Clin 26:73-115, 1986.
6. Schuman JS, Orellana J, Friedman AH, et al: Acquired immunodeficiency syndrome (AIDS). Surv Ophthalmol 31:384-410, 1987.
7. Fabricius E-M, Jäger H, Prantl F, et al: AIDS am Auge—eine Retrospektive Analyse von 70 HIV-infizierten Patienten. Fortschr Ophthalmol 85: 420-426, 1988.
8. Holland GN, Kreiger AE: Neuroophthalmology of acquired immunodeficiency syndrome. In Rosenblum ML, Levy RM, Bredesen DE (eds): AIDS and the Nervous System. New York, Raven Press, 1988, pp 103-120.
9. Kreiger AE, Holland GN: Ocular involvement in AIDS. Eye 2:496-505, 1988.
10. Martenet A-C: Manifestations oculaires du syndrome d'immunodéficience aquise. J Fr Ophtalmol 11:105-118, 1988.
11. Nussenblatt R: Ocular complications of the acquired immunodeficiency syndrome. Nat Immun Cell Growth Regul 7:131-134, 1988.
12. Culbertson WW: Infections of the retina in AIDS. Int Ophthalmol Clin 29:108-118, 1989.
13. Dennehy PJ, Warman R, Flynn JT, et al: Ocular manifestations in pediatric patients with acquired immunodeficiency syndrome. Arch Ophthalmol 107:978-982, 1989.
14. Jabs DA, Green WR, Fox R, et al: Ocular manifestations of acquired immune deficiency syndrome. Ophthalmology 96:1092-1099, 1989.
15. Jensen OA, Klinken L: Pathology of brain and eye in the acquired immune deficiency syndrome (AIDS): A comparison of lesions in a consecutive autopsy material. Acta Pathol Microbiol Immunol Scand 97:325-333, 1989.
16. Ward RC, Weiner MJ, Albert DM: The eye. In Harawi SJ, O'Hara CJ (eds): Pathology and Pathophysiology of AIDS and HIV-Related Diseases. St. Louis, Mosby, 1989, pp 363-377.
17. Bienfang DC, Kelly LD, Nicholson DH, et al: Ophthalmology. N Engl J Med 323:956-967, 1990.
18. Deschênes J, Seamone C, Baines M: The ocular manifestations of sexually transmitted diseases. Can J Ophthalmol 25:177-185, 1990.
19. Kestelyn P: Ocular problems in AIDS. Int Ophthalmol 14:165-172, 1990.
20. De Girolami U, Hénin D, Girard B, et al: Etude pathologique de l'oeil et du système nerveux central dans 25 cas de SIDA. Rev Neurol (Paris) 145: 819-828, 1989.
21. De Girolami U, Hénin D, Hauw J-J: Anatomie pathologique de l'oeil au cours du SIDA. In Le Hoang P, Rousselie F (eds): Oeil et SIDA. Paris, Doin, 1989, pp 67-71.
22. Pivetti-Pezzi P, Tamburi S, D'Offizi GP, et al: Retinal cotton-wool-like spots: A marker for AIDS? Compr Ther 14:41-44, 1988.
23. Bernauer W, Daicker B: HIV-Patient und Auge. Schweiz Med Wochenschr 120:888-893, 1990.
24. Ashton N, Harry J: The pathology of cotton wool spots and cytoid bodies in hypertensive retinopathy and other diseases. Trans Ophthalmol Soc UK 83:91-114, 1963.
25. McLeod D: Reappraisal of the retinal cotton-wool spot: A discussion paper. J R Soc Med 74: 682-686, 1981.
26. Brown GC, Brown MM, Hiller T, et al: Cotton-wool spots. Retina 5:206-214, 1985.
27. McLeod D, Marshall J, Kohner EM, et al: The role of axoplasmic transport in the pathogenesis of retinal cotton-wool spots. Br J Ophthalmol 61: 177-191, 1977.
28. Chihara E: Pathogenesis of cotton wool patches: A clinical study. Jpn J Ophthalmol 27:397-403, 1983.
29. Murata M, Yoshimoto H: Morphological study of the pathogenesis of retinal cotton wool spot. Jpn J Ophthalmol 27:362-379, 1983.

30. Newsome DA, Green WR, Miller ED, et al: Microvascular aspects of acquired immune deficiency syndrome retinopathy. Am J Ophthalmol 98:590-601, 1984.

31. Kwok S, O'Donnell JJ, Wood IS: Retinal cotton-wool spots in a patient with *Pneumocystis carinii* infection. N Engl J Med 307:184-185, 1982.

32. Tanenbaum M, Russell S, Richmond P, et al: Calcified cytoid bodies in acquired immunodeficiency syndrome. Retina 7:84-88, 1987.

33. Ammann AJ: The immunology of AIDS. Int Ophthalmol Clin 29:77-82, 1989.

34. Johnson BL: Retinal axonal swelling in patients with acquired immunodeficiency syndrome. Arch Pathol Lab Med 113:574, 1989.

35. Giangaspero F, Foschini MP: Diffuse axonal swellings in a case of acquired immunodeficiency syndrome. Arch Pathol Lab Med 112:1259-1262, 1988.

36. Freeman WR, Chen A, Henderly DE, et al: Prevalence and significance of acquired immunodeficiency syndrome–related retinal microvasculopathy. Am J Ophthalmol 107:229-235, 1989.

37. Kestelyn P, Lepage P, Van de Perre P: Perivasculitis of the retinal vessels as an important sign in children with AIDS-related complex. Am J Ophthalmol 100:614-615, 1985.

38. Pavan-Langston D: Major ocular viral infections. In Galasso GJ, Whitley RJ, Merigan TC (eds): Antiviral Agents and Viral Diseases of Man, ed 3. New York, Raven Press, 1990, pp 183-233.

39. Dhermy P, DiCostanzo P, Le Hoang P, et al: Etude histologique de la nécrose rétinienne à cytomégalovirus au cours d'un SIDA. Bull Soc Ophthalmol Fr 84:381-384, 1984.

40. Bloom JN, Palestine AG: The diagnosis of cytomegalovirus retinitis. Ann Intern Med 109:963-969, 1988.

41. Palestine AG: Clinical aspects of cytomegalovirus retinitis. Rev Infect Dis 10(suppl 3):S515-S521, 1988.

42. Cantrill HL, Henry K, Melroe NH, et al: Treatment of cytomegalovirus retinitis with intravitreal ganciclovir. Ophthalmology 96:367-374, 1989.

43. Hennis HL, Scott AA, Apple DJ: Cytomegalovirus retinitis. Surv Ophthalmol 34:193-203, 1989.

44. Jabs DA, Enger C, Bartlett JG: Cytomegalovirus retinitis and acquired immunodeficiency syndrome. Arch Ophthalmol 107:75-80, 1989.

45. Cochereau-Massin I, Le Hoang P, Lautier-Frau M, et al: Rétinite à cytomégalovirus au cours du SIDA: Traitement par injections intravitréennes de ganciclovir. Presse Med 19:1313-1316, 1990.

46. Schmitt-Gräff A, Neuen-Jacob E, Rettig B, et al: Evidence for cytomegalovirus and human immunodeficiency virus infection of the retina in AIDS. Virchows Arch [A] 416:249-253, 1990.

47. Gass JDM: Stereoscopic Atlas of Macular Diseases: Diagnosis and Treatment, ed 3, vol 2. St. Louis, Mosby, 1987.

48. Smith ME, Zimmerman LE, Harley RD: Ocular involvement in congenital cytomegalic inclusion disease. Arch Ophthalmol 76:696-699, 1966.

49. Cogan DG: Immunosuppression and eye disease. Am J Ophthalmol 83:777-788, 1977.

50. Egbert PR, Pollard RB, Gallagher JG, et al: Cytomegalovirus retinitis in immunosuppressed hosts. II. Ocular manifestations. Ann Intern Med 93:664-670, 1980.

51. Newman NM, Mandel MR, Gullet J, et al: Clinical and histologic findings in opportunistic ocular infections: Part of a new syndrome of acquired immunodeficiency. Arch Ophthalmol 101:396-401, 1983.

52. Holland GN, Pepose JS, Pettit TH, et al: Acquired immune deficiency syndrome: Ocular manifestations. Ophthalmology 90:859-873, 1983.

53. Jensen OA, Gerstoft J, Thomsen HK, et al: Cytomegalovirus retinitis in the acquired immunodeficiency syndrome (AIDS): Light-microscopical, ultrastructural and immunohistochemical examination of a case. Acta Ophthalmol 62:1-9, 1984.

54. Grossniklaus HE, Frank KE, Tomsak RL: Cytomegalovirus retinitis and optic neuritis in acquired immune deficiency syndrome: Report of a case. Ophthalmology 94:1601-1604, 1987.

55. Morgello S, Cho E-S, Nielsen S, et al: Cytomegalovirus encephalitis in patients with acquired immunodeficiency syndrome: An autopsy study of 30 cases and a review of the literature. Hum Pathol 18:289-297, 1987.

56. Fay MT, Freeman WR, Wiley CA, et al: Atypical retinitis in patients with the acquired immunodeficiency syndrome. Am J Ophthalmol 105:483-490, 1988.

57. Teich SA, Castle J, Friedman AH, et al: Active cytomegalovirus particles in the eyes of an AIDS patient being treated with 9-[2-hydroxy-1-(hydromethyl) ethoxymethyl] guanine (ganciclovir). Br J Ophthalmol 72:293-298, 1988.

58. Pomerantz RJ, Kuritzkes DR, de la Monte SM, et al: Infection of the retina by human immunodeficiency virus type I. N Engl J Med 317:1643-1647, 1987.

59. Cantrill HL, Henry K, Jackson B, et al: Recovery of human immunodeficiency virus from ocular tissues in patients with acquired immune deficiency syndrome. Ophthalmology 95:1458-1462, 1988.

60. Qavi HB, Green MT, SeGall GK, et al: Demonstration of HIV-1 and HHV-6 in AIDS-associated retinitis. Curr Eye Res 8:379-387, 1989.

61. Cheng-Mayer C, Rutka JT, Rosenblum ML, et al: Human immunodeficiency virus can productively infect cultured human glial cells. Proc Natl Acad Sci USA 84:3526-3530, 1987.

62. Fujikawa LS, Salahuddin SZ, Ablashi D, et al: HTLV-III in the tears of AIDS patients. Ophthalmology 93:1479-1481, 1986.

63. Fujikawa LS, Salahuddin SZ, Ablashi D, et al: Human T-cell leukemia/lymphotrophic virus type III in the conjunctival epithelium of a patient with AIDS. Am J Ophthalmol 100:507-509, 1985.

64. Doro S, Navia BA, Kahn A, et al: Confirmation of HTLV-III virus in cornea. Am J Ophthalmol 102:390-391, 1986.

65. Salahuddin SZ, Palestine AG, Heck E, et al: Isolation of the human T-cell leukemia/lymphotrophic virus type III from the cornea. Am J Ophthalmol 101:149-152, 1986.

66. Kestelyn P, Van de Perre P, Sprecher-Goldberger S: Isolation of the human T-cell leukemia/lymphotropic virus type III from aqueous humor in two patients with perivasculitis of the retinal vessels. Int Ophthalmol 9:247-251, 1986.

67. Culbertson WW, Blumenkranz MS, Pepose JS, et al: Varicella zoster virus is a cause of the acute retinal

necrosis syndrome. Ophthalmology 93:559-569, 1986.

68. Forster DJ, Dugel PU, Frangieh GT, et al: Rapidly progressive outer retinal necrosis in the acquired immunodeficiency syndrome. Am J Ophthalmol 110:341-348, 1990.

69. Pepose JS, Hilborne LH, Cancilla PA, et al: Concurrent herpes simplex and cytomegalovirus retinitis and encephalitis in the acquired immune deficiency syndrome (AIDS). Ophthalmology 91: 1669-1677, 1984.

70. Cole EL, Meisler DM, Calabrese LH, et al: Herpes zoster ophthalmicus and acquired immune deficiency syndrome. Arch Ophthalmol 102:1027-1029, 1984.

71. Sandor EV, Millman A, Croxson TS, et al: Herpes zoster ophthalmicus in patients at risk for the acquired immune deficiency syndrome (AIDS). Am J Ophthalmol 101:153-155, 1986.

72. Anders KH, Guerra WF, Tomiyasu U, et al: The neuropathology of AIDS: UCLA experience and review. Am J Pathol 124:537-558, 1986.

73. Navia BA, Petito CK, Gold JWM, et al: Cerebral toxoplasmosis complicating the acquired immune deficiency syndrome: Clinical and neuropathological findings in 27 patients. Ann Neurol 19: 224-238, 1986.

74. Friedman AH: The retinal lesions of the acquired immune deficiency syndrome. Trans Am Ophthalmol Soc 82:447-491, 1984.

75. Parke DW, Font RL: Diffuse toxoplasmic retinochoroiditis in a patient with AIDS. Arch Ophthalmol 104:571-575, 1986.

76. Holland GN, Engstrom RE, Glasgow BJ, et al: Ocular toxoplasmosis in patients with the acquired immunodeficiency syndrome. Am J Ophthalmol 106:653-667, 1988.

77. Holland GN: Ocular toxoplasmosis in the immunocompromised host. Int Ophthalmol 13:399-402, 1989.

78. Pillai S, Mahmood MA, Limaye SR: Herpes zoster ophthalmicus, contralateral hemiplegia, and recurrent ocular toxoplasmosis in a patient with acquired immune deficiency syndrome–related complex. J Clin Neurol Ophthalmol 9:229-233, 1989.

79. Freeman WR, Gross JG, Labelle J, et al: *Pneumocystis carinii* choroidopathy: A new clinical entity. Arch Ophthalmol 107:863-867, 1989.

80. Rao NA, Zimmerman PL, Boyer D, et al: A clinical, histopathologic, and electron microscopic study of *Pneumocystis carinii* choroiditis. Am J Ophthalmol 107:218-228, 1989.

81. Dugel PU, Rao NA, Forster DJ, et al: *Pneumocystis carinii* choroiditis after long-term aerosolized pentamidine therapy. Am J Ophthalmol 110:113-117, 1990.

82. Sneed SR, Blodi CF, Berger BB, et al: *Pneumocystis carinii* choroiditis in patients receiving inhaled pentamidine. N Engl J Med 322:936-937, 1990.

83. Carney MD, Combs JL, Waschler W: Cryptococcal choroiditis. Retina 10:27-32, 1990.

84. Macher A, Rodrigues MM, Kaplan W, et al: Disseminated bilateral chorioretinitis due to *Histoplasma capsulatum* in a patient with the acquired immunodeficiency syndrome. Ophthalmology 92:1159-1164, 1985.

85. Kurosawa A, Pollock SC, Collins MP, et al: *Sporothrix schenckii* endophthalmitis in a patient with human immunodeficiency virus infection. Arch Ophthalmol 106:376-380, 1988.

86. Friedberg DN, Stenson SM, Orenstein JM, et al: Microsporidial keratoconjunctivitis in acquired immunodeficiency syndrome. Arch Ophthalmol 108:504-508, 1990.

87. Croxatto JO, Mestre C, Puente S, et al: Nonreactive tuberculosis in a patient with acquired immune deficiency syndrome. Am J Ophthalmol 102:659-660, 1986.

88. Blodi BA, Johnson MW, McLeish WM, et al: Presumed choroidal tuberculosis in a human immunodeficiency virus infected host. Am J Ophthalmol 108:605-607, 1989.

89. Passo MS, Rosenbaum JT: Ocular syphilis in patients with human immunodeficiency virus infection. Am J Ophthalmol 106:1-6, 1988.

90. Levy JH, Liss RA, Maguire AM: Neurosyphilis and ocular syphilis in patients with concurrent human immunodeficiency virus infection. Retina 9:175-180, 1989.

91. Davis JL, Nussenblatt RB, Bachman DM, et al: Endogenous bacterial retinitis in AIDS. Am J Ophthalmol 107:613-623, 1989.

92. Shuler JD, Engstrom RE Jr, Holland GN: External ocular disease and anterior segment disorders associated with AIDS. Int Ophthalmol Clin 29: 98-104, 1989.

93. Reich H, Hollwich F, Uthoff D: Kaposi-Sarkom und AIDS. Klin Monatsbl Augenheilkd 187:1-8, 1985.

94. Shuler JD, Holland GN, Miles SA, et al: Kaposi sarcoma of the conjunctiva and eyelids associated with the acquired immunodeficiency syndrome. Arch Ophthalmol 107:858-862, 1989.

95. Brooks HL Jr, Downing J, McClure JA, et al: Orbital Burkitt's lymphoma in a homosexual man with acquired immune deficiency. Arch Ophthalmol 102:1533-1537, 1984.

96. Lauer SA, Fischer J, Jones J, et al: Orbital T-cell lymphoma in human T-cell leukemia virus-1 infection. Ophthalmology 95:110-115, 1988.

97. Hamed LM, Schatz NJ, Galetta SL: Brainstem ocular motility defects and AIDS. Am J Ophthalmol 106:437-442, 1988.

98. Zaidman GW: Neurosyphilis and retrobulbar neuritis in a patient with AIDS. Ann Ophthalmol 18: 260-261, 1986.

99. Lipson BK, Freeman WR, Beniz J, et al: Optic neuropathy associated with cryptococcal arachnoiditis in AIDS patients. Am J Ophthalmol 107:523-527, 1989.

15

MISCELLANEOUS ORGAN SYSTEMS

Jonathan W. Said

ENDOCRINE SYSTEM

Symptoms relating to the endocrine system in patients with AIDS are often masked by more dramatic sequelae of HIV infection. Nevertheless, gonadal dysfunction may be present in 50% of patients with AIDS,[1] and adrenal cortical reserve may be significantly impaired.[2] Thyroid function tests usually show no abnormalities,[1] although rarely the thyroid gland is infected by opportunistic organisms including cytomegalovirus (CMV) and *Cryptococcus.*

Adrenal Gland

Adrenal insufficiency may be easily overlooked in debilitated individuals, but chemical evidence of adrenal insufficiency may be present in AIDS patients, particularly with advanced disease.[2] Carefully controlled adrenal function tests should therefore be performed. Symptoms of adrenal insufficiency include hyponatremia, hypotension, hypocalcemia, and hypoglycemia.[3] Lipid depletion is widespread in the adrenal gland at autopsy, and CMV has been found in the adrenal gland of up to 50% of AIDS patients.[3,4] Adrenal necrosis in patients who died of AIDS has been linked to CMV infection[5] and is greater in the medulla than in the cortex.[4] Necrosis may be localized or diffuse; adrenal insufficiency may be present with diffuse necrosis. Adrenal insufficiency is not usually life threatening in AIDS

patients. *Cryptococcus, Mycobacterium avium-intracellulare,* and Kaposi's sarcoma may also involve the adrenal gland.[4]

Pituitary Gland

Pituitary involvement in AIDS patients is associated with generalized or cerebral infection by organisms including cytomegalovirus, *Pneumocystis, Cryptococcus,* and *Toxoplasma.*[6] Pathologic findings are focal or widespread necrosis and fibrosis of the anterior pituitary gland and microglial nodules in the pars nervosa.[7]

Male Genital Tract

The prostate and testis can be directly infected with HIV, and virus has been demonstrated in seminal fluid.[8] Hypogonadism may be the first endocrine abnormality in AIDS patients.[1]

HIV has been found in degenerating germ cells and Sertoli's cells in the testis.[8] Histologic changes of testicular atrophy include peritubular fibrosis, thickening of tubular basement membranes, and hyalinization of tubules. Arrest of spermatogenesis, depletion of germ cells, and a "Sertoli cell only" appearance may also occur.[9] Atrophy of interstitial cells[10] and an interstitial mononuclear inflammatory infiltrate consisting of lymphocytes and macrophages may be present.[11] Testicular blood vessels may be thickened, with intimal proliferation and luminal narrowing.[11] Possible causes of testicular atrophy in AIDS patients include chronic illness, prolonged fever, malnutrition, testicular infection by HIV and other organisms, chemotherapy, and an as yet uncharacterized immune process.[12] Specific infections of the testis include cytomegalovirus, *M. avium-intracellulare* infection, and toxoplasmosis.[10]

JOINTS

Symptoms relating to the joints (predominantly arthralgias) are common in HIV-infected individuals, and overt arthritis is reported in approximately 10%.[13-17] Reactive arthritis similar to Reiter's syndrome may precede or occur simultaneously with other manifestations of AIDS.[16,17] Joint symptoms may be severe and unresponsive to nonsteroidal antiinflammatory agents.[15] The pathogenesis and relationship of this form of reactive arthropathy to HIV infection have not been established.[13] Biopsy reveals a chronic nonspecific synovitis with mononuclear cell infiltrate.[14] The possibility of HIV infection should therefore be considered in all patients with conditions suggesting reactive arthritis.[15] Hematogenous infectious arthritis is uncommon in AIDS and may be caused by unusual organisms such as *Sporothrix schenckii, Cryptococcus neoformans*, and *M. avium-intracellulare*.[16,17]

REFERENCES

1. Dobbs AS, Dempsey MA, Ladenson PW, et al: Endocrine disorders in men infected with human immunodeficiency virus. Am J Med 84:611-616, 1988.
2. Greene LW, Cole W, Greene JB, et al: Adrenal insufficiency as a complication of the acquired immunodeficiency syndrome. Ann Intern Med 101: 497-498, 1984.
3. Pulakhandam U, Dincsoy HP: Cytomegaloviral adrenalitis and adrenal insufficiency in AIDS. Am J Clin Pathol 93:561-656, 1990.
4. Glascow BJ, Steinsapir KD, Anders K, et al: Adrenal pathology in the acquired immunodeficiency syndrome. Am J Clin Pathol 84:594-597, 1985.
5. Tapper ML, Rotterdam HZ, Lerner CW, et al: Adrenal necrosis in the acquired immunodeficiency syndrome. Ann Intern Med 100:239-241, 1984.
6. Sano T, Kovacs K, Sheithauer BW, et al: Pituitary pathology in acquired immunodeficiency syndrome. Arch Pathol Lab Med 113:1066-1070, 1989.
7. Ferreiro J, Vinters HV: Pathology of the pituitary gland in patients with the acquired immune deficiency syndrome (AIDS). Pathology 20:211-215, 1988.
8. Da Silva M, Shevchuk MM, Cronin WJ, et al: Detection of HIV-related protein in testes and prostates in patients with AIDS. Am J Clin Pathol 93: 196-201, 1990.
9. Yoshikawa Y, Truong LD, Fraire AE, et al: The spectrum of histopathology of the testis in acquired immunodeficiency syndrome. Mod Pathol 2: 233-238, 1989.
10. De Paepe ME, Waxman M: Testicular atrophy in AIDS: A study of 57 autopsy cases. Hum Pathol 20:210-214, 1989.
11. Chabon AB, Stenger RJ, Grabstald H, et al: Histopathology of testis in acquired immune deficiency syndrome. Urology 29:658-663, 1987.
12. De Paepe ME, Vuletin JC, Lee MH, et al: Testicular atrophy in homosexual AIDS patients: An immune mediated phenomenon? Hum Pathol 20: 572-578, 1989.
13. Winchester R, Bernstein DH, Fischer HD, et al: The co-occurrence of Reiter's syndrome and acquired immunodeficiency. Ann Intern Med 106:19-26, 1987.
14. Rynes RI, Goldenberg DL, DiGiacomo R, et al: Acquired immunodeficiency syndrome–associated arthritis. Am J Med 84:810-816, 1988.
15. Forster SM, Siefert MH, Keat AC, et al: Inflammatory joint disease and human immunodeficiency virus infection. Br Med J 296:1625-1627, 1988.
16. Kaye BE: Rheumatologic manifestations of infection with human immunodeficiency virus (HIV). Ann Intern Med 111:158-167, 1989.
17. Sokoloff L: A prospective necropsy study of arthritis in acquired immunodeficiency syndrome. Arch Pathol Lab Med 114:1035-1037, 1990.

Index

Note: Page numbers in *italics* refer to illustrations; page numbers followed by the letter t refer to tables.